Oxford Medical Publications

Paediatric Gastroenterology, Hepatology, and Nutrition

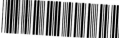

Oxford Specialist Handbooks published and forthcoming

General Oxford Specialist Handbooks

A Resuscitation Room Guide
Addiction Medicine
Day Case Surgery
Parkinson's Disease and Other Movement Disorders 2e
Perioperative Medicine, 2e
Pharmaceutical Medicine
Postoperative Complications, 2e
Renal Transplantation
Retrieval Medicine

Oxford Specialist Handbooks in Anaesthesia

Anaesthesia for Medical and Surgical Emergencies
Cardiac Anaesthesia
Neuroanaesthesia
Obstetric Anaesthesia
Ophthalmic Anaesthesia
Paediatric Anaesthesia
Regional Anaesthesia, Stimulation and Ultrasound Techniques
Thoracic Anaesthesia

Oxford Specialist Handbooks in Cardiology

Adult Congenital Heart Disease
Cardiac Catheterization and Coronary Intervention
Cardiac Electrophysiology and Catheter Ablation
Cardiovascular Computed Tomography
Cardiovascular Magnetic Resonance
Echocardiography, 2e
Fetal Cardiology
Heart Failure, 2e
Hypertension
Inherited Cardiac Disease
Nuclear Cardiology
Pacemakers and ICDs
Pulmonary Hypertension
Valvular Heart Disease

Oxford Specialist Handbooks in Critical Care

Advanced Respiratory Critical Care
Cardiothoracic Critical Care

Oxford Specialist Handbooks in End of Life Care

End of Life Care in Cardiology
End of Life Care in Dementia
End of Life Care in Nephrology
End of Life Care in Respiratory Disease
End of Life in the Intensive Care Unit

Oxford Specialist Handbooks in Infectious Disease

Infectious Disease Epidemiology
Manual of Childhood Infections 4e

Oxford Specialist Handbooks in Neurology

Epilepsy
Parkinson's Disease and Other Movement Disorders, 2e
Stroke Medicine, 2e

Oxford Specialist Handbooks in Oncology

Practical Management of Complex Cancer Pain

Oxford Specialist Handbooks in Paediatrics

Paediatric Dermatology
Paediatric Endocrinology and Diabetes
Paediatric Gastroenterology, Hepatology, and Nutrition
Paediatric Haematology and Oncology
Paediatric Intensive Care
Paediatric Nephrology, 2e
Paediatric Neurology, 2e
Paediatric Palliative Medicine, 2e
Paediatric Radiology
Paediatric Respiratory Medicine
Paediatric Rheumatology

Oxford Specialist Handbooks in Pain Medicine

Spinal Interventions in Pain Management

Oxford Specialist Handbooks in Psychiatry

Addiction Medicine, 2e
Child and Adolescent Psychiatry
Forensic Psychiatry
Medical Psychotherapy
Old Age Psychiatry

Oxford Specialist Handbooks in Radiology

Interventional Radiology
Musculoskeletal Imaging
Pulmonary Imaging
Thoracic Imaging

Oxford Specialist Handbooks in Surgery

Cardiothoracic Surgery, 2e
Colorectal Surgery
Gastric and Oesophageal Surgery
Hand Surgery
Hepatopancreatobiliary Surgery
Neurosurgery
Operative Surgery, 2e
Oral and Maxillofacial Surgery, 2e
Otolaryngology and Head and Neck Surgery
Paediatric Surgery
Plastic and Reconstructive Surgery
Surgical Oncology
Urological Surgery
Vascular Surgery, 2e

Oxford Specialist Handbook of Paediatric Gastroenterology, Hepatology, and Nutrition

Second Edition

Mark Beattie

Consultant Paediatric Gastroenterologist, University Hospital Southampton NHS Foundation Trust, and Honorary Professor of Paediatric Gastroenterology and Nutrition, University of Southampton, Southampton, UK

John WL Puntis

Consultant in Paediatric Gastroenterology and Nutrition, The General Infirmary at Leeds, Leeds, UK

Anil Dhawan

Consultant in Paediatric Hepatology and Professor of Paediatric Hepatology, King's College London, London, UK

Akshay Batra

Consultant Paediatric Gastroenterologist, University Hospital Southampton NHS Foundation Trust, Southampton, UK

Eirini Kyrana

Consultant in Paediatric Hepatology, Leeds Children's Hospital, Leeds, UK

OXFORD
UNIVERSITY PRESS

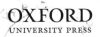

OXFORD
UNIVERSITY PRESS

Great Clarendon Street, Oxford, OX2 6DP,
United Kingdom

Oxford University Press is a department of the University of Oxford.
It furthers the University's objective of excellence in research, scholarship,
and education by publishing worldwide. Oxford is a registered trade mark of
Oxford University Press in the UK and in certain other countries

Published in the United States of America by Oxford University Press
198 Madison Avenue, New York, NY 10016, United States of America

British Library Cataloguing in Publication Data
Data available

Library of Congress Control Number: 2018940620

ISBN 978–0–19–875992–8

Printed and bound in China by
C&C Offset Printing Co., Ltd.

Foreword to the first edition

There is a romantic notion that paediatric gastroenterology in the UK began in a smoke-filled room in a pub somewhere in the 1970s. In fact, the truth is more prosaic. It did begin in the early 1970s, but in a seminar room in the Medical School in Birmingham, when a small group of leading exponents decided to form the British Paediatric Gastroenterology Group. Then, there were only a handful of tertiary specialists in paediatric gastroenterology, and only one in hepatology; nutrition was only incorporated 20 years later.

Since then, of course, paediatric hepatology has come of age, its growth helped enormously by progress in transplantation science and immunology. In Victorian households, feeding the children was usually left to the most junior and inexperienced housemaid. Perhaps as a consequence, the observation that malnutrition is bad for the child has only been formally recognized somewhat belatedly in developed economies. Indeed, we now recognize that in certain disorders, nutritional therapy is a key component of the primary treatment.

The editors and their contributors are to be congratulated for having condensed a large subject into a small format and for having left nothing of importance out; the bullet point style is particularly suited to this kind of publication. It is particularly pleasing to see clinical nutrition so comprehensively dealt with; there is much here that makes this publication relevant to all paediatric specialties. One disadvantage of clinical nutrition having been championed by gastroenterologists has been the mistaken belief that nutrition is relevant only to those patients with gastrointestinal disease.

This book provides a valuable concentrate of all the clinically relevant knowledge that we have acquired in this burgeoning field over the last 30 years. Often in paediatrics, the evidence based on which to make decisions is lacking and this specialty is no exception. The reader is therefore fortunate in having access to a pragmatic blend of evidence and clinical wisdom distilled and organized by three highly experienced specialists. The book provides a quick reference for the specialist, but is likely to be particularly useful for the non-specialist and for the trainee in paediatrics. Whatever changes may occur in the role of the doctor, they will still have to make diagnoses and initiate treatment. Moreover, all members of the large clinical team now required to look after many of these complex patients will find it helpful to have this book close to hand.

Professor Ian Booth
Dean, Leonard Parsons Professor of Paediatrics
and Child Health, The Medical School, Birmingham, UK

Foreword to the second edition

Medical textbooks are written for several reasons. Occasionally, they have appeared to be a vanity project; at other times to self-proclaim the excellence of an individual clinical department. Often in the past they have had the important function of establishing a new subspecialty and defining what it is and what it does. In paediatric gastroenterology, this was an important function of the textbooks edited by Charlotte Anderson and John Harries in the 1960s and 1970s. In contrast, many paediatricians and general practitioners in the United Kingdom struggled with the concept of community paediatrics because a textbook defining the specialty and what its practitioners were required to know was missing. So, the role of textbooks goes beyond helping to inform the management of a specific clinical problem.

This handbook has been written to impart clinical information and guidance in a specialty already firmly embedded in the practice of paediatrics. But rather than use the printed word to arrive at diagnosis and treatment, why not rely on the plethora of invited reviews and evidence-based guidelines available electronically? Photographers know that the best camera is the one that you have with you; the same applies to sources of clinical guidance. That is why the Oxford Handbook continues to be a valuable addition to patient management. It remains a distillation of information and knowledge from the impressive array of contributors assembled by the editors and one that can be accessed close to the patient. For a handbook, it is remarkably comprehensive and detailed and will provide valuable guidance to all members of the multidisciplinary team, particularly on those frequent occasions in paediatric practice when a handy evidence-based review is not available.

Professor Ian Booth
Emeritus Professor of Paediatrics and Child Health
University of Birmingham, UK

Preface to the first edition

Paediatric gastroenterology, hepatology, and nutrition encompass a wide range of paediatric practice with conditions being managed in a wide variety of settings, dependent upon their complexity. This includes primary care, secondary services, and specialist paediatric practice. Conditions such as abdominal pain and constipation can be assessed in any of these settings. Conditions such as inflammatory bowel disease, intestinal failure, and liver failure require specialist assessment but still shared care within the wider healthcare environment. Nutritional problems are seen by us all in everyday practice with nutritional support being an integral part of the management of any chronic disease.

This book is intended as a practical reference for practitioners who commonly see such conditions both in training and in clinical practice. The idea is that they can dip in for information on practical management but also background information on specific conditions. The chapters reflect common situations encountered in practice.

I have been fortunate to collaborate with Dr John Puntis (nutrition) and Professor Anil Dhawan (hepatology) in the production of the book, both of whom are well-recognized authorities in their respective areas. We have all had excellent support from Helen Liepman and the team at Oxford University Press.

We have included bullet points, lists, and managements guidelines where possible. We have limited the further reading as much of this is available through the internet, and websites have been listed where helpful. We have intentionally included only limited information about drug dosing and would refer the reader to the *British National Formulary for Children* for further information.

It is a source of great pride to produce an Oxford Handbook and I hope the book helps readers understand and enjoy the specialist areas of gastroenterology, hepatology, and nutrition in children.

RM Beattie
Southampton
February 2009

Preface to the second edition

We are delighted to have been able to produce a second edition of this handbook. All the chapters have been updated with recent developments in paediatric gastroenterology, hepatology, and nutrition and a few new ones added. We have kept the core principle which is that the text is meant to be a practical resource for clinicians and allied health care professionals who manage children with common and rare conditions, focusing on the presenting symptoms and signs, differential diagnosis, and practical management. We have included limited references, linked to relevant guidelines, and highlighted helpful websites. We have, as before, assumed clinicians will refer to the *British National Formulary for Children* for detailed information on the medications used, including indications, precise regimens, and toxicity.

The challenges of twenty-first-century medicine are immense—managing patients in teams and across networks, dealing with the complexities of medical advances, and keeping patients, families, and ourselves up to date and focused on the needs of the child. This requires careful clinical assessment, the optimum investigative approach, and careful consideration of the risks and benefits of different treatments available. We hope very much that this handbook will assist in this process and prove itself to be a useful resource.

We appreciate the time and effort given by the many contributing authors and to Dr Kyrana and Dr Batra who have joined the editorial team. We are very grateful for the commitment from Oxford University Press shown at every stage through their support in the production of this handbook.

As before, we hope the handbook helps readers understand and enjoy the specialist areas of gastroenterology, hepatology, and nutrition in children.

RM Beattie
JW Puntis
A Dhawan
August 2018

Contents

Contributors *xii*

Symbols and abbreviations *xv*

1 Congenital abnormalities of the
  gastrointestinal tract   1
2 Growth and nutritional requirements   11
3 Nutritional assessment   31
4 Breastfeeding   39
5 Formula and complementary feeding   47
6 The premature newborn   53
7 Necrotizing enterocolitis   61
8 Growth faltering (failure to thrive)   67
9 Iron deficiency   71
10 Micronutrients and minerals   75
11 Nutrition support teams   89
12 Enteral nutritional support   93
13 Refeeding syndrome   105
14 Parenteral nutrition   109
15 Intestinal failure   121
16 Intestinal transplantation   133
17 Eating disorders   143
18 Difficult eating behaviour in the young child   151
19 Food allergy   157
20 Carbohydrate intolerance   165
21 Nutritional problems in the child with
   neurodisability   173
22 Obesity   191

23 Gastrointestinal manifestations of cystic fibrosis   2(

24 Nutritional management of cystic fibrosis   2(

25 Cystic fibrosis-associated liver disease   21

26 Vomiting   22

27 Achalasia   22

28 Acute gastroenteritis   22

29 Gastro-oesophageal reflux   24

30 *Heliobacter pylori* infection and peptic ulceration   25

31 Cyclical vomiting syndrome   26

32 Pyloric stenosis   26

33 Gastrointestinal endoscopy   26

34 Gastrointestinal bleeding   27

35 Gastrointestinal polyposis   29

36 Intractable diarrhoea of infancy   29

37 Chronic diarrhoea   3(

38 Coeliac disease   31

39 Nutritional management of Coeliac disease   32

40 Bacterial overgrowth   33

41 Acute abdominal pain   33

42 Recurrent abdominal pain   33

43 Chronic constipation   35

44 Perianal disorders   37

45 Inflammatory bowel disease: introduction   37

46 Crohn's disease   38

47 Nutritional management of Crohn's disease   39

48 Ulcerative colitis   4(

49 Eosinophilic disorders   41

50 The pancreas   42

51 Liver function tests   43

52 Liver biopsy 439

53 Neonatal jaundice 445

54 Biliary atresia 459

55 Alpha-1 antitrypsin deficiency 463

56 Alagille syndrome 467

57 Familial and inherited intrahepatic cholestatic
syndromes 473

58 Drug-induced liver injury 487

59 Autoimmune liver disease 499

60 Metabolic liver disease 505

61 Non-alcoholic fatty liver disease 519

62 Wilson disease 529

63 Hepatitis B 535

64 Hepatitis C 545

65 Bacterial, fungal, and parasitic infections
of the liver 551

66 Liver tumours 565

67 Complications of chronic liver disease 569

68 Nutritional management of liver disease 583

69 Acute liver failure 601

70 Portal hypertension 619

71 Paediatric liver transplantation 629

Index 643

Contributors

Alastair Baker
Consultant in Paediatric
Hepatology and Clinical Lead
of Paediatric Hepatology
and Nutrition, King's College
London, London, UK
Chapters 56 and 57

Sanjay Bansal
Consultant Paediatric
Hepatologist, Child Health
Clinical Academic Group,
King's College London,
London, UK
Chapters 63, 64, and 69

Dharam Basude
Consultant Paediatric
Gastroenterologist, Bristol
Children's Hospital, Bristol, UK
Chapter 67

Akshay Batra
Consultant Paediatric
Gastroenterologist, University
Hospital Southampton
NHS Foundation Trust,
Southampton, UK
*Chapters 11–15, 26, 29, 38,
44–46, and 48*

Mark Beattie
Consultant Paediatric
Gastroenterologist, University
Hospital Southampton NHS
Foundation Trust, and Honorary
Professor of Paediatric
Gastroenterology and Nutrition,
University of Southampton,
Southampton, UK
*Chapters 23, 26, 29–31, 34–37,
40–46, and 48–49*

Ronald Bremner
Clinical Lead of Paediatric
Hepatology and Nutrition,
Birmingham Children's Hospital,
Birmingham, UK
Chapter 33

Anil Dhawan
Consultant in Paediatric
Hepatology and Professor of
Paediatric Hepatology, King's
College London, London, UK
Chapter 25

Emer Fitzpatrick
Clinical Senior Lecturer and
Honorary Consultant, Paediatric
Liver, GI and Nutrition Centre,
King's College London,
London, UK
Chapter 61

Tassos Grammatikopoulos
Consultant in Paediatric
Hepatology, King's College
Hospital, London, UK
Chapters 50, 60, and 70

Dino Hadzic
Consultant in Paediatric
Hepatology and Professor of
Paediatric Hepatology, King's
College London, London, UK
Chapters 54–55

Nicky Heather
Highly Specialist Paediatric
Dietitian – Gastroenterology,
University Hospital Southampton
NHS Foundation Trust,
Southampton, UK
Chapters 24, 39, and 47

Rob Hegarty
Consultant in Paediatric
Hepatology and Professor of
Paediatric Hepatology, King's
College London, London, UK
Chapters 58 and 60

Jonathan Hind
Consultant in Paediatric
Hepatology and Intestinal
Transplantation, King's College
Hospital, London, UK
Chapters 16

Lucy Howarth
Consultant Paediatric
Gastroenterologist, Oxford
University NHS Foundation
Trust, Oxford, UK
Chapter 34

Van Jain
Consultant in Paediatric
Hepatology, King's College
Hospital, London, UK
Chapter 71

Deepa Kamat
Paediatric Dietician, King's
College Hospital, London, UK
Chapter 68

Fevronia Kiparissi
Consultant Paediatric
Gastroenterologist, Great
Ormond Street Hospital for
Children, London, UK
Chapter 58

Eirini Kyrana
Consultant in Paediatric
Hepatology, Leeds General
Infirmary, Leeds, UK
Chapters 25, 51, and 53

Mich Lajeunesse
Consultant in Paediatric Allergy
and Immunology, University
Hospital Southampton
NHS Foundation Trust,
Southampton, UK
Chapter 49

Sara Mancell
Paediatric Dietician, King's
College Hospital, London, UK
Chapter 68

Lily Martin
Consultant in Paediatric
Hepatology, King's College
Hospital, London, UK
Chapter 52

Stephen Mouat
Paediatric Hepatologist and
Gastroenterologist, Starship
Child Health, Auckland, New
Zealand
Chapter 71

John WL Puntis
Consultant in Paediatric
Gastroenterology and Nutrition,
The General Infirmary at Leeds,
Leeds, UK
Chapters 2–15, and 17–22

Marianne Samyn
Consultant in Paediatric
Hepatology, King's College
Hospital, London, UK
Chapters 59 and 66

Naresh P Shanmugam
Senior Consultant in Paediatric
Hepatology, Institute of Advanced
Paediatrics, Chennai, India
Chapters 67 and 69

Michael Stanton
Paediatric Surgeon, University
Hospital Southampton
NHS Foundation Trust,
Southampton, UK
Chapters 1, 27, 32, and 42

Nancy Tan
Paediatrician, SBCC Baby & Child
Clinic, Novena, Singapore
Chapter 53

Stuart Tanner
Professor, Department of Child
Health, University of Sheffield,
Sheffield, UK
Chapter 62

Mark Tighe
Consultant Paediatrician, Poole
Hospital NHS Foundation Trust,
Poole, UK
Chapter 42

Giorgina Vergani
Director of Paediatric Liver
Science, King's College Hospital,
London, UK
Chapter 59

Anita Verma
Consultant Microbiologist,
Department of Medical
Microbiology, King's College
Hospital, London, UK
Chapter 65

Anthony Wiskin
Consultant Paediatric
Gastroenterologist, Bristol
Royal Hospital for Children,
Bristol, UK
Chapters 28, 36, and 37

Symbols and abbreviations

~	approximately
±	with or without
5-ASA	5-aminosalicylic acid
A1AT	alpha-1 antitrypsin deficiency
AD	autosomal dominant
AIE	autoimmune enteropathy
AIH	autoimmune hepatitis
AIP	autoimmune pancreatitis
ALF	acute liver failure
ALGS	Alagille syndrome
ALP	alkaline phosphatase
ALT	alanine aminotransferase
AMR	antibody-mediated rejection
AR	autosomal recessive
ASC	autoimmune sclerosing cholangitis
AST	aspartate aminotransferase
BA	biliary atresia
BMI	body mass index
BMR	basal metabolic rate
BSPGHAN	British Society of Paediatric Gastroenterology, Hepatology and Nutrition
CDG	congenital disorder of glycosylation
CF	cystic fibrosis
CFALD	cystic fibrosis-associated liver disease
CLD	chronic liver disease
CMV	cytomegalovirus
CNS	central nervous system
CRBSI	catheter-related bloodstream infection
CRP	C-reactive protein
CSF	cerebrospinal fluid
CT	computed tomography
CVC	central venous catheter
DAA	directly acting antiviral agent
DILI	drug-induced liver injury
DSA	donor-specific antibodies
DXA	dual-energy X-ray absorptiometry
EAR	estimated average requirement

EBV	Epstein–Barr virus
ECCO	European Crohn's and Colitis Organisation
ECG	electrocardiogram
EEN	exclusive enteral nutrition
ELISA	enzyme-linked immunosorbent assay
EMA	endomysial antibody
ERCP	endoscopic retrograde cholangiopancreatography
ESPGHAN	European Society of Paediatric Gastroenterology, Hepatology and Nutrition
EST	endoscopic sclerotherapy
EUS	endoscopic ultrasound
EVL	endoscopic variceal ligation
FA	fatty acids
FAOD	fatty acid oxidation disorder
FBC	full blood count
FC	faecal calprotectin
FSH	follicle-stimulating hormone
GA	general anaesthesia
GGT	gamma-glutamyl transferase
GH	growth hormone
GI	gastrointestinal
GOR	gastro-oesophageal reflux
GORD	gastro-oesophageal reflux disease
GP	general practitioner
GSD	glycogen storage disorder
HBV	hepatitis B virus
HCV	hepatitis C virus
HD	Hirschsprung disease
HLA	human leucocyte antigen
HPN	home parenteral nutrition
HSV	herpes simplex virus
IBS	irritable bowel syndrome
IBD	inflammatory bowel disease
ICP	intracranial pressure
IED	intestinal epithelial dysplasia
IF	intestinal failure
IFALD	intestinal failure-associated liver disease
Ig	immunoglobulin
IGF	insulin-like growth factor
IL	interleukin

INR	international normalized ratio
IT	intestinal transplantation
IUGR	intrauterine growth retardation
IV	intravenous
LCT	long-chain triglyceride
LH	luteinizing hormone
MCT	medium-chain triglyceride
MCV	mean cell volume
MPS	mucopolysaccharidosis
MRCP	magnetic resonance cholangiopancreatography
MRI	magnetic resonance imaging
MVID	microvillus inclusion disease
NAFLD	non-alcoholic fatty liver disease
NASH	non-alcoholic steatohepatitis
NEC	necrotizing enterocolitis
NGT	nasogastric tube
NICE	National Institute for Health and Care Excellence
NSAID	non-steroidal anti-inflammatory drug
NSBB	non-selective beta blocker
OGD	oesophagogastroduodenoscopy
ORS	oral rehydration solutions
pANCA	perinuclear antineutrophil cytoplasmic antibody
PCR	polymerase chain reaction
PEG	percutaneous endoscopic gastrostomy
PERT	pancreatic enzyme replacement therapy
PFIC	progressive familial intrahepatic cholestasis
PN	parenteral nutrition
PoPH	portopulmonary hypertension
PPI	proton pump inhibitor
PR	per rectum
PSARP	posterior sagittal anorectoplasty
PTH	parathyroid hormone
PTLD	post-transplant lymphoproliferative disorder
RAST	radioallergosorbent testing
SBS	short bowel syndrome
SCID	severe combined immunodeficiency
SIBO	small intestinal bacterial growth
SIDS	sudden infant death syndrome
TIBC	total iron binding capacity

TNF	tumour necrosis factor
TSH	thyroid-stimulating hormone
tTG	tissue transglutaminase
UGT	uridine diphosphate glucuronyl transferase
UK	United Kingdom
ULN	upper limit of normal
US	United States
USS	ultrasound scan
WD	Wilson disease
WHO	World Health Organization

Congenital abnormalities of the gastrointestinal tract

Introduction 2
Abdominal wall defects 3
Malrotation 4
Duodenal atresia 6
Distal bowel obstruction 7
Meconium ileus 7
Hirschsprung disease 8
Anorectal malformations 10

Introduction

Congenital anomalies of the gastrointestinal (GI) tract commonly present as neonatal bowel obstruction. Clinical and radiological features help to distinguish proximal and distal obstruction. Malrotation/volvulus is one of the causes of bilious (dark green) vomiting in neonates and infants. For this reason, bilious vomiting is a time-critical surgical emergency.

Development

- The embryological gut tube is formed by the end of the fourth week of gestation and is supplied by three main arterial trunks arising from the aorta (coeliac trunk, superior mesenteric artery, inferior mesenteric artery).
- The primitive foregut gives rise to the oesophagus, stomach, duodenum (proximal to the ampulla of Vater), liver, gallbladder, and pancreas.
- The midgut consists of the distal duodenum, jejunum, ileum, caecum, ascending colon, and the proximal two-thirds of the transverse colon.
- The hindgut gives origin to the rest of the colon; the rectum and urogenital sinus separate from an expansion called the cloaca.
- The rotation of the midgut is of particular importance. The primary intestinal loop (ileum) forms a physiological herniation into the umbilicus during the sixth embryonic week, returning to the peritoneal cavity during weeks 8–10. During this process there is a total of a 270-degree counter-clockwise rotation, such that the caecum lies in the right iliac fossa and the duodenojejunal (DJ) flexure is to the left of the midline.
- Malrotation (as well as 'non-rotation') occurs due to a failure in this process.

Abdominal wall defects

Gastroschisis and exomphalos result in the neonatal appearance of exteriorized abdominal contents. Both are diagnosed antenatally in the majority of cases and delivery is planned at a neonatal surgical centre.

In gastroschisis, there is no covering membrane over the bowel, although there may be significant 'peel' on the surface.

Gastroschisis

Gastroschisis is associated with preterm delivery (up to 25%) and has an incidence of 1 in 2000. Gastroschisis can be classified as 'simple' (normal bowel) and 'complex' where there can be associated volvulus or atresia. Other than intestinal atresia (10%), infants with gastroschisis usually have no other associated anomalies. Newborn management involves covering the exteriorized bowel with, e.g. cling film, placement of a nasogastric tube, and intravenous (IV) fluid resuscitation. It is common practice currently to attempt placement of a pre-formed spring-loaded silo, the base of which fits inside the umbilical defect, to cover the bowel. Sequential reduction of the external contents can then be performed over the next few days. Either sutureless umbilical closure or primary surgical closure is usually possible. A small proportion of cases may require surgical silo formation and delayed primary closure.

Long-term outcome is usually good, and survival is >95%.

Nutrition—essentially all infants will require long line placement and parenteral nutrition as return of gut function takes a median of 20 days (BAPS-CASS 2011 data). Feed intolerance is relatively common and specialized formula may be required if breastfeeding is not possible.

Exomphalos

Exomphalos (1 in 8000) results in exteriorized liver and/or bowel and can be considered as 'minor' (defect <5cm), major (defect >5cm), and 'giant'. In giant exomphalos, there is an obvious disproportion in the size of the external organs and the abdominal cavity, usually precluding abdominal closure in the neonatal period.

Neonatal management also involves covering the external contents, but surgery is not required urgently if the covering amniotic sac remains intact. Associated anomalies include cardiac, renal, and chromosomal anomalies. Beckwith–Wiedemann syndrome may result in neonatal hypoglycaemia. Echocardiography and renal tract ultrasound are undertaken. As exomphalos has significant associated anomalies, the survival rate is much lower than for gastroschisis (as low as approximately 10% in some series from the time of antenatal diagnosis). Long-term problems include gastro-oesophageal reflux and respiratory difficulties.

Minor exomphalos can usually be closed primarily in the first few days of life. Major exomphalos may require staged abdominal closure. Giant exomphalos is usually managed conservatively, with dressings to allow epithelialization over the external contents. Delayed closure can be attempted at 9–12 months.

Malrotation

Bilious vomiting in neonates/infants must be managed as a time-critical surgical emergency as the cause may be malrotation/volvulus. Left untreated, irreversible midgut infarction may occur resulting in short-gut syndrome or death. Volvulus of the bowel occurs due to twisting around the narrow mesentery, causing twisting of the entire midgut.

Incidence
1 in 2500.

Pathology
Failure of the normal process of intestinal rotation (see 'Development', p. 2). The end result of failed normal intestinal rotation is that the DJ flexure is found to the right of the midline (and below the trans-pyloric plane), with the caecum high in the midline. Ladd's bands may cross the duodenum from the caecum but are usually non-obstructive.

A narrow midgut mesentery results, which is prone to volvulus.

Associations
Trisomy 21, anorectal malformations, and cardiac anomalies.

Heterotaxy
This is abnormal positioning of thoracoabdominal organs on the left–right axis. There is debate as to whether elective correction of intestinal rotation anomalies is merited, in particular when atrial isomerism is present. The risk of elective surgery in infants with a major cardiac anomaly should be balanced with the risk of midgut volvulus.

Presentation
Bilious vomiting is the key feature. Abdominal distension may be present, with systemic upset.

Investigation
Plain abdominal X-ray—classically shows dilated stomach and duodenum, with an otherwise gasless pattern. Immediate laparotomy is indicated in this scenario if there is any associated peritonism and/or cardiovascular instability.

Upper GI series—demonstrates DJ flexure to the right of the midline, together with a 'bird-beak' narrowing at the distal duodenum, and/or corkscrew appearance of small bowel volvulus.

Ultrasound—may demonstrate inversion of the usual superior mesenteric artery/vein relationship (SMA/SMV). The SMV lies on the right in the normal anatomical situation. A corkscrew may be observed if volvulus is present. Ultrasound is not diagnostic in itself and should not be used to exclude malrotation/volvulus.

Management
Laparotomy and Ladd's procedure—bowel which has undergone volvulus is de-rotated (counter-clockwise). The duodenum is straightened, the caecum is placed in the left upper quadrant, and the small bowel on the right.

As the appendix will lie in the right upper quadrant, appendicectomy is usually removed (inversion or open excision).

If the viability of the bowel is questionable, it is de-rotated and observed to see if normal colour is restored.

In the situation of complete midgut necrosis, the options are resection (committing the infant to short-gut syndrome) or a re-look laparotomy 48 hours later.

Laparoscopic Ladd's procedure is undertaken at some centres although there is general agreement that this is not appropriate for neonates with suspected established volvulus. Laparoscopy may be useful for assessing cases where malrotation is radiologically equivocal.

Complications
- Adhesion obstruction (6%).
- Recurrent volvulus (1%).
- Short-gut syndrome.

Duodenal atresia

The incidence of duodenal atresia is 1 in 10,000, and accounts for 60% of intestinal atresias.

Presentation

- Detected at antenatal sonography in approximately 50% of cases—'double bubble' and polyhydramnios.
- Postnatally, vomiting occurs in the first 48 hours and is bilious if the obstruction is distal to the ampulla of Vater (two-thirds of cases), or non-bilious if the obstruction is proximal.

Differential diagnosis

Malrotation/volvulus—this should be suspected if there is distal gas beyond the dilated stomach and duodenum on X-ray.

Associations

Trisomy 21 (30%) and structural cardiac abnormalities (25%).

Management

Nasogastric decompression and IV fluid resuscitation. Surgery is usually not an emergency.

Surgery

Duodeno-duodenostomy (laparoscopic or open). The proximal and distal duodenal pouches are opened and joined—bypassing the atretic segment. Placement of a trans-anastomotic (nasojejunal) tube allows early enteral feeding, and avoids the need for long line/parenteral nutrition.

Long-term outcome

Usually very good in the absence of other co-morbidity. Rarely tapering duodenoplasty is required if severe proximal dilatation occurs.

Small bowel (jejuno-ileal) atresia

Four types (I–IV) are described, type IV is multiple atresias; types IIIb and IV are associated with significant loss of bowel length.

Associations

Cystic fibrosis—producing antenatal segmental volvulus (10%), prematurity, and gastroschisis.

Presentation

Antenatal (dilated bowel loops, polyhydramnios) in one-third.

Postnatally, abdominal distension, bilious vomiting, and failure to pass meconium occur.

Management

Plain X-ray is usually diagnostic—multiple dilated bowel loops with no distal gas. Nasogastric decompression and IV fluid resuscitation are commenced.

Laparotomy and primary resection/anastomosis is usually possible. Occasionally stoma formation is necessary (e.g. if multiple atresias). Postoperative parenteral nutrition is often required while gut function returns.

Long-term outcome

Usually good if bowel length is sufficient to allow enteral autonomy.

Distal bowel obstruction

- Differential includes Hirschsprung disease (HD), distal ileal atresia, meconium ileus, and small left colon syndrome.
- Typical features—abdominal distension, bilious vomiting, and failure to pass meconium.
- Initial management is directed at systemic resuscitation, with nasogastric decompression, bowel rest, IV fluids, and antibiotics. Per rectum (PR) examination and careful rectal washout will demonstrate passage of meconium and air in HD (often explosive). In meconium ileus, pellets/plugs of stool (and air) may be passed. In distal ileal atresia, small amounts of (non-pigmented) stool without air will be produced.

Meconium ileus

Abnormal inspissated meconium adheres to the bowel wall and causes a functional obstruction. 15% of neonates will present with distal bowel obstruction secondary to meconium ileus cystic fibrosis (CF). Of neonates who develop meconium ileus, nearly all will subsequently have confirmed CF.

Classification

- 'Simple' (50%)—functional obstruction only.
- 'Complicated' (50%)—associated segmental volvulus, atresia, or perforation results in obstruction.

Presentation

- *Antenatal*—dilated or echogenic bowel may be seen (echogenic bowel is non-specific).
- *Postnatal*—clinical features of distal obstruction. X-ray shows dilated loops of small bowel. Ground-glass appearance (meconium) may be present in the right iliac fossa (Neuhauser's sign). In complicated meconium ileus, calcification or evidence of a pseudocyst may be present on X-ray.

Management

Specific treatment is a contrast enema—may be diagnostic and therapeutic. Dilute Gastrografin® (Tween® 80 component emulsifies the inspissated stool).

Hirschsprung disease

Definition

HD is congenital aganglionosis of the distal colon, extending proximally from the rectum. HD usually affects the recto-sigmoid only ('short-segment'). In 25% of cases, aganglionosis extends more proximally, total colonic aganglionosis occurs in 10%.

Presentation

Classic triad is of neonatal bilious vomiting, abdominal distension, and delayed passage of meconium (>48 hours). A small proportion of cases are diagnosed in infancy with severe chronic constipation (rectal biopsy may be indicated if there is growth faltering (previously called 'failure to thrive'), significant distension, early onset, and positive family history).

Associations

Trisomy 21 (10%), Mowat–Wilson syndrome, congenital hypoventilation syndrome, and multiple endocrine neoplasia (type A and B).

Genetics

HD arises from a combination of genetic and environmental factors, >11 genes have been implicated. The *RET* gene (chromosome 10) is the most commonly associated susceptibility gene. Risk to siblings of patients with HD increases with long-segment disease.

Diagnosis

Suction rectal biopsy can be performed in the neonate without general anaesthesia (GA); open biopsy under GA is required in older infants/children. Diagnosis is confirmed by histological confirmation of absent ganglion cells (H&E stain) and hypertrophic nerve trunks on acetylcholinesterase staining. Calretinin staining (absent in HD) may be supportive.

Contrast enema may demonstrate a transition zone, and may be required to exclude other causes of distal obstruction. Anorectal manometry may show an absent recto-anal inhibitory reflex but this is not considered diagnostic without biopsy.

Management

Definitive surgical treatment is excision of the aganglionic segment and colo-anal anastomosis (pull-through) of proximal normally innervated colon. Initial management is directed at nasogastric decompression, rectal washouts (up to three times per day, retained volume should be <20mL/kg saline), and antibiotics if enterocolitis is suspected (fever, raised C-reactive protein (CRP)). Early stoma formation may be required if adequate rectal decompression cannot be achieved.

Hirschsprung-associated enterocolitis

This is most commonly defined as bilious vomiting, bloody diarrhoea, and abdominal distension. Signs of sepsis (fever, raised CRP) will usually be present. A low index of suspicion is necessary as, untreated, Hirschsprung-associated enterocolitis may be fatal. Enterocolitis may occur before or after definitive surgical treatment. Treatment is by rectal decompression, nasogastric tube/bowel rest, and IV fluids/antibiotics.

Long-term outcome

- Enterocolitis.
- Constipation/soiling.
- Worse in long-segment disease—may require long-term stoma, and/or parenteral nutrition.

Anorectal malformations

Incidence

1 in 1500 (male:female ratio 3:2).

Classification

This is a spectrum of conditions presenting in the newborn with either a 'covered anus' appearance or abnormally sited, usually narrowed, anus. The current classification relies on a descriptive terminology (Krickenback); the common variants in the male are a recto-perineal fistula or 'imperforate anus' with recto-urethral fistula. In the female, a recto-perineal or a recto-vestibular fistula are the commoner variants. Cloacal anomaly refers to a single perineal orifice in the female, with a common channel (of variable length) formed by the urethra, vagina, and ano-rectum.

Associated anomalies (present in 75%)

Urinary tract, spinal, cardiac, and central nervous system. Ultrasound of the renal tract and spine are undertaken in the newborn period, and prophylactic antibiotics used until the results of these are known. Magnetic resonance imaging (MRI) of the spine may be required if any anomalies are detected on spinal ultrasound.

Newborn management

This centres on whether a defunctioning colostomy is required for a 'high' anomaly in the male or female. With a 'low' anomaly (e.g. recto-perineal fistula), a primary anorectoplasty in the newborn is usually possible. Following colostomy formation for a high anomaly in males, a high-pressure colostogram (with micturating cysto-urethrogram) is performed at a later date to define the anatomical position of the fistula. A posterior sagittal anorectoplasty (PSARP) is usually possible.

Long-term outcome

For bowel function, constipation and soiling are the long-term problems which occur in up to 50% of patients. Continence potential is partly predicted by the type of anomaly (high vs low) and the presence or absence of spinal/sacral anomalies. Long-term difficulties with urinary and sexual function may occur if there are associated abnormalities.

Chapter 2

Growth and nutritional requirements

Growth *12*
Patterns of growth *20*
Nutritional requirements *22*
Malnutrition *26*
References and resources *30*

Growth

Growth rate in infancy is a continuation of the intrauterine growth curve, and is rapidly decelerating up to 3 years. Growth rate in childhood is a steady and slowly decelerating growth curve that continues until puberty, a phase of growth lasting from adolescence onwards. During puberty, the major sex differences in height are established, with a final height difference of ~12.5cm between males and females. Growth charts are derived from measurements of many different children at different ages (cross-sectional data). Data for growth of children are distributed 'normally' (i.e. form a bell-shaped curve). These data can be expressed mathematically as the mean and standard deviations from the mean. The centile lines delineate data into percentages: the 50th centile represents the mean (average); 25% of children are below the 25th centile. The 0.4th, 2nd, 9th, 25th, 50th, 75th, 91st, 98th, and 99.6th centiles are each two-thirds of a standard deviation away from the adjacent line.

Anthropometric indices

Weight-for-height compares a child's weight with the average weight for children of the same height, i.e. actual weight/weight-for-height at the 50th centile.
- For example, for a 2.5-year-old girl:
  - Height = 88cm.
  - Weight = 9kg.
  - 50th centile weight for a child who, at 88cm, is on the 50th centile for height = 12kg.
  - Weight-for-height = 9/12 = 75% (moderate malnutrition).
- Weight-for-height can be expressed either as % expected weight, or as a z-score (i.e. the number of standard deviations from the mean).
- Mid-upper-arm circumference (MUAC) is used for children aged 1–5 years and provides a quick population screening tool for malnutrition (i.e. more detailed assessment is required if <13.5cm).
- Skinfold thickness is measured with calipers and gives an assessment of fat stores.
- Body mass index (BMI) is derived from weight in kg divided by the square of the height in metres; it is an alternative to weight-for-height as an assessment of nutritional status.
- Growth velocity evaluates change in rate of height growth over a specified period of time (generally cm/year); it is helpful in early identification of undernutrition and standard reference charts are available.

Assessment of growth potential

- Plot height of both parents at 18-year-old end of centile chart.
- Add together parental heights and divide by 2.
- Add 7cm (male child), subtract 7cm (female) = midparental height (MPH); MPH +/− 8.5cm (girl), or +/− 10cm (boy) = target height centile range.

Normal growth—simple rules of thumb

Approximate average expected weight gain for a healthy term infant

- 200g/week in the first 3 months.
- 130g/week in the second 3 months.
- 85g/week in the third 3 months.
- 75g/week in the fourth 3 months.
- Birth weight usually doubles by 4 months and triples by 12 months.

Length

- Increases by 25cm in the first year.
- Increases by 12cm in the second year.
- By 3 years roughly half of adult height is attained.

Head circumference

- Increases by 1cm/month in the first year.
- Increases by 2cm in the whole of the second year.
- Will be 80% of adult size by 2 years.

NB Growth rates vary considerably between children; these figures should be used in conjunction with growth charts (Figs 2.1–2.6).

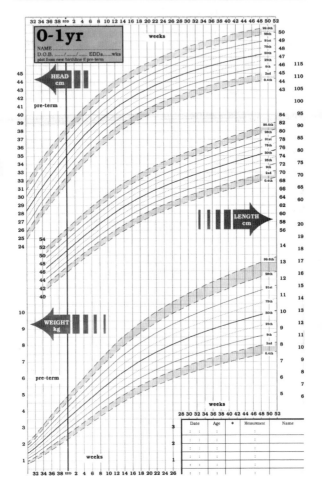

Fig. 2.1 Child Growth Foundation nine-centile growth chart for boys aged 0–1 years. Reproduced with permission from the Royal College of Paediatrics and Child Health (www.rcpch.ac.uk).

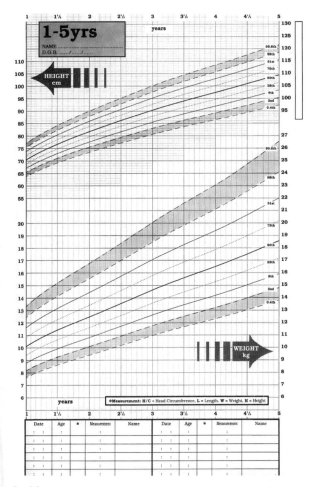

Fig. 2.2 Child Growth Foundation nine-centile growth chart for boys aged 1–5 years. Reproduced with permission from the Royal College of Paediatrics and Child Health (www.rcpch.ac.uk).

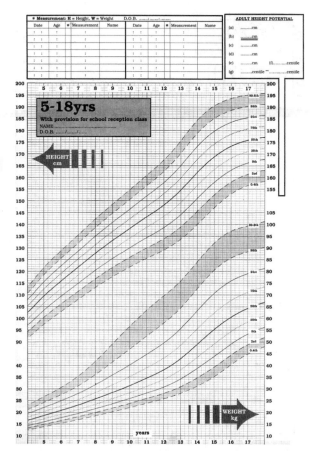

Fig. 2.3 Child Growth Foundation nine-centile growth chart for boys aged 5–18 years. Reproduced with permission from the Royal College of Paediatrics and Child Health (www.rcpch.ac.uk).

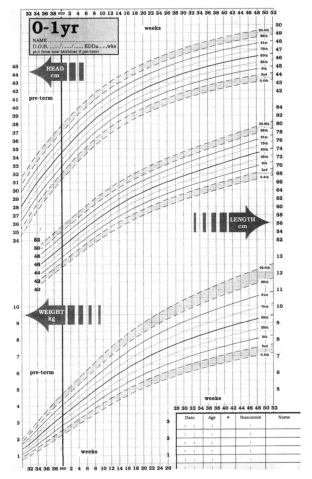

Fig. 2.4 Child Growth Foundation nine-centile growth chart for girls aged 0–1 year. Reproduced with permission from the Royal College of Paediatrics and Child Health (www.rcpch.ac.uk).

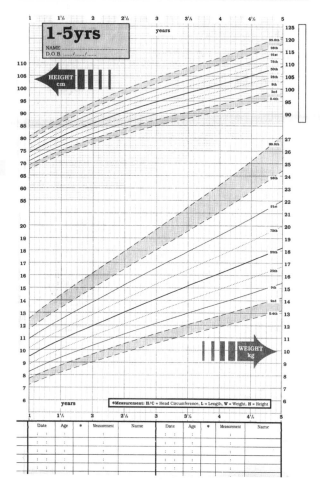

Fig. 2.5 Child Growth Foundation nine-centile growth chart for girls aged 1–5 years. Reproduced with permission from the Royal College of Paediatrics and Child Health (www.rcpch.ac.uk).

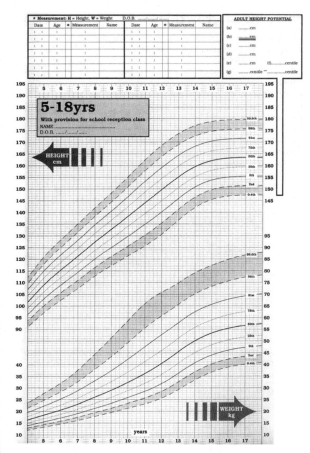

Fig. 2.6 Child Growth Foundation nine-centile growth chart for girls aged 5–18 years. Reproduced with permission from the Royal College of Paediatrics and Child Health (www.rcpch.ac.uk).

Patterns of growth

- Birth weight/centile is not always a good guide to genetic potential; some infants cross centile lines in the first few months of life ('catch-down'), but from then on continue to follow along a lower centile.
- The maximum weight centile achieved between 4 and 8 weeks is the best predictor of weight centile at 12 months.
- Infants born at <10th centile for gestational age may either have intrauterine growth retardation (IUGR), or be within the normal 10% of the population who fall below the line.
- Long-standing IUGR results in low weight and reduced head circumference and length; catch-up growth is unlikely.
- Infants with late IUGR are thin, but may have head circumference and length on a higher centile, and subsequently show catch-up in the weight centile.
- Rates of growth vary in young children, and assessments should be based on a number of serial measurements.

Abnormal growth

- Short-term energy deficit will make a child thin (low weight for height; wasting).
- Long-term energy deficit limits height gain (and head/brain growth) causing stunting (and reduced head circumference).
- Chronically undernourished children may be both thin and short.

Puberty

Growth accelerates during puberty (the sequence of physical and physiological changes occurring at adolescence culminating in full sexual maturity; Table 2.1). Average age at onset is 10–12 years in girls, and 12–13 years in boys. Age at onset is partly familial. Afro-Caribbean girls tend to have earlier puberty than white girls. Earlier puberty is seen in girls who are overweight and may be delayed in girls who are thin.

Table 2.1 Stages of puberty

Boys

Stage	Genitalia	Pubic hair	Other events
I	Prepubertal	Vellus not thicker than on abdomen	TV <4mL
II	Enlargement of testes and scrotum	Sparse long pigmented strands at base of penis	TV 4–8mL
III	Lengthening of penis	Darker, curlier, and spreads over pubes, axillary hair	TV 8–10mL
IV	Increase in penis length and breadth	Adult-type hair but covering a smaller	TV 10–15mL; peak height velocity, upper lip hair
V	Adult shape and size	Spread to medial thighs (stage VI: spread up linea alba)	TV 15–25mL
			Facial hair spreads to cheeks; adult voice

Girls

Stage	Breast	Pubic hair	Other events
I	Elevation of papilla only	Vellus not thicker than on abdomen	
II	Breast bud stage: elevation of breast and papilla	Sparse long pigmented strands along labia	Peak height velocity
III	Further elevation of breast and areola together	Darker, curlier, spreads over pubes	
IV	Areola forms a second mound on top of breast	Adult-type hair but covering a smaller area	Menarche
V	Mature stage: areola recedes and only papilla projects	Spread to medial thighs (stage VI: spread up linea alba)	

TV, testicular volume; measure by comparing with orchidometer.

Data sourced from Tanner JM. Growth at adolescence, 2nd edn, Blackwell, Oxford, 1962

Nutritional requirements

Energy metabolism

In order to maintain body weight, energy intake must equal energy expenditure. For growth to occur in children, energy intake must be greater than energy expenditure. Conversely, weight loss is achieved by increasing energy expenditure or decreasing energy intake. The energy content of food is usually expressed in kilojoules (kJ) or kilocalories (kcal). A calorie is defined as the energy needed to heat 1g of water by 1°C; 1kcal is equivalent to 4.184kJ.

Energy balance

- Total energy expenditure (TEE) is made up of:
  - basal metabolic rate (BMR) 50–75%
  - physical activity 20–40%
  - diet-induced thermogenesis (DIT) 10%.
- Growth, injury, and fever will increase energy expenditure.
- BMR is the amount of energy expended by the body to maintain normal physiological functions.
- Energy metabolism is sustained by the oxidation of fatty acids, carbohydrates, and amino acids to carbon dioxide and water, with the release of some heat.
- An individual's metabolic rate can therefore be measured from either oxygen consumption and carbon dioxide production, or from the amount of heat produced.
- For clinical purposes, *indirect calorimetry* (measurement of oxygen consumption and carbon dioxide production) is used to determine metabolic rate.

Nutrient requirements for healthy children

- The Department of Health has published recommendations regarding nutrient intakes at different ages (DHSS 1979). These can be used as a baseline for the individual child, although reference values are intended to relate to healthy groups rather than the sick (Table 2.2).
- Dietary reference value (DRV) is a term used to cover lower reference nutrient intake (LRNI), estimated average requirement (EAR), recommended nutrient intake (RNI), and safe intake.
- Recommended daily amount (RDA)—the average amount of the nutrient which should be provided per head in a group of people if needs of practically all members of the group are to be met.
- Requirement—the amount of a nutrient that needs to be consumed in order to maintain normal nutritional status.
- EAR—the mean requirement of a nutrient for a population or group of people; on average 50% will consume more and 50% less than the EAR.
- LRNI—two standard deviations below the EAR; only 2.5% of the population likely to be meeting their requirements at this level of intake.
- RNI—two standard deviations above EAR; at this level intake will be adequate for 97.5% of the group.

- Safe level—is given when insufficient information is available to derive requirements; it is believed to be adequate for most people's needs.
- Saturated fatty acids should be 11% of total dietary energy.
- Essential fatty acids—linoleic acid should be a minimum of 1% total dietary energy and α-linolenic acid a minimum of 0.2% total dietary energy.
- There are no specific recommendations for non-starch polysaccharides (NSP) or fibre in children, but the 'age + 5' rule is commonly used, e.g. a 4-year-old child should have a daily intake of 4 + 5 = 9g of NSP.
- A rough estimate of energy requirement from 1 year of age is '1000 + 100 for each year of life', e.g. a 7-year-old requires 1000 + 700 = 1700kcal/day.
- Nutritional needs of sick children will vary, and increased demands from infection, sepsis, inflammation, etc. may be offset by decreased energy expenditure.

Table 2.2 Some nutrient requirements in childhood

Age	Weight (kg)	Fluid (mL/kg)	Energy (kcal/day) EAR	Protein (g/day) RNI	Na (mmol/day) RNI	K (mmol/day) RNI	Vitamin C (mg) RNI	Ca (mmol/day) RNI	Fe (μmol/day) RNI
Males									
0–3m	5.1	150	545	12.5	9	20	25	13.1	30
4–6m	7.2	130	690	12.7	12	22	25	13.1	80
7–9m	8.9	120	825	13.7	14	18	25	13.1	140
10–12 m	9.6	110	920	14.9	15	18	25	13.1	140
1–3 y	12.9	95	1230	14.5	22	20	30	8.8	120
4–6 y	19	85	1715	19.7	30	28	30	11.3	110
7–10 y	–	75	1970	28.3	50	50	30	13.8	160
11–14 y	–	55	2220	42.1	70	80	30	25	200
15–18 y	–	50	2755	55.2	70	90	40	25	200

Females								
0–3m	4.8	150	515	12.5	9	20	25	13.1	30
4–6m	6.8	130	645	12.7	12	22	25	13.1	80
7–9m	8.1	120	765	13.7	14	18	25	13.1	140
10–12 m	9.1	110	865	14.9	15	18	25	13.1	140
1–3 y	12.3	95	1165	14.5	22	20	30	8.8	120
4–6 y	17.2	85	1545	19.7	30	28	30	11.3	110
7–10 y	–	75	1740	28.3	50	50	30	13.8	160
11–14 y	–	55	1845	42.1	70	70	35	20	260
15–18 y	–	50	2110	45.4	70	70	40	20	260

Malnutrition

Classification

There is no universally agreed definition of malnutrition in children, but the criteria shown in Table 2.3 are commonly used. Classification does not define a specific disease, but rather clinical signs that may have different aetiologies. Other nutrients such as iron, zinc, and copper may be deficient in addition to protein and energy.

The Wellcome classification of malnutrition (Table 2.4) is based on the presence or absence of oedema and the body weight deficit.

When to intervene

Malnutrition is difficult to define and quantify because of insensitive assessment tools and the challenges of separating the impact of malnutrition from that of the underlying disease on markers of malnutrition (e.g. hypoalbuminaemia is a marker of both malnutrition and severe inflammation) and on outcome.

Nutritional intervention may be indicated both to prevent and to reverse malnutrition. In general, the simplest intervention should come first, followed if necessary by those of increasing complexity: for example, give energy-dense foods and energy supplements before progressing to tube feeding. Parenteral nutrition should be reserved for children with impairment of gastrointestinal function to a degree that precludes maintaining growth and homeostasis using enteral feeding. If simple measures aimed at increasing energy intake by mouth are ineffective, tube feeding should be considered according to the criteria shown in Table 2.5.

World Health Organization (WHO) definition of severe malnutrition in children 6–60 months

- Weight for height >3 standard deviations below the mean for the population and symmetrical oedema.

WHO definition of moderate malnutrition in children 6–60 months

- Weight for height between 2 and 3 standard deviations below the mean for the population.

WHO definition of malnutrition in older children

- BMI <5th centile.

WHO treatment of acute severe malnutrition

WHO has developed guidance for management of children with acute severe malnutrition in resource-poor countries. Children with loss of appetite (check by offering ready-to-use therapeutic feed) or medical complications require admission to hospital. Children who have an appetite and are clinically well can be managed as an outpatient. Please refer to the WHO 'Pocket book of hospital care for children' for full details (http://www.who.int/maternal_child_adolescent/documents/child_hospital_care/en/)

No distinction is made between the conditions of kwashiorkor or severe wasting as the treatment is similar.

Table 2.3 Classification of malnutrition

	Obese	Overweight	Normal	Mild	Moderate	Severe
Height for age %				90–95	85–90	<85
Weight for height %	>120	110–120	90–100	80–90	70–80	<70
BMI	>30 (>98th centile)	>25 (>91st centile)				

Table 2.4 Wellcome classification of malnutrition.

Marasmus	<60% expected weight for age No oedema
Marasmic kwashiorkor	<60% expected weight for age Oedema present
Kwashiorkor	60–80% expected weight for age Oedema present
Underweight	60–80% expected weight for age No oedema

Reprinted from The Lancet 296(7667) Shattock FM Classification of infantile nutrition, 302–303 Copyright (1971), with permission from Elsevier.

Table 2.5 Criteria for tube feeding

Impaired energy consumption	Usually 50–60% recommended daily amount despite high-energy supplements
Plus	
Severe and deteriorating wasting	Weight for height >2SD below the mean
Plus	
Skinfold thickness <3rd centile	
And/or	
Depressed linear growth	Fall in height of >0.3SD/year or In early to mid-puberty, height velocity <5cm/year or Decrease in height velocity of >2cm from previous year

SD, standard deviation.

Check for:
- nutritional history
- diarrhoea
- infection history/contact
- dehydration
- shock.

Children with vitamin A deficiency are likely to be photophobic and keep their eyes closed. Children admitted for treatment should be kept separately from those with infection, and nursed in a warm environment (25–30°C). General treatment includes ten steps in two phases: initial stabilization and rehabilitation (Table 2.6).

- Give first feed of ready-to-use F-75 formula (75kcal and 0.9g protein/100mL) and continue every 2 hours for 24 hours, then every 2–3 hours day and night.
- Hypothermia is common and may indicate coexisting hypoglycaemia or serious infection.
- Dehydration is difficult to assess, but assume it is present in all children with watery diarrhoea or reduced urine output.
- Rehydrate with a special rehydration solution for malnutrition (ReSoMal) via nasogastric tube, 5mL/kg every 30 minutes for first 2 hours, then 5–10mL/kg per hour for next 4–10 hours on alternate hours with F-75 formula.
- All severely malnourished children have deficiencies of potassium and magnesium, which may take about 2 weeks to correct; give extra potassium (3–4mmol/kg/day) and extra magnesium (0.4–0.6mmol/kg/day); extra sodium is hazardous and should not be given.

Table 2.6 General treatment plan for children admitted for acute severe malnutrition

	Stabilization		Rehabilitation
	Days 1–2	Days 3–7	Weeks 2–6
Hypoglycaemia			
Hypothermia			
Dehydration			
Electrolytes			
Infection			
Micronutrients	No iron		With iron
Initiate feeding			
Catch-up feeding			
Sensory stimulation			
Prepare for follow-up			

- In severe malnutrition, the usual signs of bacterial sepsis are often absent; assume infection is present and treat with broad-spectrum antibiotics.
- All severely malnourished children have vitamin and mineral deficiencies; supplementation is included in F-75 and F-100 (100kcal and 2.9 g protein/100mL) ready-to-use feeds.
- Iron can make infections worse; don't give iron until the child has a good appetite and starts gaining weight (usually 2nd week).
- Feeds start with the lower energy and protein feed F-75, which is then gradually replaced by F-100.

Children in the catch-up phase can usually be managed as outpatients. Signs of reaching the rehabilitation phase for catch-up growth are return of appetite, no episodes of hypoglycaemia (metabolically stable), and reduced or disappearance of oedema.

References and resources

Aggett PR, Bresson J, Haschke F. Recommended dietary allowances (RDAs), recommended dietary intakes (RDIs), recommended nutrient intakes (RNIs) and population reference intakes (PRIs) are not 'recommended intakes'. J Pediatr Gastroenterol Nutr 1997;25:236–41. https://journals.lww.com/jpgn/Fulltext/1997/08000/Recommended_Dietary_Allowances__RDAs_,_Recommended.22.aspx

Department of Health and Social Security (DHSS). Recommended daily amounts of food, energy and nutrients for groups of people in the UK. Reports on Health and Social Subjects No.15. London: HMSO; 1979.

Ghosh-Jerath S, Singh A, Jerath N, et al. Undernutrition and severe acute malnutrition in children. BMJ 2017;359:j4877.

Infant & Toddler Forum. Growth and its Measurement. Factsheet and interactive tutorial. http://www.infantandtoddlerforum.org

Olsen IE, Mascarenhas MR, Stallings VA. Clinical assessment of nutritional status. In: Walker WA, Watkins JB, Duggan C (eds), Nutrition in paediatrics. London: BC Decker; 2005, pp. 6–16.

Scientific Advisory Committee on Nutrition. Application of WHO growth standards in the UK. http://www.sacn.gov.uk/pdfs/report_growth_standards_2007_08_10.pdf

World Health Organization. Severe acute malnutrition. In: Pocket book of hospital care for children, 2nd edn. Geneva: World Health Organization; 2013, pp. 197–222.

Nutritional assessment

Nutritional assessment *32*
Risk factors for undernutrition *33*
Nutritional intake *34*
Taking a feeding history ('what you eat') *35*
Basic anthropometry: the assessment of body form
    ('what you are') *36*
Nutritional screening *38*
References and resources *38*

Nutritional assessment

Nutritional status reflects the balance between supply and demand and the consequences of any imbalance. The purpose of nutritional assessment is to document objective nutritional parameters, identify nutritional deficiencies, and establish nutritional needs for an individual patient. When judging the need for nutritional support, an assessment must be made both of the underlying reasons for any feeding difficulties, and of current nutritional status. This process includes a detailed dietary history, physical examination, anthropometry (weight, length, head circumference in younger children) with reference to standard growth charts, and basic laboratory indices when possible. In addition, skinfold thickness and mid-upper arm circumference measurements provide a simple method for estimating body composition.

The multisystem consequences of protein–energy malnutrition include:
- Growth failure.
- Impaired gastrointestinal function:
  - Hypochlorhydria.
  - Reduced mucosal function.
  - Pancreatic exocrine impairment.
- Immunodeficiency:
  - Impaired cell-mediated immunity.
  - Anergy.
- Respiratory dysfunction:
  - Reduced respiratory force and minute volume
- Myocardial dysfunction.
- Reduced muscle mass.
- Increased operative morbidity/mortality.
- Delayed wound healing.
- Impaired intellectual development.
- Altered behaviour:
  - Apathy.
  - Depression.

Risk factors for undernutrition

Worldwide, the most common reasons for undernutrition are poverty and lack of access to food. Malnutrition contributes to over a third of global deaths in children <5 years of age, with one in nine people in the world not having enough food to eat to lead an active and healthy life. In the developed world, up to a third of hospital patients may be malnourished to some degree, according to the definition used.

Factors which may decrease food intake

- Age-inappropriate food being offered.
- Inadequate amount of food being offered.
- Unappetizing food.
- Too much food.
- 'Forced' feeding.
- Reduced appetite resulting from illness.
- Symptoms associated with disease or treatments, e.g. nausea, vomiting, sore mouth, pain, diarrhoea, breathlessness.
- Repeated fasting for treatments or procedures.
- Swallowing or chewing difficulties.
- Difficulty self-feeding.
- Poor child–carer interaction at meal times.
- Impaired conscious level.

Increased nutritional requirements

- Illness/metabolic stress.
- Wound or fistula losses.

Impaired ability to absorb or utilize nutrients due to:

- Disease or treatment, e.g. coeliac disease, short bowel, pancreatic exocrine insufficiency.
- Intraluminal factors, e.g. high/low pH.
- Abnormal gut motility.
- Infection, e.g. gastroenteritis, parasites; chronic suppuration.

Nutritional intake

Questions regarding mealtimes, food intake, and difficulties with eating should be part of routine history taking. This gives a qualitative impression of nutritional intake. For a more quantitative assessment, a detailed dietary history may need to be taken and can involve recording a food diary or (less commonly) weighing food intake. Use of compositional food tables or computer software allows these data to be analysed so that a more accurate assessment of intake of energy and specific nutrients can be made.

When considering if such intakes are sufficient, reference can be made to *dietary reference values* (DRV) which provide estimates of the range of energy and nutrient requirements in groups of individuals. Comparison of reported or measured average intakes against the *reference nutrient intake* (RNI), *estimated average requirement* (EAR), or *lower reference nutrient intake* (LRNI) provides an indication of whether intake is likely to satisfy demands. In a particular individual, intakes above the RNI are almost certainly adequate and those below the LRNI almost certainly inadequate (see pp. 22–3 for definitions).

Taking a feeding history ('what you eat')

A careful history is an important component of nutritional assessment. Listed below are some of the questions and 'cross checks' that are integral to an accurate feeding/diet history.

Infant
- Is the baby taking breastfeeds or formula?

For breastfed infants
- How often is the baby being fed and for how long on each breast (check positioning and technique—see Chapter 4)?
- Are supplementary bottles or other foods offered?

For formula-fed infants
- What type of formula?
- How do you make up the feed? (What is final energy concentration/ 100mL?)
- Is each feed freshly prepared?
- How many feeds are taken over 24 hours?
- How often are feeds offered—2-, 3-, 4-hourly?
- What is the volume of feed offered each time?
- How much feed is taken?
- How long does this take?
- Are you adding anything else to the bottle?

Older children
- How many meals and snacks are eaten each day?
- What does your child eat at each meal and snack (obtain 1 or 2 days' sample meal pattern)?
- How would you describe your child's appetite?
- Where does your child eat meals?
- Do you have family mealtimes?
- Are these happy and enjoyable situations?
- How much milk does your child drink?
- How much juice does your child drink?
- How often are snacks/snack foods eaten?

Basic anthropometry: the assessment of body form ('what you are')

Accurate measurement and charting of weight and height (length in children <85cm, or unable to stand) is essential if malnutrition in the hospital and community is not to be missed; clinical examination without charting anthropometric measurements ('eyeballing') has been shown to be very inaccurate. For those infants born prematurely, it is important to deduct the number of weeks born early from actual age ('chronological age') in order to derive the 'corrected age' for plotting on growth charts. This correction is usually made up to the age of 2 years. Head circumference should be routinely measured and plotted in children <2 years.

Measuring weight

- Weigh infants <2 years naked.
- Weigh older children in light clothing only.
- Use self-calibrating or regularly calibrated scales.

Measuring length

- When possible, use an infant measuring board, measuring mat (easily rolled and transported), or measuring rod.
- Two people are required to use the measuring board: one person holds the head against the headboard, the other straightens the knees and holds the feet flat against the moveable footboard.

Measuring height

- Use a stadiometer if possible (a device for standing height measurement comprising a vertical scale with a sliding horizontal board or arm that is adjusted to rest on top of the head).
- Remove the child's shoes.
- Ask the child to look straight ahead.
- Ensure that the heels, buttocks, and shoulder blades make contact with the wall.

Measuring head circumference

- Use a tape measure that does not stretch.
- Find the largest measurement around the mid-forehead and occipital prominence.

Mid-upper arm circumference (MUAC)

- Mark the mid-upper arm (half way between the acromion of the shoulder and the olecranon of the elbow) then, using a non-stretch tape measure, take the average of three readings at the mid point of the upper arm.

Measuring triceps and sub-scapular skinfold thickness

- Pinch the skin between two fingers and apply specialized skinfold calipers; experience is needed to produce accurate and repeatable measurements; take triceps skinfold thickness readings at the mid-upper arm using the relaxed non-dominant arm; the layer of skin and subcutaneous tissue is pulled away from the underlying muscle, and readings taken to 0.5mm, 3 seconds after application of the calipers; measurements can also be taken at other sites.

Measuring waist circumference

- Waist defined as mid-way point between the lowest ribcage and the iliac crest.
- Measure with steel tape.

Body composition

- The simplest way of describing body composition is to divide the body into fat mass (FM, all body fat) and fat free mass (FFM, all remaining tissue including body water muscle and bone).
- Body mass index (BMI) is often used to estimate thinness and obesity, but body composition can vary considerably between people with the same BMI.
- BMI is calculated by dividing weight in kg by height in metres squared.
- Measurement of triceps skinfold thickness provides a proxy for body fat; when combined with MUAC this can be used to calculate the upper arm muscle area (UAMA), a proxy for FFM:

$$UAMA = \frac{[MUAC - (triceps\ skinfold \times \pi)]^2}{4\pi}$$

Putting it together

Information from assessments should be combined together to inform management. A useful framework is to consider 'what you are, what you can do, and what you eat'. 'What you are' describes body habitus (e.g. underweight for height, short for age, etc.). 'What you can do' describes functional activity of the child and is particularly relevant in severe neurological handicap or obesity. Think also of the energy cost of increased respiratory activity, seizures, and decreased activity during illness. 'What you eat' describes current nutritional intake.

Nutritional screening

Screening implies that an underlying and important condition for which there is an effective intervention can be identified by applying a sensitive and specific test. As surveys of patients in hospital have shown that 'malnutrition' is often unrecognized, the concept of screening for nutritional risk has evolved. Scoring systems have been devised that take account of various factors such as anthropometry, illness severity, and reported food intake. 'Screening' for nutritional risk is clearly complicated as it seeks to identify not only children who are malnourished but also those, who in the course of an illness, are at risk of malnutrition. The aim is to be able to select those who need additional evaluation and potential intervention in terms of nutritional support. Clearly there is no one sensitive and specific test that can accomplish this.

Example of commonly used nutrition risk scores and their components include:

- STAMP—Screening Tool for the Assessment of Malnutrition in Paediatrics. Ages 2–16 years, weight and height centiles, predicted implications of current illness for nutritional status.
- STRONGkids—Screening Tool for Risk Of impaired Nutritional status and Growth, developed in the Netherlands where its use is mandatory. Ages 1 month–18 years, subjective assessment of nutritional status (no anthropometry), considers underlying illness, pain, diarrhoea, food intake.
- YPMS—Yorkhill Paediatric Malnutrition Score. Ages 1–16 years, BMI, history of recent weight loss, changes in nutritional intake, predicted effect of current illness on nutritional status.

When these three scores were compared in a large European population of hospitalized children, the identification and classification of malnutrition varied widely. A considerable portion of children with subnormal anthropometric measures were not identified with all the tools. Nutrition screening is probably best seen as a prompt for always considering nutritional issues as part of the clinical evaluation of children. Strong emphasis should be placed on routinely taking a nutritional history, making accurate measurements of weight and height, plotting these on appropriate growth charts, and considering the likely effect of current illness on nutritional status, as outlined earlier in this chapter.

References and resources

Chourdakis M, Hecht C, Gerasimidis K, et al. Malnutrition risk in hositalised children: use of 3 screening tools in a large European population. Am J Clin Nutr 2016;103:130–10.

Johnson MJ, Wiskin AE, Pearson F, Beattie RM, Leaf AA, How to use: nutritional assessment in neonates. Arch Dis Child Educ Pract Ed 2015;100:147–54.

Puntis JWL. Malnutrition and growth. J Pediatr Gastroenterol Nutr 2010;51(Suppl 3):S125–6.

Wiskin AE, Johnson MJ, Leaf AA, Wootton SA, Beattie RM. How to use: nutritional assessment in children. Arch Dis Child Educ Pract Ed 2015;100:204–9.

Further information on anthropometry

http://www.cdc.gov/nchs/data/nhanes/nhanes3/cdrom/nchs/manuals/anthro.pdf

Measuring devices

http://www.miami-med.com/Height_Measuring_Devices.htm

Breastfeeding

Benefits of breastfeeding *40*
Breastfeeding basics *42*
Contraindications to breastfeeding *43*
Promotion of breastfeeding *44*
Tongue tie and breastfeeding *45*
References and resources *45*

Benefits of breastfeeding

Breast milk is the ideal food for infants. The WHO recommends exclusive breastfeeding for at least the first 6 months of life. Until March 2001, the WHO recommended exclusive breastfeeding only for the first 4–6 months of life. This change in policy was based on a systematic review of the published scientific literature which highlighted a protective effect of prolonged breastfeeding against gastrointestinal disease, and confirmed health benefits to mothers. The applicability of these findings to developed countries has been questioned.

The Department of Health in the UK promotes exclusive breastfeeding for the first 6 months of life. In the 2010 Infant Feeding Survey, 81% of mothers started to breastfeed (up from 76% in 2005); by 6 months of age breastfeeding rate had dropped to 34%, and only 1% were exclusively breastfed at this age. Breastfeeding is more likely to occur with higher socioeconomic status. Nearly all mothers have the potential to successfully breastfeed their newborn infants. Healthcare professionals play an important role in providing consistent advice and support (Table 4.1), and in ensuring that parents are aware of the potential benefits.

For the baby
- Ideal nutrient composition, including whey casein ratio (70:30); protein of high biological value; fat 40–50% of calories; essential fatty acids; long-chain fatty acids (docosahexaenoic acid and arachidonic acid) may improve vision and cognition; cholesterol, important for central nervous system (CNS) development and intake from breast milk may influence later cholesterol metabolism.
- Low renal solute load.
- Breast milk contains beneficial immunological, antimicrobial, and anti-inflammatory agents: secretory immunoglobulin (Ig)-A, lactoferrin; lysozyme, macrophages, and lymphocytes.
- Breast milk also contains digestive enzymes: lipase and amylase.
- Reduced risk of gastroenteritis, otitis, respiratory tract infection, and in preterm infants, necrotizing enterocolitis.
- Long-term-effects include a reduction in blood pressure, cholesterol, overweight/obesity, and type 2 diabetes, and an improvement in IQ.
- Lower risk of atopy in those with a family history.
- May prevent or delay onset of coeliac disease.

For the mother
- Uterus contracts faster postpartum.
- Inexpensive and convenient compared with formula.
- Promotes bonding between mother and infant.
- More rapid return to pre-pregnant weight.
- Possible decreased risk of osteoporosis.
- Lactation amenorrhoea (and so infertility) and conservation of iron stores with less anaemia.
- Possible reduced risk of ovarian cancer and premenopausal breast cancer.

Table **4.1** Common problems during breastfeeding

Concern	Action
Engorgement	Often occurs when milk first comes in or when feedings are missed. Use warm compresses or warm shower before feeding. Hand express before feed to make it easier for baby to suck. Breastfeed frequently, every 1–2 hours; encourage baby to suck from each breast. If unable to breastfeed, use breast pump to relieve pressure. Apply ice pack to breast and underarm after feeding until swelling decreases
Inadequate supply	Offer frequent breastfeeds. Check mother's diet and fluid intake; ensure getting adequate rest; check medications
Is baby getting enough milk?	Check for 6–8 wet nappies a day, sleeping between feeds but not for an excessively long time. Good weight gain (up to 8% of birth weight lost in first week is acceptable). Frequency of bowel movements very variable, and can be after every feed or every few days
Jaundice	Feed every 2–3 hours around the clock. If breastfeeding is stopped, express to maintain supply
Leaking	It is a normal sign of 'let down', especially in the early weeks of breastfeeding. Breast pads can be worn between feeds
Mastitis	Rest, frequent breastfeeds; mother should drink plenty of fluids. Antibiotics may be needed; use one that is safe for breastfeeding. Do not stop breastfeeding
Flat or inverted nipples	Frequent breastfeeds to avoid engorgement. Use nipple rolling or stretching before breastfeeds. Express for a short period before each breastfeed
Sore nipples	Some tenderness can be normal but breastfeeding should not be painful. Check for correct latch on and positioning. Vary baby's position at breast; air dry nipples after feeding; avoid soap, alcohol wipes, and nipple creams. Shorter, more frequent feedings. Rub a little breast milk on nipples after each feed
Poor weight gain in infant	Check adequate number of feeds. Increase to 2 hourly during the day. Check position and feeding technique. Ensure baby fully completes feeding at one breast before switching to the other breast; hindmilk is high in fat. Alternate breastfeeds at each feeding. If formula feeding is necessary, give bottle at the end of each breastfeed to encourage stimulation of breast milk, with a goal to fully resume breastfeeding. Reassure mother; encourage relaxation. Seek specialist advice (e.g. lactation advisor) early

Breastfeeding basics

The following are important for successful breastfeeding:
- Infant needs to be sufficiently awake and alert for feeding.
- Coordinated suck and swallow.
- Baby needs to be correctly positioned on the breast (Fig. 4.1).
- Adequate time at the breast to provide stimulation (5–15 minutes).
- Adequate feeding frequency, usually 8–12 times a day for the first 2–3 months.
- Extra water and juice are not necessary until after weaning.
- Avoid introduction of bottle until breastfeeding well established.
- Good nutritional health of mother.
- Relaxed, positive attitude of mother and other family members.
- Social and emotional support for mother.
- Support from health professionals.

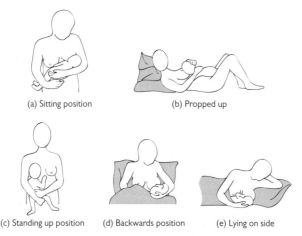

(a) Sitting position

(b) Propped up

(c) Standing up position

(d) Backwards position

(e) Lying on side

Fig. 4.1 Breastfeeding positions. Reproduced from Vinther T, Helsing E. Breastfeeding: How to support success. A practical guide for health workers (1997) World Health Organization, Geneva with permission from the World Health Organization.

Contraindications to breastfeeding

It is important to note that there are very few reasons not to breastfeed a baby.

Maternal illness

- Infection with human immunodeficiency virus (HIV), provided that formula feeding is a safe and feasible option.
- Active tuberculosis; mother can maintain milk with breast pump until treatment renders her non-infectious.
- Drug abuse, e.g. amphetamine, cocaine, heroin, marijuana, and phencyclidine.
- Excessive alcohol intake.
- NB Hepatitis B and C are *not* contraindications to breastfeeding.

Illness in baby

- Galactosaemia (use lactose-free infant formula).
- Phenylketonuria (PKU infants may alternate breastfeeds with phenylalanine-free formula).

Medications taken by breastfeeding mothers

Comprehensive information on drugs in breast milk is provided in the appendix to the British National Formulary. Sometimes alternative drugs can be substituted to allow continuation of breastfeeding, and few drugs constitute an absolute contraindication. Discuss with pharmacist before advising against continuing feeding.

Promotion of breastfeeding

Maternity hospitals may seek baby-friendly accreditation once they have adopted the 'ten steps to successful breastfeeding':
- Have a written breastfeeding policy that is routinely communicated to all healthcare staff.
- Train all healthcare staff in skills necessary to implement this policy.
- Inform all pregnant women about the benefits and management of breastfeeding.
- Help mothers to initiate breastfeeding within 1 hour of birth.
- Show mothers how to breastfeed, and how to maintain lactation even if they are separated from their infants.
- Give newborn infants no food and drink other than breast milk unless medically indicated.
- Practise rooming in, allowing mother and infant to remain together 24 hours a day.
- Encourage breastfeeding on demand.
- Give no artificial teats or dummies to breastfeeding infants.
- Foster the establishment of breastfeeding support groups and refer mothers to them on discharge from hospital.

WHO International Code of Marketing

The WHO International Code of Marketing of Breast milk Substitutes is summarized here and was published in 1981 following discussions on promotion of breastfeeding and the marketing of infant formula:
- No advertising to the public.
- No promotion of products in healthcare facilities, including no free supplies.
- No company mothercraft nurses to advise mothers.
- No gifts or personal samples to healthcare workers.
- No words or pictures idealizing artificial feeding including pictures of infants on labels of products.
- Information to health workers should be scientific and factual.
- All information on artificial infant feeding, including the labels, should explain the benefits of breastfeeding and the costs and hazards associated with artificial feeding.
- Unsuitable products such as sweetened condensed milk should not be promoted for babies.
- All products should be of a high quality and take account of the climatic and storage conditions of the country in which they are used.

Tongue tie and breastfeeding

Maternal pain during feeding and difficulty in latching the baby to the breast are the main symptoms attributed to tongue tie (ankyloglossia) but can also be caused by a number of different problems. Management remains controversial with paediatricians generally being more sceptical than 'lactation advisors' that frenotomy is the solution. This is due to lack of evidence and the subjectivity of outcome variables used to assess the efficacy of tongue tie division.

- Some national paediatric societies (Canada, Japan, Netherlands) do not support frenotomy.
- There is widespread variation in reports of prevalence (0.02–10.7%).
- Tongue function is more important than the visual appearance and a number of assessment tools have been developed.
- Complications of frenotomy are unusual but can include bleeding and haematoma.
- Feeding difficulties can resolve spontaneously so timing of intervention is important with some authors suggesting not before 2–3 weeks of age.

References and resources

Agostoni C, Braegger C, Decsi T. Breast feeding: a commentary by the ESPGHAN Committee on Nutrition. J Pediatr Gastroenterol Nutr 2009;49:112–25.

Horta BL, Bahl R, Martines JC, Victora CG. Evidence on the long-term defects of breast-feeding. Systematic reviews and meta-analysis. Geneva: World Health Organization; 2007.

Infant Feeding Survey 2010. NHS Digital. https://data.gov.uk/dataset/infant-feeding-survey-2010

Vinther T, Helsing E. Breast-feeding: how to support success. A practical guide for health workers. Copenhagen: WHO Regional Office for Europe; 1997. http://www.euro.who.int/document/e557592.pdf

World Health Organization. Protecting, promoting and supporting breast-feeding: the special role of maternity services, a joint WHO/UNICEF statement. Geneva: World Health Organization; 1989.

World Health Organization. The optimal duration of exclusive breast-feeding. Report of the expert consultation. Geneva, Switzerland, March 28–30 2001. Document WHO/NHD/0.1.09.

Formula and complementary feeding

Bottle-feeding *48*
Type of formula feed *50*
Complementary feeding *51*
References and resources *52*

Bottle-feeding

Although the WHO recommends exclusive breastfeeding for 6 months and partial breastfeeding thereafter, it is recognized that some mothers will be unable, or will choose not to breastfeed, and that these mothers deserve support to optimize their infant's nutrition.

It is important that formula feeds are made up according to instructions and that both formula milk and expressed breast milk is handled in a way that minimizes the risk of bacterial proliferation in the feed.

Some simple guidelines are given as follows:

- If using milk formula, use a modified infant formula that meets manufacturing standards.
- Clean the bottle and teat in hot soapy water as soon as possible after a feed using a bottle brush.
- Rinse before sterilizing.
- Cold water or steam sterilizing apparatus may be used; follow the manufacturer's instructions.
- Before making up a feed, clean the work surface and wash your hands.
- If using a cold-water sterilizer, shake off any fluid from the teat and bottle before rinsing in cooled, boiled water.
- Boil tap water in the kettle and allow to cool for half an hour.
- Put the water in the bottle before the milk powder, filling it just up to the desired level.
- Loosely fill the scoop with powder then level without compacting the powder.
- Only use 1 scoop of powder to 30mL (1oz) water; too much powder can cause dehydration through high renal solute load; too little powder can lead to undernutrition.
- Add the powder to the water in the bottle, put the teat in place, and shake gently until the powder is dissolved.
- It is best to make up a fresh feed each time one is required, rather than to store made-up feeds in the fridge, in order to prevent bacterial proliferation.
- Bottles of infant formula should not be heated in a microwave oven as high temperatures reached in the feed can cause severe burns.
- The feed can be cooled by holding the bottle under cold running water from the tap (keep the teat under a cap and away from the water).
- The temperature of the feed can be tested by allowing a few drops to fall on the inside of the wrist; these should be warm and not hot.
- When feeding, the baby should lie comfortably in the crook of the arm, and the bottle be held at an angle so that the teat is always full of milk; this stops excessive ingestion of air during the feed.

Guidance on the average number and volume of feeds is given in Table 5.1.

Table 5.1 Average number and volume of feeds for the formula-fed infant

Age	Approximate volume of a single feed (mL)	Number of feeds per 24 hours
1–2 weeks	50–70	7–8
2–6 weeks	75–110	6–7
2 months	110–180	5–6
3 months	170–220	5
6 months	220–240	4

These figures are for guidance; many babies will vary the volumes ingested from day to day and feed to feed. Total volume of formula milk will be around 150mL/kg/24 hours.

Type of formula feed

The composition of infant formula is closely regulated in terms of the acceptable range of nutrient content. Formula must satisfy all the nutritional needs of an infant. Recommendations for the composition of infant formula have been adopted in the Codex Alimentarius of the Food and Agricultural Organization of the United Nations (FAO) and the WHO. There are two main types of infant formula that differ mainly in their protein composition. These are whey-dominant formula (60% whey, 40% casein) and casein-dominant formula (20% whey, 80% casein). Whey proteins are quickly eliminated from the stomach whereas casein forms curds which are more slowly digested. Full-term normal infants readily digest both types of formula. Although casein-based formula is promoted as being more satisfying for hungry babies, there is little evidence to support this.

- Some formula feeds have long-chain polyunsaturated fatty acids added as these are important for development of the brain and retina. The European Food Safety Authority now recommends that infant formula in Europe should contain 20–50mg docosahexaenoic acid/100kcal.
- Prebiotics (oligosaccharides), probiotics, or both together ('synbiotics') are now added to some milks; these appear to be safe but there is little convincing clinical evidence of any benefit and they are not recommended for routine use.
- Follow-on formula is designed for infants from 6–12 months of age; it contains less protein, calcium, and phosphorus than cow's milk but more than standard infant formula.
- Most follow-on milks contain almost twice as much iron as standard infant formula and 45% more vitamin C.
- Follow-on formula can be used for older infants if breastfeeding has been stopped, and may have a role in the prevention of iron-deficiency anaemia.
- Follow on milks aimed at 1–3-years-olds are not necessary if a balanced and good quality diet is being eaten.
- Soy protein can be used in infant formula as an alternative to cow milk protein; generally some free amino acids are added as the digestibility and biological value of soy protein is less than cow milk protein. Phytate content may reduce the bioavailability of some nutrients, and phytoestrogens in soy feeds mean they are not recommended before 6 months.
- Soy formula can be used for cow milk-allergic children >6 months (there is, however, around a 10% risk of cross reactivity), lactose intolerance, and when parents wish for a vegan diet.
- Other 'special' formula feeds include those containing a thickener (e.g. starch or carob bean) for infants with gastroesophageal reflux. These should not be used for simple reflux, but may have a role in infants showing growth faltering from regurgitation.
- Formula for infants with cow milk protein allergy are based on extensive protein hydrolysates or amino acids; these may also have a role in allergy prevention in the first 4–6 months of life in infants with a family history of allergy or atopy who are not fully breastfed.
- Changing from one type of milk to another is seldom helpful in resolving feeding difficulties or symptoms, and should be avoided unless there are specific indications such as lactose intolerance or cow milk allergy.

Complementary feeding

Complementary feeding embraces all solid and liquid food other than breast milk and infant formula. There is considerable variation between different countries with regard to introduction of complementary food, reflecting the absence of scientific data regarding optimal practice. In general, complementary foods should not be introduced before 17 weeks of age, and should not be delayed beyond 26 weeks. Cultural and economic factors influence timing of introduction of solid foods. For example, in the 2005 UK Infant Feeding Study, 51% of infants had received complementary foods before 4 months, and earlier introduction was associated with formula feeding, lower maternal age, and maternal smoking.

The following points are relevant to weaning practices:

- Kidneys and gastrointestinal tract are sufficiently physiologically mature by 4 months to metabolize nutrients from complementary food.
- From around 6 months, most infants can sit with support and can 'sweep' food off a spoon with their upper lip; by around 8 months they can chew and swallow more lumpy foods; from 9–12 months they have developed the manual skills to feed themselves.
- Continued breastfeeding is recommended along with the introduction of complementary feeding; infant formula or follow-on formula may be used in addition to or instead of breast milk.
- Unmodified cow's milk should not be used as the main drink before 12 months as it may be associated with iron deficiency; during complementary feeding, more than 90% of iron requirements in a breastfed infant may be met by complementary food.
- There is little evidence that delaying or avoiding the introduction of allergenic foods (e.g. egg, fish, nuts, and seafood) prevents or delays the development of allergy.
- The most effective measure for the prevention of allergic diseases is exclusive breastfeeding for 4–6 months.
- Although there is evidence for an adverse effect of rapid infant growth on later cardiovascular outcomes, little is known about diet in the complementary feeding period as a mediator of these effects; given the effect of salt intake on blood pressure, additional salt should not be added to foods during infancy.
- Both breastfeeding during the introduction of dietary gluten and increasing duration of breastfeeding are associated with a reduced risk of developing coeliac disease; it is not clear whether breastfeeding delays the onset or permanently reduces the risk.
- There is an innate preference for sweet-tasting food at birth; this can subsequently be modified by dietary experience; offering complementary foods without added sugars and salt may therefore have long-lasting effects on taste preferences.

References and resources

Agostoni, C, Decsi T, Fewtrell M, et al. ESPGHAN Committee on Nutrition: Complementary Feeding: a commentary by the ESPGHAN Committee on Nutrition. J Pediatr Gastroenterology Nutr 2008;46:99–110. http://www.espghan.med.up.pt/position_papers/con_28.pdf

Codex Alimentarius Commission: Standard for infant formula and formulas for special medical purposes intended for infants. CODEX STAN 72/1981. Rome: Codex Alimentarius Commission; 2007, pp. 1–21.

Koletzko B, Baker S, Cleghorn G, et al. Global standards for the composition of infant formula: recommendations of an ESPGHAN coordinated international expert group. J Pediatr Gastroent Nutr 2005;41:584–99.

The Association of UK Dietitians. Food Fact Sheet: Complementary feeding (weaning). https://www.bda.uk.com/foodfacts/WeaningYourChild.pdf

Chapter 6

The premature newborn

Introduction *54*
General principles *55*
Parenteral nutrition *55*
Enteral feeding *56*
References and resources *60*

Introduction

Developments in care for the premature newborn have led to increasing survival (40% of infants born at 24 weeks' gestation, 65% at 25 weeks, and 80% at 26 weeks) and an increased awareness of the importance of nutritional support. Many have difficulty tolerating enteral nutrition in the early weeks of life until gastrointestinal motility has matured. Some develop necrotizing enterocolitis (NEC) which carries a high risk of morbidity and mortality, and may be regarded as a failure of adaptation to postnatal life. Optimum nutrition should allow adequate growth in the short term, free of metabolic and other complications, with long-term fulfilment of both genetic growth and developmental potential.

General principles

- Low nutritional reserve and high energy requirements underlie the importance of providing timely and effective nutritional support (particularly in infants <1500g) (Table 6.1).
- Ideally, *in utero* growth and nutrient accretion would be replicated, but in practice this is difficult to achieve and early temporary growth cessation is common, with a variable degree of later catch-up.
- Undernutrition in the early weeks of life may have a lasting adverse effect on neurodevelopment and increase the risk of chronic disease in adulthood.
- Parenteral nutrition (PN) is used more widely in the premature newborn than in any other group of paediatric patients.
- The principal indication for PN is immaturity of gastrointestinal function since gastric stasis, abdominal distension, and infrequent stooling impede advancement of enteral feeding.
- Rapid incrementation of milk feeds (>25mL/kg/24 hours) is associated with the development of NEC in case–control studies.
- In terms of enteral feeding regimen, the most appropriate strategy for prevention of NEC remains undefined, but breast milk appears to confer some protection compared with formula feeds; feed volumes should be increased cautiously over the first 10 days of life.
- There is considerable variation in the practice of neonatal nutritional support, reflecting a lack of evidence base; however, there has been a trend towards providing the best possible nutrition as soon after delivery as feasible.

Parenteral nutrition

- Significant risks of PN include glucose intolerance (with osmotic diuresis), bloodstream infection related to a central venous catheter, cholestasis, and hypertriglyceridaemia.
- Variable fluid and electrolyte requirements mean that individualized PN prescriptions are often desirable, although there is an increasing role for standard bags driven both by increasing demand and by the need to have PN readily available (e.g. at weekends).
- Aim to begin PN within the first 24 hours of life if possible; also begin 'minimal enteral feeding' (use mother's or banked breast milk if available); start at 0.5mL/hour in infants <1kg, and 1mL/hour in those >1kg.
- Parenteral nutrient intake may be built up over a number of days; glucose and fat tolerance needs to be monitored carefully with blood glucose and plasma triglyceride measurements.

Enteral feeding

- Respiratory disease or immaturity of suck and swallow mechanisms mean that most premature infants (<37 weeks' gestation) will be tube fed, usually nasogastrically.
- In some units, orogastric tubes are favoured for infants with respiratory distress.
- When fully established, daily milk feeds are of the order of 150–180mL/kg.
- Continuous feeds may be better tolerated in infants with immature gastrointestinal motor function, and are associated with lower energy expenditure than bolus feeds, and possibly improved weight gain.
- Bolus feeds are thought by some to be more 'physiological' and may be better than continuous feeds at stimulating gut hormone release, promoting motor development, and stimulating bile flow.
- A mother's milk appears to be protective against NEC and tolerated better than formula feed in sick infants; it may be expressed breast milk from the infant's own mother or donor breast milk, collected by feeding mothers in the community and given to a milk bank.
- Breast milk is associated with neurodevelopmental advantage, possibly because of its omega-3 fatty acid content, or through an effect of its various biologically active peptides.
- Enthusiasm for milk banking waned in the late 1980s because of concerns regarding nutritional adequacy (low energy and mineral content) and the potential for viral transmission; there has been a recent resurgence of interest in part related to the availability of breast milk fortifiers that can be used to make up the nutritional deficiencies.
- Breast milk fortification with human milk or bovine proteins, minerals, and vitamins has been shown to influence short-term outcomes including growth, nutrient retention, and bone mineralization.
- Fortified human milk may not produce as much weight gain as preterm formula milk, but is associated with a reduction in late-onset sepsis and NEC.
- When breast milk is not available, a preterm formula milk should be used; this has a higher energy, protein, and mineral content than a term formula.
- Infants are often discharged from the neonatal unit a little before their expected date of delivery; they often weigh much less than a term infant, and their nutritional requirements for catch-up growth are now being taken into account through provision of nutrient-enriched post-discharge formula.
- Recent evidence suggests that either low birthweight or rapid early weight gain (or the combination) may predispose to adverse long-term effects, including increased risk of hypertension, cardiovascular disease, type 2 diabetes, and osteoporosis.
- Poorer neurodevelopmental outcomes have been documented both in infants small for gestational age who remained small at 9 months of age, and in those appropriately grown infants who had crossed down weight centiles.
- Nutrient-enriched post-discharge formula have been shown to improve growth but not to enhance neurodevelopment; in the formula-fed infant; these should be used until a post-conceptional age of 40 weeks, and possibly up to 3 months post term.

- Careful growth monitoring must be part of routine follow-up of all premature infants, and both over- and under-feeding avoided.
- See Table 6.1 for recommendations for nutrient intake in newborns.
- Nutritional assessment can be approached in a logical manner (ABCDE—Box 6.1); infants at highest risk of malnutrition include those with birth weight <1kg, those with poor growth (<10g/kg/day after 2 weeks of age), and infants with NEC, chronic lung disease, or gastrointestinal surgical conditions.

Box 6.1 ABCDE approach to nutritional assessment in premature infants

Anthropometry
- Weight.
- Head circumference.
- Length.
- Plot measurements on growth chart.

Biochemistry
- Serum glucose.
- Serum triglycerides (should be <2.8mmol/L if tolerating parenteral lipid).
- Serum electrolytes (to enable adjustment of PN).
- Urea <1.6mmol/L may indicate inadequate protein intake.
- Bone markers: serum phosphate levels a good reflection of intake, and phosphate <1.8mmol/L and ALP >900IU/L may indicate metabolic bone disease.
- Vitamins and trace elements useful if on long-term PN.

Clinical assessment
- Hydration status, oedema, and fluid needs.
- General health.
- Diseases that may affect nutritional requirements or tolerance/absorption of nutrition.

Dietary assessment
- Calculate intakes of energy and protein (and any other nutrients of interest) from parenteral and enteral intakes.
- Compare intakes with recommended amounts.

Evaluation
- Take into account findings from all of above and decide if intakes and growth are adequate.
- Formulate plan to address shortfalls or excesses.

ALP, alkaline phosphatase; PN, parenteral nutrition.

Table 6.1 Nutritional requirements for neonates (for fully enterally fed infants, amounts are per kg per day unless otherwise stated)

	Energy (kcal)	Protein (g)	Fat (g)	Sodium (mmol)	Potassium (mmol)	Calcium (mmol)	Phosphate (mmol)	Magnesium (mmol)	Iron (mg)	Vitamin A (IU)	Vitamin D (IU)	Vitamin E (IU)
Term infants (UK Department of Health)*	115	2.1	Not specified	9 (per day)	13.1 (per day)	13.1 (per day)	13.1 (per day)	2.2 (per day)	1.7 (per day)	1166 (per day)	340 (per day)	Not specified
Very low birthweight infants (<1500g). (Nutrition of the Preterm Infant 2014)**	110–130	3.5–4.5	4.8–6.6	3.0–5.0	2.0–5.0	3.0–5.0	1.9–4.5	0.3–0.6	2.0–3.0	1332–3663	400–1000	3.3–16.4
Preterm infants <1800g at birth (ESPGHAN 2010)†	110–135	3.5–4.5	4.8–6.6	3.0–5.0	1.7–3.4	3.0–3.5	1.9–2.9	0.3–0.6	2.0–3.0	1332–3300	800–1000	3.3–16.4
Low birthweight infants (<2500g, WHO)‡	105–135	3.0–3.6	4.5–6.6	2.5–4.0	2.5–3.5	4–6	2.5–3.8	0.2–0.4	2.0–3.0	700–1500	400	6–12

ESPGHAN, European Society of Paediatric Gastroenterology, Hepatology and Nutrition.

* Dietary reference values for food energy and nutrients for the United Kingdom. HMSO, London, 1991.

** Koletzko B, Poindexter B, Uauy R. Nutritional care of preterm infants: scientific basis and practical guidelines. S. Karger AG, Basel, 2014.

† Agostoni C, Buonocore G, Carnielli VP, et al. Enteral nutrient supply for preterm infants: commentary from the European Society of Paediatric Gastroenterology, Hepatology and Nutrition Committee on Nutrition. J Pediatr Gastroenterol Nutr 2010;50:85–91.

‡ Edmond K, Bahl R. Optimal feeding of low-birth-weight infants. World Health Organization, 2006.

References and resources

Cleminson JS, Zalewski SP, Embleton ND. Nutrition in the preterm infant: what's new? Curr Opin Clin Nutr Metab Care 2016;19:220–5.

Hay WW. Aggressive nutrition in the preterm infant. Curr Pediatr Rep 2013;1:229–39.

Johnson MJ, Wiskin AE, Pearson F, Beattie RM, Leaf AA. How to use nutritional assessment in neonates. Arch Dis Child Educ Pract Ed 2015;100:147–54.

Klein CJ, Heird WC. Summary and comparison of recommendations for nutrient content of low-birth-weight infant formulas. Bethesda, MA:Life Sciences Research Office,; 2005. http://www.lsro.org/articles/lowbirthweight_rpt.pdf

Singhal A. The role of infant nutrition in the global epidemic of non-communicable disease. Proc Nutr Soc 2016;75:162–8.

Necrotizing enterocolitis

Necrotizing enterocolitis 62
Disease management 63
Pathogenesis 64
References and resources 66

Necrotizing enterocolitis

Necrotizing enterocolitis (NEC) is a common and serious disease among premature newborns with an incidence, mortality, and morbidity that has remained unchanged over several decades. Around 7% of infants with a birth weight of 500–1500g are affected; the disease often manifests around 8–10 days of age. The inflammatory response initiated in the gastrointestinal tract may become systemic and affect organs including the brain with long-term adverse neurodevelopmental effects. Some cases of NEC occur in term or near-term infants and are associated with disorders such as maternal illicit drug use, intestinal anomalies, congenital heart disease, and perinatal stress that may affect mesenteric blood flow.

Presenting signs and symptoms

- Feed intolerance; bilious aspirates/vomits.
- Abdominal distension.
- Blood in stools.
- Shiny, distended abdomen with periumbilical erythema.
- Palpable mass (phlegmon) in abdomen.

Radiological features

- Pneumatosis intestinalis (gas in the bowel wall; occasionally seen in other conditions and not by itself pathognomonic of NEC).
- Portal venous gas.
- Free gas on either side of the falciform ligament.
- Free gas on a lateral abdominal film (both sides of bowel wall visible).
- Central free gas shadow on supine anteroposterior film.
- Dilated loops of intestine.
- Ascitic fluid.
- Bowel gas pattern unchanging on serial films (aperistaltic bowel).
- Air/fluid levels in obstruction.

Symptoms can progress rapidly from subtle signs to abdominal distension, intestinal perforation, peritonitis, and hypotension. Laboratory investigations may show acidosis, falling platelet count, raised inflammatory markers, and deranged clotting.

Clear diagnostic criteria are needed, not least to develop effective preventive strategies. A staging system for NEC was described by Bell et al. in 1978 and although imperfect, is still commonly used[*]:

- Stage 1 (non-specific): feed intolerance, abdominal distension.
- Stage 2 (radiographic): e.g. pneumatosis intestinalis.
- Stage 3: perforated viscus.

* Staging reproduced from Bell MJ et al. Neonatal necrotizing enterocolitis. Therapeutic decisions based upon clinical staging. Ann Surg. 1978 Jan; 187(1):1–7 with permission from Wolters Kluwer.

Disease management

Medical management
- Abdominal decompression via nasogastric tube (NGT).
- Broad-spectrum IV antibiotics.
- Bowel 'rest'; total parenteral nutrition (PN).

Surgical management
- Generally required for intestinal perforation or deteriorating clinical condition despite medical treatment.
- Decision to intervene should be based on serial observations.
- About 20% of patients operated on will die; the predominant morbidity is short bowel syndrome with PN dependency.
- Laparotomy is considered in perforation, severe disease, rapid progression, or those who fail to respond to increasing medical intervention.
- Surgery aims to save life and preserve sufficient intestinal length for survival.
- If there is a perforation, abdominal toilet and repair or a stoma are appropriate.
- Resection and primary anastomosis is an option in some patients.
- In patients weighing less than 1.5kg, a peritoneal drain may stabilize the patient before surgery or be a sufficient intervention on its own.
- In extensive disease, a proximal defunctioning stoma and second laparotomy at 24–48 hours can assist in deciding which parts of the bowel can be preserved.
- Affected bowel left behind can stricture after 6–8 weeks and cause obstruction; a distal contrast study may be needed before closure.
- Adhesive obstruction is most common in the first year after surgery.
- Long-term PN dependency should be managed by an experienced intestinal rehabilitation team.

Pathogenesis

Likely to be multifactorial including genetic predisposition, gastrointestinal immaturity, imbalance in microvascular tone, abnormal intestinal microbial colonization, and a highly immunoreactive intestinal mucosa.

Intestinal immaturity

- Immature motility, digestion, absorption, immune defences, barrier function, and circulatory regulation.
- Reduced gastric acid secretion (additional risk from treatment with H_2 blockers).
- Excessive inflammatory response to luminal microbial stimuli (enterocytes in the preterm infant have been in a germ-free environment before birth, and are not prepared for excessive stimulation of initial postnatal colonization).

Microbial colonization

- Experimental NEC does not occur in germ-free animals.
- Specific pathogens have been cultured in outbreaks of NEC, but no one organism has been consistently implicated.
- Molecular methods suggest NEC is associated with both unusual intestinal microbial species, and overall reduction in the diversity of microbiota, especially when there has been prolonged antibiotic therapy.

Hypoxia–ischaemia

- Less emphasis now placed on perinatal hypoxic–ischaemic events as a major contributor to NEC.
- Hypoxia-ischaemia modulates microvascular tone related to production of vascular regulators such as nitric oxide and endothelin; likely to play a downstream role in pathogenic cascade leading to NEC.

Prevention

- Cautious incrementation of enteral feeding.
- Breast milk appears to be protective.
- Enteral aminoglycoside may be helpful, but disadvantages (emergence of resistant organisms) likely to outweigh advantage.
- Probiotic possibly helpful, but does not appear to decrease mortality, may increase sepsis, and questions about safety, dosing, and type of organism remain.
- Prebiotics in feeds (e.g. the oligosaccharides inulin, galactose, fructose, and lactulose) enhance growth of potentially beneficial flora; no strong evidence of benefit in prevention of NEC.

Modulation of inflammation

- Animal models suggest specific microbial components that affect toll-like receptor signalling could modulate excessive inflammatory stimuli.
- Potential area for future therapeutic intervention.

Case study

A male infant with a birth weight of 800g was delivered vaginally at 30 weeks' gestation following spontaneous onset of premature labour. He required ventilatory support, and an umbilical artery catheter was inserted for blood sampling and pressure monitoring. His condition remained stable over the next few days, and small volumes of enteral feed were introduced. Weaning from the ventilator occurred on day 8 of life, from which time enteral feed volumes were further advanced. On day 11, he had a sudden collapse requiring reintubation; aspiration of the NGT showed large gastric residuals, and this was followed by abdominal disten-sion, leading to the discontinuation of milk feeds. An increasing metabolic acidosis was noted on blood gas analysis, and widespread pneumatosis seen on abdominal radiograph. Initial treatment was with IV fluids and broad-spectrum antibiotics. Despite this, his clinical condition continued to deteriorate and a laparotomy was performed. This confirmed NEC with extensive involvement of the small bowel. Non-viable bowel was resected and a jejunostomy fashioned; 40–50cm of potentially viable small bowel was left behind, including the last few centimetres of ileum and the ileocaecal valve. PN was commenced and after 10 days 1mL/kg per hour of formula milk* was introduced. Over the following 3 months, feed volumes were slowly advanced unless unacceptably high stoma losses (>20mL/kg per day) occurred. Subsequently, the jejunostomy was closed and after 4 months of PN, full enteral feeding was established.

* When possible, maternal or donor breast milk should be used; however, lactose intolerance may be a problem post NEC and a hydrolysed formula or amino acid-based feed are alternatives.

References and resources

Bell MJ, Ternberg JL, Feigin RD, et al. Neonatal necrotizing enterocolitis. Therapeutic decisions based upon clinical staging. Ann Surg 1978;187:1–7.

Duthie G, Lander A. Necrotizing enterocolitis. Paed Surg 2013;31:119–22.

Mihatsch WA, Braegger CP, Decsi T, et al. Critical systematic review of the level of evidence for routine use of probiotics for reduction of mortality and prevention of necrotising enterocolitis and sepsis in preterm infants. Clin Nutr 2012;31:6–15.

Growth faltering (failure to thrive)

Introduction 68
Factors influencing growth 69
Pitfalls 69
Management 69
References and resources 70

Introduction

Growth faltering (previously called 'failure to thrive') is a descriptive term implying failure not only of growth, but also impairment of other aspects of a child's well-being. It is a dynamic process involving a failure to meet expected potential, and there is no universally accepted definition. Weight crossing down two major centile lines is often taken as an indicator of need for referral to a paediatrician. In the absence both of symptoms suggesting specific organ dysfunction (e.g. vomiting, diarrhoea, breathlessness, etc.) and physical findings other than poor growth, an underlying organic cause is unlikely. It is important to bear in mind common factors influencing growth, such as parental size and *in utero* growth retardation.

Epidemiological work has demonstrated associations between poor early growth and several adult diseases such as stroke, coronary heart disease, and type 2 diabetes. More recently, attention has also focused on the role of childhood growth patterns in this association. Rather than small size itself predisposing to later disease, there is increasing evidence that it is the disparity between early and later size that is important.

Growth faltering may result from a combination of dietary, organic, and social factors leading to undernutrition; the aetiology includes:

- Unintentional inadequate energy intake.
- Inappropriate feeding, e.g. failure to progress with solids, force feeding, dietary restriction.
- Subtle oromotor problems impairing food intake.
- Behavioural feeding difficulties/food refusal.
- Disturbed parent–child interaction.
- Neglect by parents or carers.
- Abuse by parents or carers.
- Chronic illness or disability adversely affecting nutritional status (the minority, ~5%).

Factors influencing growth

- Familial height (familial short stature).
- Genetic abnormality (e.g. Turner syndrome, Down syndrome).
- Birth size (intrauterine growth retardation).
- Chronic illness (e.g. cystic fibrosis, heart failure, inflammatory bowel disease).
- Psychological factors (psychosocial deprivation).
- Environmental factors (poverty).
- Endocrine factors (e.g. growth hormone deficiency, hypothyroidism).

Investigations should generally be determined by symptomatology or abnormal physical findings (e.g. chromosome analysis if dysmorphic features).

In attempting to rule out or confirm underlying disease, it is reasonable to perform some basic investigations, although the precise choice will depend upon the individual clinical circumstances. Initial investigations might include:
- Inflammatory markers (platelets, CRP, albumin).
- Liver, renal (including bicarbonate and chloride), and thyroid function.
- Full blood count.
- Calcium, phosphate.
- Sodium, potassium, chloride, bicarbonate.
- Ferritin.
- Albumin.
- Urine culture, pH, and test for blood and protein.
- IgA anti-tissue transglutaminase (coeliac disease) if eating gluten-containing food.
- Wrist radiograph for bone age if >18 months.

Pitfalls

- Coeliac disease can cause growth faltering without associated symptoms; the IgA anti-tissue transglutaminase antibody test may be negative in children who are IgA deficient.
- Infants with renal tubular acidosis may present with growth faltering; there will be a hyperchloraemic metabolic acidosis on investigation, with a urine pH <5.8.
- Occasionally, Crohn's disease can manifest as growth failure with little in the way of reported symptoms; clinical signs such as finger clubbing or perianal skin tags/fissures may sometimes be found on examination.

Management

Multidisciplinary assessment including a paediatrician, dietician, psychologist, social worker, speech and language therapist, specialist nurse, etc., is often required to fully assess growth faltering and coordinate effective intervention. Accurate monitoring of growth parameters including length is vital.

Visits to the home and video recordings of interactions at mealtimes by a specialist health visitor or speech and language therapist can be extremely enlightening.

References and resources

Homan GJ. Failure to thrive: a practical guide. Am Fam Physician 2016;94:295–9.

Infant and Toddler Forum. Growth and its measurement. Factsheet and interactive tutorial available from http://www.infantandtoddlerforum.org/measurement

National Institute for Health and Care Excellence (NICE). Faltering growth: recognition and management of faltering growth in children. London: NICE; 2017. https://www.nice.org.uk/guidance/ng75

Raynor P, Rudolf MCJ. Anthropometric indices of failure to thrive. Arch Dis Child 2000;82:364–5.

Raynor P, Rudolf MCJ, Cooper K, Marchant P, Cottrell D, Blair M. A randomised controlled trial of specialist health visitor intervention for failure to thrive. Arch Dis Child 1999;80:500–6.

Iron deficiency

Introduction 72
Diagnosis 72
Management 73
References and resources 74

Introduction

Iron deficiency is the most common nutritional deficiency in the world, affecting around 5 billion people, most of them from developing countries. The prevalence of iron deficiency anaemia in UK preschool children is ~8%, increasing considerably in inner city children; ~9% of under 5s in the US are thought to be iron deficient. Depletion of iron stores is followed by the development of anaemia, initially with a normal mean cell volume (MCV). Continuing deficiency leads to impairment of erythropoiesis, with hypochromia and microcytosis apparent on blood film. Iron is essential in haemoglobin for oxygen transport, and is also found in myoglobin, and some enzymes (peroxidase, catalase, and cytochromes). Iron from red blood cell breakdown is recycled and excess iron stored as ferritin and haemosiderin. Risk factors for iron deficiency anaemia in infants include low birthweight, high cow's milk consumption, low intake of iron containing complementary foods, low socioeconomic status, and immigrant status.

Complications of iron deficiency include:

- Pallor, koilonychia, angular stomatitis, glossitis.
- Tiredness; irritability.
- Poor appetite.
- Impaired exercise tolerance.
- Increased risk of infections (impaired lymphocyte and polymorph function).
- Developmental delay.
- Poor educational achievement.
- Dysphagia (pharyngeal web).
- Breath-holding attacks.
- Pica (e.g. licking newspapers; eating soil, carpet underlay, wood, etc.).

Diagnosis

- Anaemia (haemoglobin <110g/L in children aged 1–2 years, <112g/L in older children).
- Microcytic red cells, hypochromia, anisocytosis, occasional target cells.
- Increased red cell distribution width (>20%).
- Low MCV and mean cell haemoglobin.
- Low plasma ferritin concentration (<10µg/L), can be increased as part of the acute phase response.
- Other causes of anaemia excluded (e.g. β-thalassaemia trait).
- Rise in haemoglobin with therapy.

Other indices of iron status

- Serum iron; unreliable as a measure of iron deficiency, can be depressed as part of the acute phase response.
- Total iron binding capacity (TIBC); a measure of total transferrin; as serum iron decreases, TIBC increases.
- Transferrin saturation—ratio of serum iron:TIBC × 100; low percentage suggestive of iron deficiency.
- Transferrin receptor; bound to transferrin in circulation and relates to concentration of cellular transferrin receptor, increases with iron deficiency.
- Erythrocyte protoporphyrin, increased.
- Zinc protoporphyrin, increased.

Management

Prevention

- Breastfeed: high bioavailability of iron in breast milk.
- If breast milk not available, use an iron-fortified formula (12mg Fe/L).
- Use iron-fortified weaning foods.
- Encourage iron-rich foods, e.g. red meat, egg yolk, iron-fortified breakfast cereals, beans and pulses, dark green vegetables, and dried fruit.
- Give vitamin C-rich fruit/fortified juices with meals as this promotes iron absorption.
- Avoid whole cow's milk during the first year of life, and then restrict intake to <750mL/day.

Treatment and response

- 3–6mg/kg body weight (max. 200mg) of elemental iron daily in two or three divided doses (1mg elemental iron = 0.3mg ferrous sulfate or 9mg ferrous gluconate).
- Increase in reticulocytes 5–10 days after starting treatment.
- Haemoglobin should rise by 10–20g/L over 3–4 weeks; continue treatment for further 3 months once anaemia corrected to replenish iron stores.
- Poor compliance is the most likely cause of non-response in children (but consider other pathologies such as coeliac disease, blood loss, malignancy, inflammation, etc.).
- Persistently positive testing for faecal occult blood (when off iron medication) suggests gastrointestinal blood loss; further investigation may be required including upper and lower gastrointestinal endoscopy, and wireless endoscopy (to identify unusual causes of blood loss such as vascular anomalies in the small bowel).
- Parenteral iron rarely needed unless severe intolerance to oral iron, gastrointestinal disease preventing absorption or exacerbated by oral iron, chronic bleeding, refractory non-compliance. (Rare risk of anaphylaxis.)

NB Side effects of oral iron medication include nausea, epigastric pain (gastric irritation—try lowering dose), constipation or diarrhoea, and turning stools black; accidental overdose is a medical emergency.

References and resources

Baker RD, Greer FR, Committee on Nutrition. Diagnosis and prevention of iron deficiency and iron deficiency anaemia in infants and young children (0–3 years of age). Pediatrics 2010;126:1040–50.

Domellöf M, Braeggar C, Campoy C, et al. Iron requirements of infants and toddlers. J Pediatr Gastroenterol Nutr 2014;58:119–29.

Micronutrients and minerals

Introduction 76
Vitamin deficiency 78
Mineral deficiency 82
Trace element deficiency 84
Vitamin supplementation for infants and young children 86
References and resources 88

Introduction

The term 'micronutrients' includes two main classes of nutrient substances required in the diet in very small amounts: the essential organic micronutrients (vitamins) and the essential inorganic micronutrients (trace elements). Vitamin and mineral deficiencies may complicate malnutrition arising from underlying disease or inadequate diet. Key features are given in the following sections in this chapter. Micronutrients have wide-ranging physiological effects; effects of deficiency can manifest before the development of typical deficiency states.

In children with restricted diets, a detailed dietary assessment by an experienced dietitian may help identify likely vitamin or mineral deficiencies. Children with cow's milk allergy maintained on a strict dairy-free diet, for example, are likely to require calcium supplements unless they are drinking adequate volumes of calcium-containing milk substitute. Fat-soluble vitamin supplementation may be necessary in any chronic condition where there is impairment of fat digestion or absorption (e.g. previous small bowel resection).

Plasma concentrations of vitamins and trace elements do not always accurately reflect tissue stores and should be interpreted with caution, particularly when paediatric reference ranges are not well defined (e.g. selenium). Plasma zinc falls during an acute phase response, whereas plasma copper increases.

Vitamin deficiency

Vitamin A
- Xerophthalmia; cornea becomes dry and hazy and may progress to necrosis and scarring (keratomalacia), occasionally to perforation.
- Major cause of preventable childhood blindness worldwide.
- Subclinical deficiency associated with increased mortality.
- Sources: vegetables (carrots); fish oils; liver.
- Assessment: plasma vitamin A; retinol-binding protein.

Vitamin B$_1$ (thiamine)
- The deficiency syndrome (beriberi) is mainly seen in South-east Asia, and associated with polished rice diet.
- Acute cardiomyopathy at a few months of age.
- Hoarseness, aphonia, encephalopathy, apathy, drowsiness, convulsions, death in older children.
- Sources: germ of cereals, pulses, yeast.
- Assessment: red cell transketolase, blood thiamine.

Vitamin B$_2$ (riboflavin)
- Usually associated with other nutritional defects, rather than occurring by itself.
- Angular stomatitis, fissuring of lips, nasolabial seborrhoea, magenta-coloured tongue.
- Sources: liver, milk, eggs, vegetables.
- Assessment: red cell glutathione reductase.

Nicotinic acid (niacin)
- Together with nicotinamide makes up vitamin B$_3$ complex.
- Deficiency causes pellagra (children eating maize diet; toddlers with kwashiorkor).
- Child usually of school age; symmetrical, desquamating pigmented dermatitis affecting exposed areas of skin.
- Dementia and diarrhoea (more common in adults).
- Sources: meat, fish, cereals, yeast, tryptophan.
- Assessment: urine N-methyl nicotinamide, blood niacin.

Vitamin B$_6$ (pyridoxine)
- Deficiency rare; reported in association with use of infant formula deficient in pyridoxine.
- Convulsions; abnormal electroencephalogram.
- Consider in any newborn with persistent seizures.
- Features in children include weakness, depression, stomatitis, diarrhoea, and dermatitis.
- Sources: animal products, milk.
- Assessment: red cell transaminase, blood pyridoxal phosphate.

Vitamin B$_{12}$

- Deficiency may occur in infants of strict vegetarians, B$_{12}$-deficient mothers, feeding with unfortified artificial milks.
- Pernicious anaemia (intrinsic factor deficiency associated with autoantibodies against gastric parietal cells causing B$_{12}$ malabsorption) may occur in older children.
- Complication of ileal resection; may take years to become apparent.
- Pallor, fatigue, glossitis.
- Subacute combined degeneration of spinal cord (diminished tendon reflexes, loss of vibration sense, ataxia, extensor plantar response).
- Megaloblastic anaemia on blood film; neutropenia, hypersegmentation of neutrophil nuclei, thrombocytopenia.
- Sources: animal products, milk.
- Assessment: serum vitamin B$_{12}$.

Biotin

- Scaly dermatitis and hair loss.
- Sources: most foods, intestinal bacteria.
- Assessment: serum biotin, urine biotin.

Vitamin C

- Scurvy; rarely before 6 months of life.
- Associated with extremely limited dietary intake (e.g. in a child with severe neurological handicap) or tube feeding with special formula or homemade 'blended' diet.
- Petechial haemorrhage into the skin, impaired growth, irritability; painful joints with 'pseudoparalysis'.
- Radiologically may be mistaken for rickets; long bones show thinning of cortex; 'eggshell' calcification around epiphysis; periosteal elevation; occasionally epiphyseal separation.
- Sources: fresh fruit and vegetables, particularly citrus fruits.
- Assessment: leucocyte vitamin C, plasma vitamin C.

Vitamin D

- The main functions of vitamin D are the regulation of calcium and phosphate metabolism; it is essential for bone health. If deficient in childhood, rickets and osteomalacia will develop.
- The term vitamin D (calciferol) refers to a group of fat-soluble secosteroids with endocrine function. The two major forms are vitamin D$_2$ (ergocalciferol) and vitamin D$_3$ (cholecalciferol). Both are synthesized in the skin and are inactive prohormones that bind to vitamin D-binding protein to be transported to the liver where they are converted to 25-hydroxyvitamin D which undergoes further hydroxylation in the kidney to become the active metabolite 1,25 dihydroxy vitamin D. This second hydroxylation step is regulated by calcium and phosphate concentrations via parathyroid hormone (PTH).
- Vitamin D status depends not only on oral supply but also, to a greater extent for most humans, on sun exposure.

- Risk factors for deficiency include inadequate exposure to sunlight, those that live at high latitude particularly if dark skinned, and prolonged exclusive breastfeeding.
- Dietary sources of vitamin D are scarce and include fatty fish and to a lesser extent egg yolk and certain fungi. In some European countries, foods such as milk dairy products, margarine, breakfast cereals, and fruit juices are supplemented with vitamin D.
- Defining vitamin D deficiency is difficult since there are substantial interassay variations and only scant evidence on the correlation of serum concentrations and health outcomes. Most commonly, vitamin D deficiency is considered to be present at 25(OH)D serum concentrations <50 nmol/L, whereas severe vitamin D deficiency is defined by a threshold <25 nmol/L.
- The importance of vitamin D for bone health is well established. Vitamin D supplementation during infancy prevents rickets and osteomalacia and is recommended.
- There is no evidence supporting vitamin D supplementation in children and adults with normal vitamin D concentrations to improve bone health and linear growth. Although many conditions have been associated with vitamin D deficiency, there is insufficient evidence for supplementation in healthy children in respect of improving muscle function, reducing infection, prevention of allergy, reduction in risk of type 1 diabetes, or preventing ischaemic heart disease, cerebrovascular disease, or cancer.

Clinical features of deficiency
- Rickets; impaired bone formation and growth.
- Decreased calcium absorption, low plasma calcium; raised alkaline phosphatase.
- Raised PTH mobilizes calcium from bone, but also leads to phosphaturia and hypophosphataemia; ultimately, PTH effect on bone is impaired and plasma calcium falls.
- Hypotonia and impaired linear growth in infancy, delayed closure of anterior fontanelle; prominent forehead.
- Rarely, symptomatic hypocalcaemia (e.g. stridor, seizures); cardiomyopathy.
- Swelling of costochondral junctions ('rachitic rosary').
- Bowing of tibia in weight-bearing children; swelling over growing end of long bones (e.g. wrists).
- Enamel hypoplasia and delayed appearance of teeth.
- Coxa vara, kyphoscoliosis, pelvic deformity in long-standing cases.
- Radiologically: poor mineralization, delayed development of epiphyses; cupping, fraying, and splaying of metaphyses; radiolucent transverse bands (Looser's zones).
- Sources: fish oil; vegetable oil; skin synthesis.
- Assessment: serum Ca, PO_4, alkaline phosphatase, serum 25OH-vitamin D.

Vitamin E

- Deficiency may be seen in preterm infants and children with malabsorption.
- Haemolytic anaemia in the preterm.
- Progressive neuropathy and retinopathy in severe, prolonged deficiency.
- Sources: vegetable oils.
- Assessment: serum vitamin E.

Folic acid

- Nutritional deficiency mainly in developing countries; may occur in prematurity, malignant disease and its treatment, chronic haemolytic anaemia; malabsorption; drugs (e.g. methotrexate, anticonvulsants); B_{12} deficiency.
- Megaloblastic anaemia on blood film, macrocytosis, neutropenia with hypersegmentation of polymorph nuclei, thrombocytopenia.
- Supplementation in pregnancy reduces risk of neural tube defects.
- Sources: green vegetables, liver.
- Assessment: serum folate, red cell folate.

Vitamin K

- Haemorrhagic disease of newborn (breastfed infants at increased risk).
- Gastrointestinal haemorrhage or bleeding from cord; intracranial haemorrhage.
- Prevented by routine prophylactic vitamin K administration after birth (usually multiple oral doses).
- Sources: green vegetables, gut flora.
- Assessment: prothrombin time.

Mineral deficiency

Calcium
- Absorbed from proximal small bowel.
- Nutritional deficiency in isolation very unusual.
- Absorption affected by other nutrients, e.g. fat malabsorption.

Phosphorus
- Isolated deficiency very unlikely.
- Prolonged treatment with aluminium or magnesium hydroxide: bind to phosphorus resulting in non-absorption.
- Deficiency leads to osteoporosis or rickets.

Magnesium
- Deficiency may be encountered in protein–energy malnutrition, after small-bowel resection or with protracted diarrhoea.
- Rare selective inability to absorb magnesium managed by magnesium supplementation.

Trace element deficiency

Iron

- Deficiency from poor intake (common), impaired absorption, or excessive losses.
- Anaemia, pallor, tiredness, loss of appetite, increased infection, impaired development, pica.
- Assessment: serum iron/iron binding capacity; serum ferritin.

Zinc

- Growth retardation, hypogonadism, hepatosplenomegaly, and anaemia.
- Delayed wound healing, pica, diminished taste.
- Symmetrical, peri-orificial erythematous rash.
- May occur in preterm newborn receiving PN (particularly after bowel resection).
- Assessment: plasma zinc, leucocyte zinc, alkaline phosphatase (low, zinc-dependent enzyme).

Copper

- May occur in infants with protein–energy malnutrition or malabsorption (or during PN with inadvertent omission of trace elements).
- Hypochromic anaemia unresponsive to iron; neutropenia.
- Skeletal changes can resemble scurvy or non-accidental injury.
- Assessment: plasma copper, caeruloplasmin.

Fluoride

- Important for reducing risk of dental caries.
- Assessment: urine excretion.

Iodine

- Hypothyroidism with poor growth and development.
- Assessment: serum T_4, T_3, thyroid-stimulating hormone (TSH).

Chromium

- Deficiency may impair glucose tolerance; weight loss.
- Assessment: plasma chromium; glucose tolerance.

Cobalt

- Essential component of vitamin B_{12}.

Manganese

- Role in human metabolism uncertain.
- Deficiency in animals results in growth impairment, neonatal ataxia, chondrodystrophy, and impaired fertility.
- Assessment: plasma manganese.

Molybdenum
- Essential component of xanthine oxidase.
- Assessment: urine xanthine, plasma molybdenum.

Selenium
- Deficiency implicated in Keshan disease (cardiomyopathy, China) and Kashin–Beck disease (osteoarthropathy, Siberia), but other environmental factors likely to be important.
- Skeletal myopathy and pseudo-albinism described during PN without selenium.
- Assessment: plasma selenium, red cell glutathione peroxidase

Vitamin supplementation for infants and young children

Precise daily requirements for vitamins are not well established (Table 10.1) but supplementation is regarded as important in early life (children <4 years).

- The fetus acquires vitamins from its mother, with fat-soluble vitamins being transferred towards the end of pregnancy.
- Breast milk from mothers with adequate nutritional status supplies sufficient amounts of all vitamins other than K and D.
- The UK Department of Health recommends either a single intramuscular dose of 1mg vitamin K at birth to newborn babies, or an alternative oral regimen of three 2mg doses during the first 6–8 weeks.
- Infant formula is fortified with vitamin K.
- Dark skin and low sunlight exposure increase the risk of vitamin D deficiency.

Risk factors for vitamin deficiency should be identified in the child and in the diet.

- In the UK there is strong evidence that vitamin D deficiency exists.
- In addition, large surveys have suggested that ~50% of children may have a suboptimal vitamin A intake, although clinical deficiency is not seen except with underlying disease (e.g. short bowel syndrome/ malabsorption).
- The key steps in ensuring adequate vitamin status in children are giving vitamin K at birth, promoting a healthy, balanced diet in early life, and maintaining a low threshold for giving supplementary vitamin D (5µg/ day; 200IU).

Use of vitamin and mineral supplements

This may also be required in children with a poor diet, those on therapeutic diets, and to replace increased losses. Expert dietetic assessment is appropriate and vitamin and mineral supplementation should go together with dietary advice.

- Children with eating difficulties, or those on vegan or vegetarian diets, may be short of iron and zinc.
- Children on exclusion diets for food allergy, and low-protein diets for inborn errors of metabolism or renal disease, may need comprehensive supplementation.
- Diets excluding or reducing specific items such as milk or fructose or sucrose may need supplementation with calcium or vitamin C respectively.
- Low-fat diets should routinely be supplemented with fat-soluble vitamins.
- A complete trace element and vitamin supplement is needed for children being fed a modular feed.

Table 10.1 Nutrient intakes for vitamins (units/day)

Vitamin	Reference Nutrient Intake	Reference Nutrient Intake	Reference Nutrient Intake	Tolerable upper intake
	0–6 months	7–12 months	1–3 years	
A (μg)[a]	350	350	400	800μg/day (1–3 yr)
D (μg)[b]	8.5	7	7	25μg/day (0–24 m)
E (mg)[c]	0.4mg/g PUFA[d]	0.4mg/g PUFA	0.4mg/g PUFA	10mg/100 kcal formula
K (μg)	10	10	10	not given
B1 (thiamine) (mg)	0.2	0.2/0.3	0.5	not given
B2 (riboflavin) (mg)	0.4	0.4	0.6	not given
Niacin (equivalents mg)	3	4/5	8	2 mg/day (1–3 yr)
B6 (pyridoxine) (mg)	0.2	0.3/0.4	0.5	not given
B12 (μg)	0.3	0.4	0.5	not given
Biotin (μg)[e]	not given	not given	not given	7.5/100 kcal
Pantothenate (mg)	1.7	1.7	1.7	1.2/100kcal
Folic acid (μg)	50	50	70	200μg/day (1–3 yr)
C (mg)[f]	25	25	30	30mg/100 kcal

[a] 1μg vitamin A retinol equivalent (RE) = 3.33IU.

[b] Vitamin D (calciferol); 1μg = 40IU.

[c] Vitamin E, A-tocopherol equivalent, 1mg = 1IU.

[d] PUFA, polyunsaturated fatty acids.

[e] No daily reference value given for biotin; an intake between 10 and 200μg/day considered safe and sufficient.

[f] Vitamin C as ascorbic acid.

Reproduced from Leaf AA. Vitamins for babies and young children. Arch Dis Child 2007;92:160–164, Copyright © 2007, BMJ Publishing Group Ltd and the Royal College of Paediatrics and Child Health with permission from BMJ Publishing Ltd.

References and resources

Braegger C, Campoy C, Colomb V, et al. Vitamin D in the healthy European paediatric population. J Pediatr Gastroenterol Nutr 2013;56:692–701.

Leaf AA. Vitamins for babies and young children. Arch Dis Child 2007;92:160–4.

NHS choices. Vitamins for children. http://www.nhs.uk/conditions/pregnancy-and-baby/pages/vitamins-for-children.aspx

Reid IR. What diseases are causally linked to vitamin D deficiency? Arch Dis Child 2016;101:185–9.

Nutrition support teams

Introduction *90*
Malnutrition *90*
Suggested core composition of the NST *91*
Roles of the NST *91*
References and resources *92*

Introduction

There has been a considerable increase in the use of intensive nutritional support (both parenteral and enteral) in the management of children with chronic disorders at risk of malnutrition. In addition, awareness of overt or potential malnutrition among hospital inpatients has increased. The identification of those with (or at risk from) malnutrition, and provision of effective nutritional intervention requires a multidisciplinary team approach since the skills required to deal with the details of assessment, prescription, administration, and monitoring of treatment frequently fall outside the remit of a single practitioner.

Malnutrition is common among hospitalized children with a reported prevalence of 15–30%. An expert report from the Council of Europe published in 2002 highlighted shortcomings in nutritional care throughout European hospitals, and provided recommendations for improving the situation, including the implementation of nutrition support teams (NSTs). The overall aim of a multidisciplinary NST is to provide safe up-to-date appropriate nutritional support to an individual patient, who is malnourished or at risk of malnutrition, in a coordinated fashion.

Malnutrition

- Is a continuum that starts with a nutrient intake inadequate to meet physiological requirements, followed by metabolic and functional alterations and later by changes in body composition.
- Is associated with an increase in morbidity and mortality in hospitalized children.
- Is a consequence of imbalance between low nutrient supplies and high substrate needs.
- In childhood, especially during infancy and adolescence, an increase in nutritional demands imposed by illness will compete with the specific needs of growth; however, increased energy requirements during acute illness may be balanced by a decrease in energy expenditure.
- Careful measurements and use of appropriate growth charts are essential for the diagnosis of malnutrition in children and for nutritional monitoring.

Suggested core composition of the NST

- Paediatric gastroenterologist.
- Nutrition nurse specialist.
- Dietician.
- Pharmacist with specialist training in prescribing PN.
- Paediatric surgeon.

For managing problems associated with central venous access, impaired oromotor function, feeding difficulties, and ongoing need for PN the team should develop close working links with:

- Microbiologists.
- Interventional radiologists.
- Cardiologists.
- Speech and language therapists.
- Clinical psychologists.
- Occupational therapists.
- Radiologists.
- Clinical biochemists.

Roles of the NST

- To implement patient screening for nutritional risk.
- To identify patients who require nutritional support.
- To ensure effective nutritional management.
- To plan home nutritional support following discharge when required.
- To liaise with community staff and sources of social support.
- To facilitate teaching parents and carers how to undertake home nutritional support (enteral and parenteral).
- To educate hospital staff with respect to identification and management of nutritional problems.
- To audit practice.

References and resources

Agostoni C, Axelson I, Colomb V, et al. The need for nutrition support teams in pediatric units: a commentary by the ESPGHAN committee on nutrition. J Pediat Gastroent Nutr 2005;41:8–11.

Beck AM, Balknäs UN, Camilo ME, et al. Practice in relation to nutritional care and support: report from the Council of Europe. Clin Nutr 2002;21:351–4.

Nightingale J. Nutrition support teams: how they work, are set up and maintained. Frontline Gastroenterol 2010;1:171–7.

Wales PW, Allen N, Worthington P, et al. A.S.P.E.N. clinical guidelines: support of pediatric patients with intestinal failure at risk of parenteral nutrition-associated liver disease. JPEN J Parenter Enteral Nutr 2014;38:538–57.

Enteral nutritional support

Introduction 94
Access routes for enteral tube feeding 96
Liquid feed composition and choice of feed 100
Complications of enteral nutritional support 102
References and resources 104

Introduction

Assessment of a patient needing nutritional support will include a decision regarding the most appropriate method of feeding. The enteral route is preferred for children who have an adequately functioning gastrointestinal tract. Oral intake can simply be increased by use of food fortification, sip feeds, or energy supplements. If oral intake is poor or contraindicated, tube feeding may be used.

Tube feeding is used to prevent or correct malnutrition in the following groups of conditions:

- Impaired suck, chew, and swallow:
  - Prematurity.
  - Cerebral palsy.
  - Neurodegenerative disorders.
  - Orofacial malformations.
  - Intensive care/impaired conscious level.
- Breathlessness on feeding:
  - Respiratory disease.
  - Congenital heart disease.
- Disordered appetite:
  - Cachexia associated with chronic disease/malignancy.
  - Primary appetite disorder.
- Increased energy requirements:
  - Cystic fibrosis
  - Advanced liver disease.
  - AIDS.
- Continuous supply of nutrients needed:
  - Short-bowel syndrome.
  - Protracted diarrhoea.
  - Glycogen storage disease.
- Unpalatable liquid diet used as primary therapy:
  - Crohn's disease.
  - Multiple food intolerance/allergy.

Access routes for enteral tube feeding

Short-term feeding (<6 weeks)
- Fine-bore nasoenteral tubes (e.g. Silk tube):
  - Nasogastric.
  - Nasojejunal (e.g. if vomiting from severe gastro-oesophageal reflux).

Longer-term feeding (>6 weeks)

Gastrostomies
- Percutaneous endoscopic gastrostomy (PEG): a feeding tube placed endoscopically into the stomach while under a GA.
- Balloon gastrostomy (button): a low-profile feeding device placed into the stomach and held in place by a balloon.
- Balloon gastrostomy tube (BGT): a feeding tube placed into the stomach held in place by a balloon.
- Surgical gastrostomy (e.g. when PEG is technically not feasible/contraindicated).
- Fluoroscopic percutaneous gastrostomy (interventional radiologist).
- Laparoscopic gastrostomy.

Jejunostomies
- Percutaneous endoscopic gastrostomy with jejunal insert: (PEGJ): a feeding tube placed endoscopically into the stomach with a coaxial tube placed into the small bowel via the pylorus.
- Transgastric double lumen jejunostomy (GJ button): low-profile device place into the stomach with a jejunal extension. The device is held in with a balloon and is fitted by radiology once a gastric stoma has been formed.
- Surgical jejunostomy: a feeding tube placed surgically into the jejunum.
- Surgical jejunostomy (e.g. Roux-en-Y).

How to place a nasogastric tube (NGT)

Use a tape measure to determine the length of NGT to be inserted (see Fig. 12.1 and Table 12.1). For gastric placement in children, measure from ear to nose, then to tip of xiphisternum (Fig. 12.1a). For newborns and infants, measure from ear to nose, then to the mid-point between the xiphisternum and umbilicus (Fig. 12.1b). The tube can be marked with a small piece of tape or permanent marker pen. Remember to record the external length of the tube.

When to check the safe positioning of a NGT
- After initial insertion.
- Before a bolus feed.
- After a bout of vomiting.
- After paroxysm of coughing.
- If symptoms suggest feed aspiration (coughing, choking, tachypnoea, wheezing, etc.).
- When receiving a child moved from another clinical area.
- 12-hourly for children on continuous nasogastric feeds.
- 4-hourly in infants and newborns on continuous feeds.

(a)

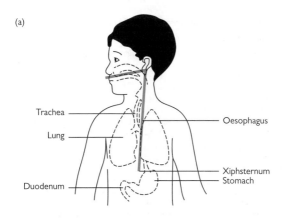

Trachea

Oesophagus

Lung

Xiphsternum
Stomach

Duodenum

(b)

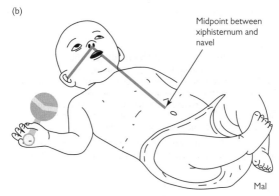

Midpoint between
xiphisternum and
navel

Mal

Fig 12.1 Measuring a NGT: (a) for children; (b) for infants and newborns.

Table 12.1 How to confirm correct NGT position

Confirmatory test result	Action
Positive aspiration of gastric contents (pH <5.5 using pH paper) and correct length of tube	Accept placement as correct
Unable to obtain aspirate of gastric contents despite correct external length of tube	1. If possible, offer drink to child and re-aspirate 2. Inject 2–5mL of air and re-aspirate 3. Inject 2–5mL 0.9% saline, position child on their side, and re-aspirate
Unable to obtain aspirate of gastric contents and incorrect external length of tube	Reposition tube to correct length and re-aspirate; if no aspirate, follow steps 1–3 above.
Unable to obtain aspirate of gastric contents and correct external length of tube	Confirm satisfactory placement by chest/abdominal X-rayor Remove tube and re-site, then repeat confirmatory tests

Giving medicines via an enteral feeding tube

- If possible, give medicines by mouth or other route than tube.
- Use liquid preparation, or thoroughly crush tablets and mix with water.
- Dissolve contents of gelatin capsules in warm water.
- Do not give enteric-coated and slow-release tablets via the tube.
- Flush tube with water before and after each medication.
- Avoid adding medication directly to liquid feed.

For details of gastrostomy care, replacement of a PEG button, management of a leaking stoma, and treatment of over-granulation, see Chapter 21.

Liquid feed composition and choice of feed

- Carbohydrates in enteral formula are derived from different starches, including corn and tapioca; maltodextrin and hydrolysed corn starch, glucose-derived saccharides, and corn syrup are most commonly used.
- Formula for children usually contain little or no lactose.
- Protein is often derived from casein, soy, or whey protein, with a nitrogen:non-nitrogen energy ratio of ~1:150.
- Lipids are supplied predominantly as triglycerides, either as long-chain (LCT) or medium-chain triglycerides (MCT).
- MCT come mainly from coconut oil, and are rapidly hydrolysed and effectively absorbed even at low concentrations of pancreatic enzymes or bile acids.
- A high intake of MCT may cause osmotic diarrhoea; essential fatty acids need to be added to the feed.
- LCT promote intestinal motility and stimulate biliary and pancreatic secretions; however, when there is maldigestion, hydroxylation by bacteria can induce secretion into the bowel, worsening diarrhoea.
- Some enteral formulas contain fibre, which may be useful to prevent constipation; fibre is also a substrate for bacterial production of short-chain fatty acids that are trophic to colonic mucosa and a source of energy.
- Most enteral formula contain sufficient micronutrients to meet increased needs associated with stress and wound healing; L-carnitine, taurine, and inositol are commonly added.

Nutrient density and osmolarity

- The nutrient density of an enteral feed clearly depends on fluid content; at standard dilution, the energy content of infant formula is usually 0.67kcal/mL, and standard paediatric enteral formula 1kcal/mL.
- More concentrated enteral formula are also available (1.3–2kcal/mL) for patients with increased energy requirements or with restricted fluid intake.
- Osmolality refers to the concentration of osmotically active particles per litre of a liquid formula, expressed as mOsm/L; the osmolality is affected by the concentration of all constituents such as amino acids, carbohydrates, lipids, and electrolytes. Formula with a higher osmolality than normal body fluids may produce an osmotic diarrhoea; this is particularly important in children with severe small intestinal disease, or with jejunal feeds; isotonic formula with an osmolality of around 300mOsm/L are preferred.

Selection of enteral formula

Enteral formula feeding must result in delivery of an adequate nutrient intake in a form and volume that the child can tolerate. In selecting an appropriate formula, the following factors are relevant to choice:

- Nutrient and energy requirements suitable for the age and clinical condition of the child.
- History of food intolerance or allergy.

- Intestinal function.
- Site and route of delivery.
- Osmolality.
- Taste.
- Cost.

For the great majority of paediatric patients, a standard paediatric polypeptide-based enteral formula will be appropriate. There are, however, many specialized and disease-specific products designed for those with particular needs (see the British National Formulary for Children). In some children, a ready-made formula is not suitable and a 'modular' feed must be made up in the diet kitchen, or by parents at home once suitably trained. This allows flexibility with type and concentration of macronutrients so that the feed can be adjusted to suit individual requirements and tolerance. A modular feed is most commonly used in severe enteropathy (e.g. post-gastroenteritis syndrome) or short-bowel syndrome complicating NEC.

Hygiene and enteral tube feeding

Points to remember

- A non-touch technique must be used when preparing a feed, transferring it to another container, and when priming and connecting the giving set to the feeding tube. Extra care must be taken to avoid touching key parts of the system that will be in contact with the feed.
- Discard any open/hanging feed after a 24-hour period.
- Throw away any refrigerated feed that has been open for 24 hours or more.
- Throw away any used feed containers and giving sets after 24 hours.

Bolus or continuous feeding

Delivery methods include bolus or continuous feeding. The feeding regimen will need to be adjusted depending on the child's lifestyle, rehabilitation activities, social activities, and treatments or medication.

- *Bolus feeding*: this involves a volume of feed given by gravity or by a feeding pump at regular intervals, mimicking meals and snack times. Bolus feeding should only be considered for gastric feeding (not jejunal).
- *Continuous feeding*: this is less physiological than bolus feeding but may be appropriate for patients unable to tolerate large volumes of feed. This should also be used for all children with any form of jejunal feeding.

Jejunal feeding

- Jejunal feeding is used in children where feeding into the stomach is contraindicated (e.g. severe gastro-oesophageal reflux with risk of aspiration) or not tolerated (e.g. gastroparesis).
- Tubes are normally passed either at the bedside (confirmation of a tube placed post pylorus should be by abdominal X-ray) or in radiology under screening.

Complications of enteral nutritional support

It is important to consider and regularly review the objectives of nutritional support in individual patients. Monitoring will include regular review of nutritional intake, anthropometry, biochemical and haematological status, general clinical state, gastrointestinal function, and tube integrity. Potential complications are shown in Table 12.2.

Table 12.2 Complications associated with tube feeding

Cause	Possible solution
Diarrhoea	
Unsuitable feed in a child with impaired gut function	Change to hydrolysed formula or modular feed
Excessive infusion rate	Slow rate and increase as tolerated
Intolerance of bolus feeds	Frequent, smaller feeds, or change to continuous feeds
High feed osmolarity	Build up strength of feed slowly and give by continuous infusion
Microbial contamination of feed	Use sterile, commercially produced feeds when possible; prepare other feeds in clean environment
Drugs (e.g. antibiotics, laxatives)	Review drug prescription
Nausea/vomiting	
Excessive infusion rate	Slowly build up feed infusion
Slow gastric emptying	Encourage lying on right side; prokinetics
Constipation	Maintain regular bowel habit with adequate fluid intake, fibre-containing feed, and/or laxatives
Medicines given at the same time as feed	Allow time between giving medicines and giving feed, or stop continuous feed for a short time
Psychological factors	Review feeding behaviour; consider referral to psychologist
Regurgitation/aspiration	
Gastro-oesophageal reflux	Correct positioning; feed thickener; drugs; continuous feeds; jejunal tube; fundoplication
Dislodged tube	Secure tube adequately and regularly review position
Excessive infusion rate	Slow infusion rate
Intolerance of bolus feeds	Smaller, more frequent feeds, or continuous infusion

Dumping syndrome

Feeding can only be done via a feeding pump as bolus feeding in the jejunum can cause dumping syndrome. Dumping syndrome is characterized by a set of vasomotor and gastrointestinal symptoms associated with sudden nutrients exposure to the small intestine. Early dumping (within 30 minutes of a meal) is a result of a vasomotor response to intravascular volume being drawn into the gut lumen by hyperosmolar feed. It presents as palpitations, hypotension, tachycardia, fatigue, dizziness, sweating, headache, flushing, epigastric pain and fullness, diarrhoea, nausea, and vomiting. Late dumping is in response to excessive insulin secretion secondary to high serum glucose due to rapid absorption. It presents with sweating, tremors, and loss of consciousness.

References and resources

Braegger C, Decsi T, Dias JA, et al. Practical approach to Paediatric Enteral Nutrition: a comment by the ESPGHAN committee on Nutrition. J Paed Gastro Nutr 2010;51:110–22. http://www.espghan.org/fileadmin/user_upload/guidelines_pdf/EN.practical_approach.2010.pdf

British National Formulary for Children. https://www.medicinescomplete.com/about/publications.htm

National Institute for Health and Care Excellence (NICE). Nutritional support for adults: oral nutrition support, enteral tube feeding and parenteral nutrition. London: NICE; 2017. http://guidance.nice.org.uk/CG32

Refeeding syndrome

Refeeding syndrome *106*
References and resources *108*

Refeeding syndrome

- Defined as severe fluid and electrolyte imbalances with metabolic abnormalities that occur in malnourished patients as a result of reinstituting enteral nutrition or PN. The hallmark biochemical feature of refeeding syndrome is hypophosphataemia and there may be associated abnormal sodium and fluid balance, thiamine deficiency, hypokalaemia, and hypomagnesaemia.
- During starvation, there is a change in the hormonal milieu in addition to a reduction in basal metabolic rate, conservation of protein, prolongation of organ function, preferential catabolism of skeletal muscle, and loss of visceral cell mass. The concentration of insulin is decreased while that of glucagon increases, resulting in the conversion of glycogen to glucose in addition to gluconeogenesis from lipid and protein stores. Free fatty acids and ketone bodies replace glucose as the primary sources of energy. As feeds (parenteral or enteral) are initiated in a starving child, the protective mechanisms against starvation (ketosis) are disrupted. There is a rapid shift from fat metabolism (ketosis) to the utilization of carbohydrate. Excess glucose evokes a release of insulin, which acts as a driving mechanism causing an increased uptake of glucose, phosphate, potassium, magnesium, and water into the cell in addition to stimulating protein synthesis. This often results in a precipitous drop in serum electrolytes and fluid shifts. Fluid shifts may result in congestive cardiac failure, dehydration or overload, hypotension, pre-renal failure, and sudden death. Carbohydrate can result in the retention of sodium and water. The complications arising from this can be life-threatening, so judicious use of protein and calories is advised.

Refeeding syndrome is likely to occur in patients who have had:

- Prolonged periods of suboptimal nutrition intake over days or weeks prior to hospital admission.
- Experienced significant weight loss prior to hospital admission in both the obese or underweight patient.
- Experienced significant diarrhoea or vomiting in the week leading up to institution of nutrition support.
- Prolonged period of nil by mouth for >7–10 days, or poor nutrition intake during hospital stay with evidence of stress and depletion.
- Anorexia nervosa.
- Classic severe malnutrition with or without oedema.
- Some critically ill patients.

Management of refeeding syndrome

- All patients at risk should have close monitoring in a hospital setting before feeds are started.
- A complete anthropometrical assessment, including measurement of weight, height, and BMI, should be completed before commencing feeds.

- Fluid and electrolyte status should be assessed and any abnormalities corrected before enteral nutrition or PN is started.
- Enteral nutrition or PN should be started at 60% of the total requirement for current weight and increased gradually over a period of 5–7 days.
- Daily monitoring of the following is required over this period:
  - Weight.
  - Urine specific gravity.
  - Serum electrolytes especially sodium, potassium, phosphate, and magnesium.
  - Acid–base balance.
- Oral replacement of electrolytes such as magnesium, phosphorus, and potassium may cause diarrhoea and if levels are very low would need replacing intravenously.
- In children fed enterally, lactose- and sucrose-free feed should be considered if milk-based feeds induce diarrhoea.
- Multivitamins and thiamine should be started to prevent deficiency. Thiamine is an essential coenzyme in carbohydrate metabolism and its requirements are increased with utilization of carbohydrate for metabolism.

References and resources

Braegger C, Decsi T, Dias JA, et al. Practical approach to paediatric enteral nutrition: a comment by the ESPGHAN committee on nutrition. J Pediatr Gastroenterol Nutr 2010;51:110–22.

Mehanna HM, Moledina J, Travis J. Refeeding syndrome: what it is, and how to prevent and treat it. BMJ 2008;336:1495–8.

Royal College of Psychiatrists. Junior MARSIPAN: Management of really sick patients under 18 with anorexia nervosa. CR168. London: Royal College of Psychiatrists; 2012. http://www.rcpsych.ac.uk/pdf/CR168summary.pdf

Chapter 14

Parenteral nutrition

Introduction *110*
Indications for parenteral nutrition *111*
Monitoring of parenteral nutrition *112*
Complications and their management *114*
Home parenteral nutrition *118*
References and resources *119*

Introduction

- Parenteral nutrition (PN) is the mainstay of treatment for intestinal failure and is required to preserve nutritional status, provide for growth and development, and ensure maintenance of fluid and electrolyte balance.
- The time when PN should be initiated will depend on the underlying disease, background nutritional status, and the age of the child. Well-nourished children who are predicted to be unable to achieve enteral autonomy by 5 days should be started on PN. This duration would be shorter for neonates, small preterm infants, and undernourished children.
- The main indication for PN is when nutritional status cannot be maintained or restored to normal using enteral feeding.
- The first case report of successful long-term PN (in an infant with small-bowel atresia) was published in 1968; since that time products for PN have been developed and refined with the result that metabolic complications are less common, and use in clinical practice has become widespread.
- PN fluids contain glucose solution, synthetic crystalline amino acids, fat emulsion, electrolytes, minerals, vitamins, and trace elements.
- Details of regimens appropriate for different age groups are readily available (e.g. see ESPGHAN guidelines).
- Vascular access—PN fluids are usually hyperosmolar and cause phlebitis as well as tissue injury if extravasation occurs. Peripherally inserted central lines are very effective means of providing PN over a short to medium term. Patients requiring prolonged duration of PN require more definitive central venous access which is usually via a central venous catheter (CVC) inserted surgically and with the tip just outside the right atrium.
- Estimating calorie requirement—this will be variable and dependent on needs but can be estimated in most cases based on the patient's corrected age, degree of undernutrition, and underlying disease. Energy requirements can be calculated by estimating their basal metabolic rate/resting energy expenditure, and requirements for growth. Children who are undernourished at the time of starting PN will need additional calories for catch-up growth. This can be estimated by calculating their requirements at expected rather than current weight.
- Suboptimal nutrition results in poor growth, impaired immunological responses, and poor adaptation. Overfeeding can cause hyperglycaemia, hyperinsulinism with resultant hypertriglyceridemia, and liver disease.
- The principal unsolved problems associated with PN are CVC-related bloodstream infection (CRBSI), and intestinal failure-associated liver disease (IFALD), both of which are life-threatening.
- Mechanical CVC-related problems such as blockage and fracture are also relatively common, and may sometimes be resolved without removal of the catheter.

Indications for parenteral nutrition

- The decision to commence PN will be based on an assessment of nutritional reserve, and the nature of the underlying illness; in tiny premature infants, death from starvation may occur in under a week, and nutritional support is an urgent necessity; in a much older child with a postoperative ileus, PN may be unnecessary.
- The principal indication for PN is 'intestinal failure' (see Chapter 14), i.e. normal growth, nutritional status, and homoeostasis cannot be maintained using enteral nutrition. This can be short term (e.g. postoperatively), medium term secondary to inability to feed enterally (e.g. after bowel surgery), or long term (e.g. after resection of small bowel).
- The most common causes of intestinal failure are extreme prematurity with immaturity of gastrointestinal motor function; necrotizing enterocolitis; short bowel syndrome (e.g. ileal atresia, neonatal volvulus, extensive bowel resection for NEC); chronic intestinal pseudo-obstruction; and severe, persistent diarrhoea (e.g. congenital enteropathy; immunodeficiency).

Monitoring of parenteral nutrition

Serious and unexpected biochemical side effects of PN are uncommon, although particular care must be taken with children who are poorly nourished and may be at risk of refeeding syndrome. Table 14.1 provides a suggested schema for monitoring.

Table 14.1 Suggested monitoring protocol during PN in clinically stable patients

	Before PN	Daily	Twice weekly	Once weekly	Monthly	6-monthly
Plasma						
Na	x		x			
K	x		x			
Bilirubin	x			x		
Ca				x		
PO$_4$	x			x		
Alk phos				x		
Glucose		x week 1		x		
Cu, Zn, Se, Mn					x	
Cholesterol triglyceride			If fat >3g			x
Full blood count; ferritin; PT/PTT						x
Al, Cr						x
Folate; Vitamins A, E, D						x
Urine						
Na	x					
K	x					
Glucose		x				
Other						
CXR						x
ECG						x
Cardiac echo						x

CXR, chest X-ray; ECG, electrocardiogram; echo, echocardiogram; PT, prothrombin time; PTT, partial thromboplastin time.

Complications and their management

Diagnosis and management of catheter-related complications

Administration of long-term PN requires placement of an indwelling CVC. The problems associated with central lines include infections, mechanical damage, blockages, and thrombosis. From Infections are the commonest complication with the incidence being around 2 per 1000 days of PN. Prevention is based on optimal catheter placement and strict hand hygiene. Taurolidine, a derivative of the amino acid taurine, has been shown to have a role in reducing catheter-related sepsis.

- Suspect in any child with an indwelling CVC who develops fever/signs of sepsis.
- Additional features may include hyperglycaemia, diarrhoea, and/or vomiting.
- Exclude tunnel/exit site, wound, urine, respiratory infection, and meningitis.
- Take 'through CVC' and/or peripheral blood samples for microbial culture.
- Start antibiotic treatment through the CVC as soon as possible if temperature >38.5°C or other strong indication of sepsis.
- First-line antibiotics should provide broad-spectrum cover against likely organisms.
- Discuss treatment with microbiologist.
- Bear in mind the possibility of yeast infection if no clinical response within 48 hours (send blood cultures direct to mycology laboratory; ophthalmic examination).
- Remove CVC if overwhelming sepsis (unless little prospect of alternative venous access for giving essential drugs); yeast isolated; continuing positive blood cultures despite appropriate antibiotics; septic embolism.

Occlusion of the CVC is another common problem complicating long-term PN. For prevention and management of partial or complete CVC occlusion:
- Use a suitable infusion pump for PN, with appropriate alarm settings.
- For flow rates <20mL/hour, pressure should be set at 30–40mmHg greater than the resting pressure.
- For flow rate ≥20mL/hour, infusion pumps may be used with occlusion alarms at 100mmHg.
- The infusion pressure should be recorded 4-hourly.
- A trend of increasing pressure measurements indicates developing occlusion; early intervention at this point may prevent complete blockage.

If the pump alarms repeatedly
- Are the clamps open?
- Are there kinks or twists in the tubing?
- Is the flow rate too high for the catheter being used?

If none of these apply
- Flush the CVC with saline/heparin sodium (10 units/mL).
- If the CVC resists flushing, an unblocking agent is required (see following section).

When attempting to unblock a CVC
- Use a small syringe (delivers greater pressure).
- Start with a 5mL syringe, and work down to 2mL, then 1mL.
- NB Excessive force may rupture the CVC.
- Repeated gentle 'pull and push' on the syringe may clear the obstruction.
- If required, use the following treatments in turn until occlusion is cleared (the CVC lumen is filled with the solution and aspiration/flushing attempted after a short period of time).

Urokinase lock
- Add 1mL of water for injection (WFI) to a vial of 25,000 units of urokinase:
  - Child <1 year: take 0.1mL (2500 units) and make up to 1mL with WFI; instil 1mL into CVC.
  - Child >1 year: take 0.2mL (5000 units) and make up to 2mL with WFI; instil 2mL into CVC.
- Leave for 2 hours, then aspirate and flush with 0.9% sodium chloride.

Urokinase infusion
- Use only for patients with normal coagulation and platelets.
- Not suitable for a CVC that is completely blocked to manual flush.
- Make a 200 units/mL solution of urokinase in dextrose 5%.
- Infuse at 1mL/kg/hour for 6 hours.

Management of IFALD

Liver disease is the most frequent and severe complication of IF, developing in 40–60% of infants. The clinical spectrum includes hepatic steatosis, cholestasis, cholelithiasis, and hepatic fibrosis. Progression to biliary cirrhosis and the development of portal hypertension and liver failure occurs in a small proportion.

The aetiology of IFALD is multifactorial and risk factors include:
- Prematurity and low birth weight.
- Duration of PN.
- Underlying diagnosis and severity of intestinal failure.
- Lack of enteral feeding.
- Recurrent sepsis.
- Excessive intake of long-chain polyunsaturated fatty acids.
- Inadequate calories or micronutrients in PN.
- Deficiencies of essential fatty acids (FAs).

PN can be adapted to reduce the risk of liver injury. The changes that can be made include the following:
- Using appropriate type of fat emulsion. The recent development of emulsions with balanced concentrations of omega (ω)-6/ω-3 lipids reduce liver damage. SMOF lipid is an intravenous lipid emulsion

containing soybean oil, medium-chain triglycerides, olive oil, and fish oil developed to provide energy, essential FAs, and long-chain ω-3 FAs as a mixed emulsion containing α-tocopherol. It has been shown to decrease plasma bilirubin, increase ω-3 FA, and α-tocopherol status without changing lipid peroxidation.

- Limit the amount of glucose in PN and cycling of PN to reduce hepatic fat accumulation secondary to hyperinsulinism.
- Providing adequate nutrition in PN to ensure growth.
- Prevention and treatment of catheter-related infections has also been shown to significantly improve outcome in these children.
- Bacteria in the small bowel deconjugate bile salts and produce hepatoxic metabolites thus prevention and early treatment of small bowel bacterial overgrowth reduces liver damage.
- To improve bile flow and reduce the formation of biliary sludge, oral ursodeoxycholic acid may be advantageous and is commonly prescribed although there is no clear evidence of efficacy.

Metabolic complications of PN

The metabolic complications include metabolic bone disease, hyperlipid-aemia, hypercalciuria with risk of nephrocalcinosis, manganese hepato- and neurotoxicity, and other nutrient deficiencies. The frequencies of these complications are reduced with increased experience in managing these patients.

Renal complications

Colonic oxalate absorption is increased in patients with short bowel syndrome, resulting in hyperoxaluria and the risk of calcium oxalate nephrolithiasis. The risk of stone formation is reduced if all or part of the colon is removed.

Social implications

Transferring care of these children from hospital to home has a positive influence on CVC infections, social circumstances, as well as reducing the cost of treatment. At the same it also puts a significant burden on the family, who will have to spend a lot of time caring for the child and have difficulty in maintaining gainful employment.

Home parenteral nutrition

In infants who do not need hospitalization but are dependent on long-term PN, home parenteral nutrition (HPN) is an alternative. HPN can be used for children with irreversible intestinal failure or those who are expected to achieve the transition from PN to full enteral nutrition over weeks to months rather than a shorter time period. Patients eligible for HPN should be in a medically stable condition and require PN for at least 3 months. When possible, PN is infused for 12 hours overnight and the CVC 'locked' with anticoagulant (± antimicrobial) during the day. Cyclical PN helps to prevent liver complications as well as freeing the child from the infusion pump during the day. Parents or carers need to be highly motivated and trained in delivering PN.

Teaching in preparation for HPN

The following topics should be covered:
- The child's underlying diagnosis and prognosis.
- Placement and function of the CVC.
- Potential complications (e.g. infection, embolism, cholestasis).
- General overview of nutrients.
- How to set up PN infusions.
- How to adjust flow rates.
- Maintenance and problem-solving re infusion pumps.
- Aseptic technique.
- Emergency management of the CVC: air, blockage, infection, rupture.
- Management of hypoglycaemia.
- Monitoring urine and blood glucose.
- Understanding social implications of therapy.
- Emergency contact numbers.
- Support group contacts.

Parent-held records

Parents/carers should have an up-to-date set of health records for any health professionals they might encounter at different times who are unfamiliar with their child's care. These should include:
- Medical summary of condition.
- CVC history and care protocols.
- Feed prescription information.
- Techniques for heparinizing CVCs.
- Unblocking a CVC.
- Treatment of suspected sepsis.
- How to respond to emergency situations.
- List of hospital and community contacts.
- Growth charts.
- Record of biochemical monitoring.

References and resources

British National Formulary for Children. https://www.medicinescomplete.com/about/publications. htm

Kelly DA. Intestinal failure-associated liver disease: what do we know today? Gastroenterology 2006;130:S70–7.

Koletzko B, Goulet O, Hunt J, et al. Guidelines on paediatric parenteral nutrition of the European Society of Paediatric Gastroenterology, Hepatology and Nutrition (ESPGHAN) and the European Society for Clinical Nutrition and Metabolism (ESPEN), supported by the European Society of Paediatric Research (ESPR). J Pediatr Gastroenterol Nutr 2005;41(Suppl 2):S1–S4. https://journals.lww.com/jpgn/Fulltext/2005/11002/1__Guidelines_on_Paediatric_Parenteral_Nutrition.1.aspx

Wales PW, Allen N, Worthington P, et al. A.S.P.E.N. clinical guidelines: support of pediatric patients with intestinal failure at risk of parenteral nutrition-associated liver disease. JPEN J Parenter Enteral Nutr 2014;38:538–57.

Intestinal failure

Introduction *122*
Short bowel syndrome *124*
Motility disorders *126*
Mucosal disorders *127*
Practical management *128*
Intestinal transplantation *132*
References and resources *132*

Introduction

The main function of the intestinal tract is to absorb fluids, electrolytes, and nutrients to sustain growth in children. Inability to perform this role as a result of various reasons is called intestinal failure. This can be a result of short bowel syndrome (SBS), mucosal disorder, or neuromuscular motility disorder. See Box 15.1.

> **Box 15.1 Causes of intestinal failure**
>
> **Short bowel syndrome**
> *Congenital*
> *Acquired:*
> - NEC
> - Gastroschisis
> - Intestinal atresias
> - Volvulus
> - Vascular thrombosis
> - Apple peel syndrome
> - Intussusception
> - Inflammatory bowel disease
> - Post-trauma resection
>
> **Mucosal disorders**
> *Congenital enteropathies:*
> - Primary epithelial disease:
>   - Microvillus inclusion disease
>   - Intraepithelial dysplasia
>   - Phenotypic diarrhoea
> - Immune mediated:
>   - Severe combined immunodeficiencies
>   - Autoimmune enteropathies (e.g. IPEX)
>
> *Acquired mucosal disease:*
> - Radiation enteritis
> - Post chemotherapy
> - Severe extensive Crohn's disease
> - Post-enteritis protracted diarrhoea
>
> **Neuromuscular motility disorders**
> *Chronic intestinal pseudo-obstruction*
> *Aganglionosis:*
> - Hirschsprung disease
>
> *Primary visceral myopathies:*
> - Familial myopathy with megaduodenum
> - Megacystis microcolon
> - Hollow visceral myopathy
>
> *Primary neuropathies:*
> - Familial visceral neuropathies
> - Ganglioneuromatosis with MEN type IIb
> - Disorders of interstitial cells of Cajal
>
> IPEX, immunodysregulation polyendocrinopathy enteropathy X-linked syndrome; MEN, multiple endocrine neoplasia

Short bowel syndrome

SBS is the result of the alteration of intestinal digestion and absorption that occurs as a result of extensive bowel resection or congenital absence of bowel. It represents a complex disorder that affects normal intestinal physiology with nutritional, metabolic, and infectious consequences. In a large population-based study, the overall incidence of SBS was 22.1 per 1000 neonatal intensive care unit (NICU) admissions and 24.5 per 100,000 live births, with a much greater incidence in premature infants.

Causes

These include:
- Congenital atresia of small bowel.
- Gastroschisis with associated atresia, or bowel infarction (typically territory of superior mesenteric artery: from proximal small bowel to splenic flexure in colon).
- Malrotation with volvulus (may present with yellow or green vomit in the newborn period; symptoms may be intermittent).
- NEC (usually in the preterm infant).
- Crohn's disease with resection.

The small bowel measures ~250cm at birth in term babies, being shorter in preterm infants. Nutritional consequences are likely to follow loss of >50% of small bowel. After massive gut resection, there is a process of adaptation, ultimately resulting in an increased absorptive capacity, such that many children are dependent on PN for a time (sometimes years) but eventually manage to make the transition to full enteral feeding. Favourable factors for intestinal adaptation include >30cm of residual small bowel, presence of the ileocaecal valve, and preservation of the colon.

Adaptation involves mucosal hyperplasia, increasing surface area fourfold. Enteral nutrition is essential for this process, and should be given to the maximum tolerated without provoking severe diarrhoea. Intraluminal nutrition stimulates hyperplasia through contact of epithelial cells with nutrients, stimulation of secretion of trophic gastrointestinal hormones, and upper gastrointestinal secretions. The process of adaptation can go on over a number of years. Failure to achieve full enteral feeding after 5 years of PN suggests there will be lifelong dependency on PN (but this is not invariable).

Ultrashort bowel syndrome

Ultrashort bowel syndrome (USBS) is a group of heterogeneous disorders where the length of small bowel is <10cm or 10% of expected for the age. It is caused by massive loss of the gut which in the neonatal period can be a result of vanishing gastroschisis or surgical resection following midgut volvulus, jejuno-ileal atresia, and/or extensive NEC. The exact prevalence of USBS is not known although there is a clear trend towards increasing numbers because of increased incidence and improved survival. Long-term PN is the mainstay of treatment and is best delivered by a multidisciplinary intestinal rehabilitation team.

Outcome

Outcome in SBS is dependent on many factors including the primary condition leading to resection. The survival of children on HPN has improved considerably with long-term survival rates at 2, 5, 10, and 15 years of 97%, 89%, 81%, and 72%, respectively.

Motility disorders

- Neuromuscular motility disorders are disorders of intestinal motility leading to intestinal failure.
- The commonest cause of motility disorder is gastroschisis which is the evisceration of the fetal intestine through a defect in the paraumbilical anterior abdominal wall with herniation of gastrointestinal structures into the amniotic cavity. Its incidence has been increasing over the last two decades and is reported around 2.4 per 10,000 births. A higher incidence is seen in women <20 years of age. Despite significant improvement in antenatal detection and neonatal management of gastroschisis, ~15% of children need to have a resection of the bowel leading to SBS and chronic intestinal failure. This is because of associated intestinal anomalies including malrotation, midgut volvulus with necrosis, and intestinal atresia.
- Chronic idiopathic intestinal pseudo-obstruction (CIPO) is a heterogeneous group of rare disorders, presenting with signs and symptoms of intestinal obstruction in the absence of an identifiable mechanical obstruction.
- Most cases present in infancy.
- There may be abnormalities in the enteric nervous system or gut musculature ('neuropathic' or 'myopathic').
- Sometimes other hollow viscera such as the bladder are involved, e.g. megacystis microcolon and intestinal hypoperistalsis syndrome.
- Hirschsprung disease and fabricated illness should always be considered as possible diagnoses.
- Manometric studies and full-thickness bowel biopsy may be necessary to fully clarify the diagnosis.
- Long-term management especially in severe cases with use of HPN.

Mucosal disorders

- Congenital enteropathies are a common cause of intestinal failure in children and present as intractable diarrhoea of infancy—see Chapter 36.
- This can be due to primary epithelial disease or immune-mediated damage of mucosal lining.
- Management is with use of long-term PN to maintain growth and promoting enteral intake.
- Microvillus inclusion disease (MVID) is a congenital disorder of intestinal epithelial cells. The diagnosis is based on histology which reveals a variable degree of villous atrophy and presence of intracytoplasmic inclusions that are lined by intact microvilli on electron microscopy.
- Intestinal epithelial dysplasia (IED) is related to abnormal development and differentiation of enterocytes and is characterized by histological abnormalities including villous atrophy, disorganization of the surface epithelium, and basement membrane abnormalities.
- Autoimmune enteropathy (AIE) and enteropathies due to primary immune deficiencies are relatively uncommon. It involves most of the small bowel and sometimes the large bowel as well. AIE is a T-cell-mediated disorder which histologically is characterized by villous atrophy and mononuclear infiltration of the lamina propria. There is also presence of elevated circulating serum immunoglobulins, the antibody reported to be most commonly associated is anti-enterocyte antibody and this can be used for both diagnosis and monitoring of treatment. Initially children are dependent on PN and definitive treatment is in the form of immunosuppressants or a bone marrow transplant.

Practical management

The main aims in management of intestinal failure are:
- Maintaining growth and development.
- Promoting intestinal adaptation.
- Preventing complications.
- Optimizing quality of life.

Management

- Management should be by a multidisciplinary nutritional care team in a unit experienced in caring for such patients, and is a multistage process, starts with correction of fluid and electrolyte abnormalities and followed with cautious enteral feeding (1mL/kg/hour in newborn) with breast milk if available, or with hydrolysed protein/lactose-free feed. Feeds are increased slowly as tolerated unless unacceptably high stool losses or stoma losses (i.e. >6 stools per day, >20mL/kg/day from stoma), while maintaining nutrition and hydration with PN.
- High stool output is seen mainly as a result of high stoma, i.e. jejunostomy. Management of high stool output with antisecretory agents such as proton pump inhibitors or antimotility agents such as loperamide.
- Gastric acid hypersecretion may occur for 3–6 months after resection due to a lack of inhibitory hormones from the intestine and antisecretory agents such as proton pump inhibitors may be needed to control output.
- Antimotility agents such as loperamide (up to 0.2mg/kg four times daily) or codeine (1mg/kg four times daily) work by slowing transit through the bowel and increasing luminal contact to help absorption. They are very effective, especially in cases where colon is in continuity.
- Other causes of high output should be considered such as sepsis, partial/intermittent bowel obstruction, enteritis, residual bowel disease, drugs, and bacterial overgrowth.
- May involve consideration of HPN in those patients in whom dependency is anticipated for >4 months (e.g. <30cm small bowel in newborn).

Surgical interventions

- Aim to maximize mucosal contact with enteral nutrients without disturbing motility or reducing total absorptive surface area.
- Strictures should be removed and where possible, stomas closed.
- Intestinal tapering or plication is sometimes used to improve motility and in turn, absorption; bowel lengthening procedures are also used; these including the Bianchi procedure (longitudinal division of the bowel along its mesenteric and anti-mesenteric border), and more recently the serial transverse enteroplasty procedure (STEP). The precise indications and potential benefits of tapering, plication, and lengthening remain poorly defined.

Complications

Intestinal failure-associated liver disease (IFALD)

Liver disease is the most frequent and severe complication of intestinal failure and the clinical spectrum includes hepatic steatosis, cholestasis, cholelithiasis, and hepatic fibrosis. Progression to biliary cirrhosis and the development of portal hypertension and liver failure occurs in a small proportion. IFALD is multifactorial and risk factors include:

- Prematurity and low birth weight.
- Duration of PN.
- Lack of enteral feeding.
- Recurrent sepsis.
- Excessive intake of long-chain polyunsaturated FAs.
- Inadequate calories or micronutrients in PN.
- Deficiencies of essential FAs.

Catheter-related complications (including bloodstream infection)

Administration of long-term PN requires placement of an indwelling CVC. The problems associated with central lines include infections, mechanical damage, blockages, and thrombosis. Infections are the commonest complication with incidence being around 2 per 1000 days of PN. Prevention is based on optimal catheter placement and strict hand hygiene. Taurolidine, a derivative of amino acid taurine, has been shown to have a role in reducing catheter-related sepsis. With advances in type of catheters used and insertion techniques, there has been a significant reduction in complications. This still is the largest group of preventable complications which significantly affect the outcome of children with intestinal failure.

Metabolic complications of PN

The metabolic complications include metabolic bone disease, hyperlipidaemia, hypercalciuria with risk of nephrocalcinosis, manganese hepato- and neurotoxicity, and other nutrient deficiencies. The frequencies of these complications are reduced with increased experience in managing these patients.

Renal complications

Colonic oxalate absorption is increased in patients with SBS, resulting in hyperoxaluria and the risk of calcium oxalate nephrolithiasis. The risk of stone formation is reduced if all or part of the colon is removed.

Small bowel bacterial overgrowth (SBBO)

There is a high risk of SBBO because of increased amount of unabsorbed carbohydrates providing substrate for bacterial growth, intestinal dysmotility, and potentially the absence of the ileo-caecal valve.

In severe forms it can present with D lactic acidosis from bacterial fermentation of dietary carbohydrate, causing confusion, ataxia, dysarthria, etc. Early treatment of SBBO helps improve uptake of enteral nutrients, limits damage to liver, and improves intestinal function. The most effective treatment for SBBO is to improve enteral intake. Other treatments include the use of antibiotics which are not absorbed from the intestinal mucosa (e.g. gentamycin) and using probiotics to alter gut flora. There is usually an incomplete or inadequate response to these, necessitating frequent courses of treatment.

Gallstones
Disordered enterohepatic bile salt circulation.

Vitamin B$_{12}$ deficiency
Loss of terminal ileum; may take years to develop.

Social implications
Transferring care of these children from hospital to home has a positive influence on CVC infections, social circumstances, as well as reducing the cost of treatment. At the same it also puts a significant burden on the family who have to spend a lot of time caring for the child and have difficulty in maintaining gainful employment

Intestinal transplantation

- See Chapter 16.
- Indications are essentially life-threatening complications of PN, including:
  - Liver failure from IFALD (small bowel and liver transplantation, or isolated liver).
  - Venous thrombosis/occlusion jeopardizing continued venous access.
  - Recurrent overwhelming CRBSI.
- Relative contraindications include:
  - Severe congenital or acquired immunological deficiencies.
  - Multisystem autoimmune disease.
  - Insufficient vascular patency to guarantee vascular access for up to 6 months after transplant.
  - Chronic lung disease of prematurity.

References and resources

Batra A, Beattie RM. Management of short bowel syndrome in infancy. Early Hum Dev 2013;89:899–904.

Burghardt KM, Wales PW, de Silva N, et al. Pediatric intestinal transplant listing criteria – a call for a change in the new era of intestinal failure outcomes. Am J Transplant 2015;15:1674–81.

Colomb V, Dabbas-Tyan M, Taupin P, et al. Long-term outcome of children receiving home parenteral nutrition: a 20-year single-center experience in 302 patients. J Pediatr Gastroenterol Nutr 2007;44:347–53.

D'Antiga L, Goulet O. IF in children. The European view. J Pediatr Gastroenterol Nutr 2013;56:118–26.

Goulet O, Ruemmele F, Lacaille GF, Colomb V. Irreversible intestinal failure. J Pediatr Gastroent Nutr 2004;38:250–69.

Guarino A, De Marco G; Italian National Network for Pediatric Intestinal Failure. Natural history of intestinal failure, investigated through a national network-based approach. J Pediatr Gastroenterol Nutr 2003;37:136–41.

Gupte GL, Beath SV, Kelly DA, Millar AJW, Booth IW. Current issues in the management of intestinal failure. Arch Dis Child 2006;91:259–64.

Heneyke S, Smith VV, Spitz L, Milla PJ. Chronic intestinal pseudo-obstruction: treatment and long term follow up of 44 patients. Arch Dis Child 1999;81:21–7.

Khan FA, Squires RH, Litman HJ, et al. Predictors of enteral autonomy in children with intestinal failure: a multicenter cohort study. Pediatric intestinal failure consortium. J Pediatr 2015;167:29–34.

Nightingale J, Woodward JM, Small Bowel and Nutrition Committee of the British Society of Gastroenterology. Guidelines for management of patients with short bowel. Gut 2006;55(Suppl IV):iv1–12.

Quiros-Tejeira RE, Ament ME, Reyen L, et al. Long-term parenteral nutritional support and intestinal adaptation in children with short bowel syndrome: a 25-year experience. J Pediatr 2004;145:157–63.

Stanger JD, Oliveira C, Blackmore C, Avitzur Y, Wales PW. The impact of multi-disciplinary intestinal rehabilitation programs on the outcome of pediatric patients with intestinal failure: a systematic review and meta-analysis. J Pediatr Surg 2013;48:983–92.

Intestinal transplantation

Introduction *134*
Current status *134*
Indications *135*
Nomenclature *135*
Techniques *136*
Postoperative management *137*
Complications *138*
Outcomes *142*
Summary *142*
References and resources *142*

Introduction

Intestinal transplantation (IT) is the least common form of organ transplantation, but has shown improved survival figures over the past two decades and is now an established option for children with irreversible intestinal failure (IF) and life-threatening complications.

IF is defined as the reduction of functional gut mass below the minimal amount necessary for digestion and absorption of adequate nutrients and fluids for survival and growth. IF occurs secondary to either anatomical or functional loss of a portion of the intestine. The leading cause of paediatric IF is short bowel syndrome followed by dysmotility syndromes and mucosal enteropathies. IF prognosis has improved dramatically in recent years due to advances in medical and surgical techniques, better PN solutions, and the development of intestinal rehabilitation programmes, but ~15% of children with IF develop life-threatening complications despite optimal medical and surgical treatment. When these complications are present, or where quality of life on PN is severely impaired, then referral for IT should occur. Mortality on the waiting list for IT is higher than for other organs, so to improve outcomes, the referral should occur early.

Current status

The IT registry is estimated to include 95% of worldwide activity in the field. The database currently includes patient information from 82 contributing centres that provided data on 2887 transplants in 2699 patients who were transplanted on or before 2 February 2013. The majority of transplants and the centres with the largest case volumes are in the US, with North America accounting for 76% of world activity. Most of the other activity occurs in Europe, followed by small but growing centres in South America and Asia. 47 centres worldwide remain active.

Overall transplant activity has declined since 2008. This may be due to the improved prognosis of IF with multidisciplinary intestinal rehabilitation programmes, surgical advances in autologous bowel reconstruction, and new medical therapies including CVC locks to reduce catheter-related sepsis and novel lipid management strategies.

Indications

Indications

- Irreversible IF *plus*
- Life-threatening complication of PN:
  - Progressive IFALD.
  - Severe or recurrent CRBSI.
  - Loss of >50% of standard central venous access sites.
- Very poor quality of life thought to be reversible by IT.
- Congenital intractable mucosal disorders such as microvillus inclusion disease or tufting enteropathy, which can lead to early death in infancy/prolonged PN.
- Complete porto-mesenteric thrombosis.
- Tumours involving the hepatic hilum or root of the mesentery.

Contraindications

- Irreversible damage to a non-abdominal organ such as the lung.
- Severe and progressive neurological conditions.
- Loss of adequate vascular access required for transplantation.
- Underlying disease expected to progress despite transplant.

Nomenclature

Nomenclature to describe IT has historically not been consistent but a more widely accepted terminology has been agreed since 2007. This system describes whether a liver is included in the graft and whether foregut organs are included.

- Isolated intestinal transplant (small bowel).
- Combined liver–intestine transplant (liver plus small bowel).
- Multivisceral transplant (liver plus small bowel and stomach/duodenum).
- Modified multivisceral transplant (small bowel and stomach/duodenum):
  - The pancreas is usually included in liver and/or foregut-containing grafts.
  - The colon may be included in multivisceral or modified multivisceral grafts.
  - Other abdominal organs transplanted at the same time such as the kidney are described individually.

Techniques

Isolated intestinal transplant

- Indicated in irreversible IF without liver disease, e.g. ultrashort gut or microvillus inclusion disease.
- Consists of the entire jejunum and ileum.
- Proximal anastomosis between native and donor jejunum.
- Distal ileum brought out as an ileostomy with or without anastomosis to the remnant colon.
- Arterial inflow supplied by the superior mesenteric artery.
- Venous drainage via the superior mesenteric vein.
- This graft can be removed without damage to other organs, should failure occur.
- There has been a worldwide trend with increasing numbers of this type of graft.

Combined liver intestine transplant

- Indicated in IFALD, with irreversible IF.
- If there is >50% of calorie requirement enterally then an isolated liver transplant should be considered.
- Consists of liver plus jejunum and ileum.
- Organs can be procured and transplanted en bloc to avoid dissection of the liver hilum and biliary tree. In this case the graft will contain duodenum and pancreas.
- Alternatively, organs can be transplanted separately, which means the intestine could be removed safely should it fail in future.
- Proximal bowel anastomosed end to end at the ligament of Treitz
- Distal bowel brought out and anastomosed as per isolated intestinal transplant.

Multivisceral and modified multivisceral transplant

- Indicated in disease of the whole bowel, such as pseudo-obstruction or motility disorders.
- Consists of small bowel plus other organs in continuity, in particular the stomach and duodenum.
- Full multivisceral includes the liver.
- Modified multivisceral does not include the liver.
- The colon may be included:
  - Addition of the colon may increase the risk of infection, but may also have the benefit of better fluid balance after transplant.
  - There has been an increasing trend to include the colon in the last decade.

Postoperative management

Postoperative management is challenging and consists of supportive intensive care in the first days followed by rehabilitation on the ward. The average hospital stay after IT is 44 days. During this time there must be strict monitoring of the patient's parameters and lab results, with treatment given to maintain normal values. The graft is closely monitored by clinical examination, and surveillance endoscopy up to twice weekly or when symptoms develop. Donor specific antibodies should also be monitored as they may be a risk factor for antibody-mediated rejection. There is no non-invasive marker for acute cellular rejection.

Immunosuppression

Advances in immunosuppression, and in particular the introduction of the calcineurin inhibitor tacrolimus, have made intestinal transplant successful. Protocols vary between centres, but all follow a similar pathway with induction then maintenance immunosuppression.

- Induction:
  - Interleukin (IL)-2 blocker, anti-lymphocyte agent, or monoclonal anti-CD52 antibody.
  - Methylprednisolone at a high dose then wean.
  - Tacrolimus at high level with gradual reduction over weeks and months.
- Maintenance:
  - Lifelong tacrolimus maintenance.
  - A second agent such as a mTOR (mammalian target of rapamycin) inhibitor may be added.
  - Prednisolone may be continued at a low dose.

Nutrition

- PN continued after transplant until enteral nutrition is achieved.
- Enteral nutrition started between days 3 and 7 then slowly increased.
- Choice of formula varies between centres.
- Once formula is tolerated, solid food can be eaten (although some patients eat earlier).
- Normal carbohydrate and protein absorption is achieved within 3 months.
- Micronutrient supplementation may be required in the longer term.

Complications

Acute cellular rejection
See Table 16.1.

The bowel is a highly immunogenic organ. Recipient immune cells populate the transplanted gut, but the epithelium genotype remains largely that of the donor, leading to a highly chimeric and immunogenic graft.
- The risk of both acute and chronic rejection after IT is high.
- Acute rejection is a cellular and humoral immune-mediated injury.
- Occurs in up to 50% of grafts.
- Most common within the first 90 days.
- Can happen at any time after transplant.

Signs and symptoms
- Raised (or lowered) stoma output.
- Bloody stoma effluent.
- Fever.
- Abdominal pain and tenderness.
- Raised inflammatory markers.

Table 16.1 Pathological criteria for acute cellular rejection (ACR)

No evidence of ACR—Grade 0	The tissue from the bowel allograft demonstrates unremarkable histological changes that are essentially similar to normal native bowel or pathologic changes are separate from ACR
Indeterminate ACR	Minor amount of epithelial cell injury or destruction is present, principally manifested in the crypts
	Increased crypt epithelial apoptosis but <6 apoptotic bodies/10 crypt cross section
Mild ACR—Grade 1	Crypt injury
	Increased mitotic activity, and/or crypt destruction with apoptosis (>6 apoptotic bodies/10 crypt cross sections)
	Villus blunting and architectural distortion
Moderate ACR—Grade 2	Focal or diffuse crypt injury and destruction
	>6 apoptotic bodies as described for/10 crypt cross sections, with foci of confluent apoptosis
	There can be focal superficial erosions of the surface mucosa
Severe ACR—Grade 3	A marked degree of crypt damage and destruction with crypt loss, there is diffuse mucosal erosion and/or ulceration with marked diffuse inflammatory infiltrate
	If extended severe rejection exists, there is complete loss or the morphology of the bowel with granulation tissue and even fibropurulent exudate, with mucosal sloughing
	The latter changes would be endoscopically defined as 'exfoliative' rejection (ER)
	ER has high risk for graft loss and increased mortality in children

Reproduced from Martinez Rivera, A. & Wales, P.W. Intestinal transplantation in children: current status Pediatr Surg Int (2016) 32: 529–540 with permission from Springer.

Diagnosis
Made on histology from biopsy samples taken at endoscopy.

Treatment
- Mild to moderate: pulse high-dose methylprednisolone and increase of tacrolimus.
- Moderate to severe: as above plus antithymocyte globulin.
- Severe rejection may necessitate graft enterectomy.

Antibody-mediated rejection
- Sensitized patients are at risk of developing donor-specific antibodies (DSA).
- These are a risk factor for antibody-mediated rejection (AMR).
- AMR may be responsible for refractory acute rejection, chronic rejection and graft loss.
- Development of DSA and AMR is associated with a poor outcome.
- Diagnosis is difficult as the findings on histology are not well defined. Injury to mesenteric vessel structures occurs but these are not present in mucosal biopsies. Staining for complement deposition is possible but the results are non-specific.
- Treatment is directed at removing or inhibiting the circulating antibodies. Anti B-lymphocyte CD20 monoclonal antibody, plasmapheresis and immunoglobulin as well as complement inhibitor have been used.

Chronic rejection
- The most common cause of late-onset graft dysfunction.
- Manifest by slow deterioration in the gut function.
- Endoscopy shows reduced mucosal folds, mural thickening, and ulceration.
- Imaging may demonstrate pruning of the mesenteric arterial tree.
- Diagnosis made on histology, which shows the obliterative arteriopathy changes in the submucosa, subserosa, and in the mesentery.
- No treatment is available, and graft enterectomy may become necessary.

Infection
- Sepsis is the leading cause of death after IT.
- High risk of bacterial, viral, and fungal infections.
- Bacterial infection occurs in two-thirds of IT recipients.
- Common viral infections include cytomegalovirus (CMV), Epstein–Barr virus (EBV), and adenovirus.
- CMV viraemia is reported in 11%.
- CMV can cause severe enteritis, diagnosed on histology as symptoms may be similar to acute rejection.
- Prophylaxis is given against CMV with ganciclovir.
- EBV leads to the risk of post-transplant lymphoproliferative disease (PTLD).

Malignancy

- The most common malignancy after IT is PTLD.
- A proliferative disorder of B lymphocytes driven by EBV.
- Occurs in 13% of recipients.
- Prevented by polymerase chain reaction (PCR) monitoring of EBV DNA, and reducing immunosuppression when EBV count rises.
- Presents with weight loss, adenopathy, and diarrhoea.
- Treated with reduction of immunosuppression, escalation to anti-B-lymphocyte CD20 monoclonal antibody, and possibly chemotherapy.

Quality of life

- Health-related quality of life after IT is good, improves from before transplantation, and improves after the first year post transplant.
- Recent work comparing post-transplant quality of life to that on HPN showed higher scores in many domains after transplant.

Outcomes

Patient and graft survival after IT have improved over time, although long-term graft survival still remains an issue. The reasons for graft and patient loss remain the same, with sepsis accounting for >50% followed by rejection.

Individual experienced transplant centres have reported 1-year patient survival of up to 93%. The overall international registry figures are:

- 1-year patient survival 77%.
- 1-year graft survival 71%.
- 5-year graft survival 60%.
- Re-transplantation rate 8%.

Factors associated with improved graft survival:

- Younger age at transplant (with paediatrics having significantly better survival than adults).
- Transplantation from the recipient waiting at home rather than hospitalized.
- Maintenance immunosuppression including sirolimus.
- Having a liver-containing graft.

Summary

IT remains an uncommon type of transplant, but with improved outcomes over time it has become an important option on the treatment continuum for patients with irreversible IF and life-threatening complications.

The best outcomes are achieved when a patient has been cared for in a setting with a multidisciplinary intestinal rehabilitation team who have a close relationship with the transplant centre. This enables a transplant to be offered to the correct patients, and in a timely fashion before they become too unwell.

After the transplant, the recipient is likely to achieve enteral autonomy and have improved quality of life. However, issues with long-term graft survival remain.

References and resources

Grant D, Abu-Elmagd K, Mazariegos G, et al. Intestinal transplant registry report: global activity and trends. Am J Transpl Off J Am Soc Transpl Am Soc Transpl Surg 2015;15:210–19.

Kyrana E, Hind J. Intestinal transplantation in children. Paediatr Child Health 2013;23:521–5.

Martinez Rivera A, Wales PW. Intestinal transplantation in children: current status. Pediatr Surg Int 2016;32:529–40.

Ruiz P, Bagni A, Brown R, et al. Histological criteria for the identification of acute cellular rejection in human small bowel allografts: results of the pathology workshop at the VIII International Small Bowel Transplant Symposium. Transplant Proc 2004;36:335–7.

Sudan D. The current state of intestine transplantation: indications, techniques, outcomes and challenges. Am J Transpl Off J Am Soc Transpl Am Soc Transpl Surg 2014;14:1976–84.

Eating disorders

Introduction *144*
Anorexia nervosa *146*
Bulimia nervosa and binge eating disorder *148*
Avoidant-restrictive food intake disorder *149*
References and resources *150*

Introduction

Feeding and eating disorders are associated with impairment of physical health and social, emotional, and cognitive development. If untreated, the outcome is poor. Diagnosis is based on clinical assessment using a combination of patient history, parent report, and clinical observation. Eating disorders are about ten times more common in girls than boys. Assessment and treatment should be a through a multidisciplinary team (psychiatrist, family therapist, psychologist, paediatrician, nurse, dietitian, etc.).

Whatever the eating or feeding disorder, the primary aim is to establish regular meals and snacks spread throughout the day. Food choices should be appropriate in type and quantity for normal healthy eating and the importance of fluids emphasized. Higher-energy foods allow for weight gain without volume. Severely malnourished children are at risk of refeeding syndrome; detailed advice on management is given in the Junior MARSIPAN report (see References and resources as this is at the end of this chapter).

Anorexia nervosa

- Aetiology complex and multifactorial.
- Involves heritability, neuropsychological risk (cognitive inflexibility and weak central coherence), and the role of perfectionism and deficits in social cognition.
- Autism spectrum traits may influence the response to treatment.
- Genetic factors appear to play an important role in adolescent-onset anorexia nervosa.

Diagnostic criteria for anorexia nervosa (based on ICD-10 and DSM-5)

- Intentional restriction or avoidance of food intake leading to significantly low body weight, or in young people, failure to make expected weight gain.
- Distorted view of weight and shape, fear of fatness, or lack of insight into the seriousness of low body weight.
- Emergence of behaviours such as avoidance of foods perceived as fattening, excessive exercise, use of weight-control medications, or purging.
- Endocrine dysfunction that might cause loss of periods in females or sexual potency in males; in young people, pubertal development may be delayed or arrested.

Diagnosis

- Parents' concerns are usually that young people are restricting energy-dense (fatty or sugary) foods, with increasingly rigid eating patterns.
- Social withdrawal and low mood with progressive weight loss; excessive exercise, self-induced vomiting.
- Underweight should be quantified by calculating BMI and expressing this as a percentage of the median BMI for that age and gender (<70% = severe underweight).
- Medical differential diagnoses to be considered include hyperthyroidism, glucocorticoid insufficiency, diabetes, inflammatory bowel disease, coeliac disease, gastritis, peptic ulcer, CNS tumour or other malignancy, chronic infection (e.g. tuberculosis).
- Comorbidities are common and include anxiety and depression.

Additional features

- Amenorrhoea (with long-term risk of severe osteoporosis if >6 months).
- Hyperactivity.
- Feeling asexual.
- Binge eating.
- Preoccupation with appearance and body.
- Distorted body image.
- Low self-esteem.
- Denial of illness.
- Misjudgement of food requirements.
- Obsessional behaviour.

- Rigid thought patterns.
- Perfectionist.
- Eating rituals.
- Hypotension.
- Bradycardia.
- Cyanosis of extremities.
- Increased growth of fine hair (lanugo).

Biochemical features

- Deficiency of gonadotrophin-releasing hormone (GnRH), low luteinizing hormone (LH) and follicle-stimulating hormone (FSH), normal prolactin, low oestrogen in females, and low testosterone in males.
- Elevated plasma cortisol.
- Low normal thyroxine, reduced T_3, and normal TSH.
- Elevated resting plasma growth hormone (GH).
- Hypokalaemia, hyponatraemia, low magnesium, phosphorus, zinc, and copper are common.

Treatment

- As an outpatient, if medically stable and psychiatric risk can be managed
- Inpatient if medically unstable (either paediatric or psychiatric setting; NB there are concerns that inpatient management may worsen outcome and is no more effective than outpatient treatment).
- Occasionally severe weight loss gives rise to duodenal compression causing persistent vomiting: the 'superior mesenteric artery syndrome'. Radiologically there is dilatation of the proximal duodenum and narrowing of the third part of the duodenum, apparently by the superior mesenteric artery. Weight gain is often followed by resolution of this problem; transpyloric tube feeding or occasionally PN may be required.
- Weekly weight gain target 0.5–1kg inpatient, 0.5kg outpatient.
- Family-based therapy: focused on behavioural change with parents as 'experts' of their family empowered to take charge.
- Adolescent-focused therapy: adolescent taught to identify and cope with negative emotions and developmental challenges thought to be driving eating disorder.
- Enhanced cognitive behavioural therapy: focuses on the cognitive processes maintaining the eating disorder to drive changes in eating behaviour.
- Antipsychotics and selective serotonin reuptake inhibitors often prescribed but little evidence of benefit.

Outcome

- 50–75% of adolescents receiving a family-based treatment approach reach a healthy weight; at follow-up, 60–90% will have partially or fully recovered.
- A proportion of patients will relapse, are treatment resistant, and at increased risk of psychiatric disorders in adulthood.

Bulimia nervosa and binge eating disorder

- Binge eating involves regular episodes of eating much more than most people would in a similar situation over a short period of time; 'loss of control' while eating; eating alone due to shame or disgust about quantities eaten, eating when not hungry and until uncomfortably full, and feeling depressed or guilty afterwards.
- Psychological and environmental factors interact with and influence the expression of genetic risk causing eating pathology.
- Anxiety and depression are common co-morbidities.
- Treatment is usually outpatient based.
- Family-based therapy and cognitive behavioural therapy are effective treatments; fluoxetine may have a role.
- Following treatment, about 40% of patients recover, but with a high relapse rate at follow-up.

Avoidant-restrictive food intake disorder

- Avoidant-restrictive food intake disorder (ARFID) encompasses a heterogeneous group of disorders with likely multiple aetiologies.
- A large proportion have primary medical problems underlying the eating difficulty, most commonly neurological or gastrointestinal disease and it also occurs in autism spectrum disorders.
- Clinical presentations include lack of interest in food, heightened sensitivity to textures of food, and fears of the consequences of eating, such as choking.
- Diagnosis only made when eating behaviour results in significant weight loss or growth faltering, when there is dependence on nutritional supplementation (e.g. tube feeding), or when the problem markedly interferes with psychosocial functioning.
- Treatment individualized on the basis of the main feeding or eating difficulty and the factors contributing to aetiology.

Case study

A 16-year-old girl was referred to the eating disorders clinic because of anorexia. She displayed many features of anorexia nervosa, but by hiding weights in her dressing gown at outpatient review managed to conceal the true extent of her condition. She was admitted to hospital after becoming drowsy and developing bilious vomiting; admission weight was only 22kg (BMI = 13). Radiological findings were consistent with a superior mesenteric artery syndrome (compression of the duodenum just to the right of the midline). Attempts at nasojejunal feeding were unsuccessful due to vomiting back of the tube. She was parenterally fed, initially to actual weight with a cautious increase in energy intake over a number of weeks and close monitoring of serum biochemistry (particularly potassium and phosphate). A multivitamin supplement including thiamine was given prior to nutritional intervention in case her altered conscious level was symptomatic of deficiency; she needed additional supplementation with sodium, potassium, phosphate, zinc, and magnesium. As her weight increased, vomiting ceased and from 40kg, enteral tube feeding was re-established and PN discontinued. She required 24-hour 'one-to-one' nursing to prevent removal of CVC and NGT. While she was on the acute paediatric ward, medical and psychiatric teams liaised closely on a daily basis. Subsequently she was transferred to an inpatient psychiatric unit and made a full recovery, returning to school a year after admission. She subsequently completed a university degree course but complained of some mild problems with memory, possibly relating to structural changes in the brain seen on her cranial imaging during the period of severe illness.

References and resources

Mairs R, Nicholls D. Assessment and treatment of eating disorders in children and adolescents. Arch Dis Child 2016;101:1168–75.

Marikar D, Reynolds S, Moghraby OS. Junior MARSIPAN (Management of Really Sick Patients with Anorexia Nervosa). Arch Dis Child Educ Pract Ed 2016;101:140–3.

Royal College of Psychiatrists. Junior MARSIPAN: Management of really sick patients under 18 with anorexia nervosa. CR168. London: Royal College of Psychiatrists; 2012. http://www.rcpsych.ac.uk/pdf/CR168summary.pdf

Street K, Costelloe S, Wootton M, Upton S, Brough J. Structured, supported feeding admissions for restrictive eating disorders on paediatric wards. Arch Dis Child 2016;101:836–8.

Difficult eating behaviour in the young child

Introduction *152*
Appetite *153*
Common feeding problems in 1–5-year-olds *154*
How to increase energy intake *155*
References and resources *156*

Introduction

Food refusal is common in early life. During the first year, infants will try food because they are hungry, or because they are using their mouths to explore the environment. Later on, there has to be motivation to try new foods, and this usually comes from imitation of other people eating. In early childhood it is the presentation of safe and socially appropriate foods and their repeated ingestion that leads to them being liked.

Children may refuse food because of:
- Lack of appetite.
- Lack of experience at certain developmental stages.
- Poor oromotor skills.
- Onset of the neophobic response in the second year (a 'biologically protective' dislike of new foods).
- Distaste or disgust at some foods.
- Individual differences in food acceptance.
- Parental anxiety and forced feeding.

Appetite

- From ~6 weeks of age, infants regulate energy intake in accordance with energy needs.
- Well toddlers will take the amount of energy they need for normal growth.
- Children get hungry at the time they usually eat a meal, for the energy load they would usually eat.
- From around 5 years, food intake is modified by social rules, e.g. 'clearing the plate', eating as a social or comfort activity.

Development

- At birth there is a preference for sweet-tasting food (sweet = biologically safe).
- At 3–5 months, ready acceptance of new tastes based on taste and smell; lack of experience at this stage may mean limited range of tastes accepted.
- At 6–12 months, start of self-feeding with more solid foods; lack of experience at this stage may lead to poor acceptance of different textures.
- At 12–18 months, fear of new foods ('neophobia') develops; local features of food become important (e.g. biscuit must be whole, not broken).
- At 18 months–5 years, neophobic response strengthens, but overcome by imitation of adults and other children.

Modification of eating behaviour

- Move from mash to 'bite and dissolve' foods from 7 months.
- Encourage self-feeding as soon as possible, by the end of the first year.
- Allow the child to be messy at mealtimes and to enjoy eating.
- Putting a disliked food on a plate next to a liked food may lead to rejection of the liked food ('contamination').
- If one food is the reward for eating another, the food first offered is understood to be less nice.
- Repeated exposure to a food is the best way of it becoming accepted.
- Imitation (of adults or other children) also leads to an acceptance of new foods.
- If parents/carers do not eat particular foods, it is unlikely that the child will want to eat them.

The 'picky' child

Simple faddy eating is most likely to occur around 18 months.
- Take notice of satiety signals (e.g. closing mouth, turning away).
- Give frequent small meals.
- Take uneaten food away without comment.
- Give positive attention/encouragement when the child is eating.
- Don't force feed.
- Don't use one food as a reward for eating another.
- Don't give attention for not eating.
- Don't put liked and disliked food on the same plate.
- Don't expect all children to eat as well as each other.

(With grateful acknowledgement to Gill Harris.)

Common feeding problems in 1–5-year-olds

Table 18.1.

Table 18.1 Common feeding problems in 1–5-year-olds

Problem	Solutions
Food refusal	Structured meal pattern; 3 meals and 2–3 small, nutritious snacks
	Offer variety of foods, with some favourites
	Small portions (second helpings if wanted)
	Do not 'force feed'
	Family mealtimes
	Happy, relaxed environment
	Do not offer sweets/other foods as reward
Excessive milk drinking	Limit milk intake to 500–600mL/day
	Give milk after meals or at snack time
	Give water if thirsty between meals
	Use cup not bottle
	Offer milk in small cups
Excessive juice drinking	Limit juice to no more than 1 cup/day
	Give drinks after meals
	Give plain water if thirsty
	Encourage milk; limit to 500–600mL/day
Refuses to drink milk	Offer in small 'fun' cup through straw
	Add milk or cheese to foods, e.g. mashed potato, scrambled egg
	Include other milk containing foods, e.g. yoghurt, custard, porridge
	Try flavoured milk or milk shakes
Refuses to eat fruits or vegetables	Try mixing vegetables into other foods such as soups or stews
	Add grated fruits and vegetables to other foods
	Include small amount of fruit and vegetable at each mealtime to allow opportunity to try
	Children learn by example; other family members to eat fruit and vegetables
	Some children prefer raw rather than cooked vegetables
	Try fruits cut into small pieces with yoghurt dips
	Make blended fruit drinks or milk shakes with added fruits

How to increase energy intake

Increasing the nutrient density of food can improve growth rate; some suggestions are listed here.

Weaning foods

- Add infant formula to dried baby foods or home-made puréed foods.
- Include puréed meats, add to vegetables.
- Spread butter or margarine on finger foods.

Normal table foods

- Add whole milk to mashed foods.
- Add extra dried milk powder to whole milk and milk puddings.
- Add oil or butter to mashed or puréed foods.
- Add cream to desserts and porridge.
- Add grated cheese or cream cheese to savoury foods such as mashed potato or scrambled egg.
- Encourage three meals a day and nutritious snacks between meals.

Case study

A 2-year-old child was referred to the dietitian because of parental concern regarding eating. As a baby he had been reluctant to feed and had vomited with solids, taking only formula milk until 9 months of age. Subsequently, dry breakfast cereal, toast, crisps, chips, chocolate, orange juice, and certain biscuits were accepted. At mealtimes he would refuse to try any new foods and continued to request warmed milk from a bottle. He began to ask for help with feeding at mealtimes which had become increasingly stressful for the family. Height and weight had dropped from the 25th to the 10th centile, and a dietary assessment indicated that his intakes of energy and iron were suboptimal. Iron was prescribed together with an energy-dense supplement drink; both were refused by the child. A video recording was made of a family mealtime, with analysis focusing on the interaction between child and carers. Guidance was then given to parents on behavioural modification; they were also encouraged to adopt a consistent approach to feeding and mealtimes.

References and resources

Cole NC, An R, Lee SY, Donovan SM. Correlates of picky eating and food neophobia in young children: a systematic review and meta-analysis. Nutr Rev 2017;75:516–32.

Green C. New toddler taming. London: Vermilion; 2006.

Infant and Toddler Forum. Health and childcare professionals, Factsheets. http://www.infantandtoddlerforum.org

NHS Choices. Fussy eaters. 2018. http://www.nhs.uk/Conditions/pregnancy-and-baby/Pages/fussy-eaters.aspx

Puntis JWL. Specialist feeding clinics. Arch Dis Child 2008;93:164–7.

Wright CM, Parkinson KN, Shipton D, Drewett RF. How do toddler eating problems relate to their eating behavior, food preferences, and growth? Pediatrics 2007;120:e1069–75.

Food allergy

Introduction *158*
Definitions (World Allergy Organization) *158*
Types of allergic reaction *159*
Diagnosing and managing food allergy *160*
References and resources *164*

Introduction

Food allergy is one of the earliest manifestations of the 'allergic march' and its presence is strongly correlated with other atopic disorders. It appears to be increasingly common, and may be life-threatening as well as adversely affecting quality of life. For certain foods, allergy is likely to be long term, if not lifelong.

* Food allergy is an adverse immune response to food. It can be classified into IgE- and non-IgE-mediated reactions.
* Non-IgE reactions are believed to be T-cell mediated.
* Food allergy most commonly affects preschool children.
* It should be considered in children with gastroesophageal reflux disease or constipation who do not respond to conventional treatment. Careful history taking is central to making the diagnosis.
* Milk (2.5%), egg (1.3%), peanut (0.8%), tree nuts (0.2%), and fish (0.2%) are among the most prevalent causes of food allergy; soya and wheat allergy are also common.
* Food allergy resolves in most affected children, although peanut allergy may persist; 85% of children with cow milk allergy in the first 2 years of life are tolerant by the age of 3, and 80% of children with egg allergy by 5 years.
* 20% of children under 2 years with peanut allergy are tolerant by school age; children with peanut-specific IgE of 5kU/L or less have around a 50% chance of losing their allergy.
* Risk of death from fatal allergic reactions to food is around 1 in 800,000 per year, with asthmatic children being at highest risk.

Definitions (World Allergy Organization)

* *Hypersensitivity*: objectively reproducible symptoms or signs initiated by exposure to a defined stimulus at a dose tolerated by normal persons.
* *Intolerance*: abnormal physiological response to an agent, which can be certain foods or additives; not immune mediated.
* *Atopy*: a characteristic that makes one susceptible to develop various allergies; it is defined as a personal and/or familial tendency, usually in childhood or adolescence, to become sensitized and produce IgE antibodies in response to ordinary exposures to allergens, usually proteins; as a consequence, these persons can develop typical symptoms of asthma, rhino-conjunctivitis, or eczema.
* *Allergen*: an antigen causing allergic disease.
* *Allergy*: a hypersensitivity reaction initiated by specific immunological mechanisms. When other mechanisms can be proved, the term *non-allergic hypersensitivity* should be used.
* *Food allergy* is thus a term applied to a group of disorders characterized by an abnormal or exaggerated immunological response to specific food proteins that may be IgE or non-IgE mediated.
* *Psychologically based food reaction (aversion)* is food avoidance for psychological reasons, or when there is an unpleasant bodily reaction caused by emotions associated with the food (rather than by the food itself); it does not occur when the food is given in an unrecognizable form.

Types of allergic reaction

Reactions to allergens can be mild, moderate, or severe in nature.
- A mild reaction may involve itchy rash, watering eyes, and nasal congestion.
- Moderate reactions may spread to different parts of the body and include difficulty breathing.
- A severe reaction presents as anaphylaxis.
- IgE-mediated reactions cause symptoms almost immediately after food is ingested, with swelling of the lips and tongue sometimes together with vomiting, diarrhoea, asthma, and rarely anaphylaxis.
- When IgE-mediated reactions are suspected, skin tests (by trained professionals, with facilities to deal with anaphylactic reaction) and blood tests for specific IgE antibodies may be offered.
- Food-dependent, exercise-induced anaphylaxis occurs typically in atopic young adults after vigorous exercise within several hours of eating an implicated food.
- Oral allergy syndrome involves itching, irritation, swelling, and urticaria in or around the mouth after ingestion of fresh fruit or vegetables.
- Non-IgE reactions (e.g. atopic dermatitis, eosinophilic gastroenteropathy, asthma) are mediated by allergen-specific lymphocytes and IgG antibodies.

Diagnosing and managing food allergy

In the history, enquire about the following:
- What foods are under suspicion?
- Time between ingestion and reaction?
- Amount of food needed to cause a reaction?
- Frequency and reproducibility of reactions?
- Signs and symptoms?
- Was food raw or cooked?
- Could there have been any cross contamination with other foods?

Skin prick testing with standardized allergen extracts can be positive in the absence of allergy, but are rarely negative in someone with true IgE-mediated allergic reactions. Quantitative measurements of food-specific IgE antibodies have a high predictive value for allergic reactions to certain foods.

Elimination diets and subsequent dietary challenges should be instituted with the help and supervision of a dietitian. Antihistamines and corticosteroids are useful for symptomatic relief of mild to moderate allergies. Adrenaline is used for severe reactions including anaphylaxis.

Cow milk protein allergy (CMPA)
- CMPA is the clinical syndrome(s) resulting from sensitization to one or more proteins in cow's milk.
- It frequently resolves spontaneously within the first 2 years of life, and almost always by 5 years of age.
- In most affected children, gastrointestinal symptoms (vomiting, diarrhoea, colic, constipation) develop in the first 6 months of life.

Other presentations
- Respiratory: wheeze, rhinitis, asthma, laryngeal oedema.
- Dermatological: atopic dermatitis, urticaria.
- Behavioural: irritability, crying, milk refusal.

Diagnosis is based mainly upon clinical history
- Definite disappearance of symptoms after each of two dietary eliminations of cow's milk.
- Recurrence of identical symptoms after one challenge.
- Exclusion of lactose intolerance and coincidental infection.

Major foods to be excluded in a cow milk protein-free diet
- Cow's milk—all types, including modified (infant formula), skimmed, low fat, whole, dried, condensed and evaporated, buttermilk.
- Butter, ghee, some margarines, and low-fat spreads (check labels).
- Yoghurt, fromage frais, cream, ice cream.
- Cheese, cottage cheese, cream cheese, curds.
- Chocolate and other sweets containing milk solids.
- Check label of manufactured products and avoid 'non-fat milk solids', 'whey', 'casein', 'sodium caseinate', 'lactoglobulin', 'lactalbumin'.
- Goat's or sheep's milk should not be used as substitutes for infant formula as they are no less allergenic than cow's milk, contain a high solute load, and are deficient in vitamins.

- An extensively hydrolysed infant formula may be given as a milk substitute; cow milk protein allergens are secreted in breast milk, and breastfeeding mothers may need to exclude cow's milk from their diet.
- Although more palatable than hydrolysed feeds, soya milk is not a suitable milk substitute since around 5–10% of infants who react to cow's milk will do so to soya; in addition, soya is not recommended for infants <6 months of age because of concerns regarding phytoestrogen content.

NB For children on a cow milk-free diet, care must be taken to provide adequate calcium from other sources, such as cow milk-free formula, soya products fortified with calcium, or calcium supplements.

Food challenges

- Food challenges have a pivotal role in the diagnosis of food allergy.
- Unit protocols should be available for those foods commonly implicated.
- Challenges should be carried out in an appropriately staffed and equipped facility.

Challenges may be performed if:
- There is diagnostic uncertainty despite an allergy focused history, skin prick and specific IgE testing.
- There are signs of resolution of a food allergy such as a change in skin prick tests or specific IgE or there is a history of recent uneventful dietary exposure.
- Parents or adolescent seek clarification of need for antigen avoidance (often pre-school entry or prior to leaving school). These challenges often carry a higher risk of generalised allergic reaction and should be conducted by experts.

Prevention of food allergy

- Food avoidance strategies advocated in the past do not appear effective in preventing food allergy.
- In infants who can't be given breast milk and are at high risk of allergy, use of partially or extensively hydrolysed formula feeds may have a role.
- Introduction rather than avoidance of commonly allergic foods at 3–6 months alongside continued breastfeeding may be effective in preventing food allergy.
- Although there is now consensus that avoidance strategies are ineffective, there is insufficient evidence for guidelines to set out an alternative strategy with established benefit.

Pseudo-intolerance/allergy

- some parents attribute functional gut symptoms to a mistaken belief that their child has food allergy.
- Alternative diagnostic techniques such as hair analysis, Vega and pulse testing, and Specific IgG blood tests may reinforce such beliefs.
- Unsupervised dietary restriction can lead to nutritional deficiency states and occasionally even to faltering growth and death.
- In such cases, safeguarding issues arise and detailed multidisciplinary assessment is required.

Adrenaline injection

For patients who have had a life-threatening allergic reaction to food, or who have food allergy and severe asthma emergency adrenaline treatment should be carried in the form of an autoinjector. These devices deliver adrenaline intramuscularly. Examples include EpiPen®, Emerade® or Jext® 0.3mg (>30kg), or EpiPen® Junior/ Jext® 0.15mg (15–30kg), Emerade® 0.5mg (>50kg). Provision of an Adrenaline Autoinjector should always be part of an integrated management plan. It is important for patients, carers, and doctors to be thoroughly familiar with their use.

In the event of anaphylaxis

EpiPen®
- Remove the EpiPen® from its packaging.
- Remove the blue safety cap.
- Hold the EpiPen® with the orange tip at right angle to the thigh and press hard until the auto-injector mechanism functions (there should be a click); hold in place for 3 seconds.
- Remove the EpiPen® and massage the area for 10 seconds.

Emerade®
- Remove the needle shield.
- Hold Emerade® against outer thigh and press for 5 seconds.
- Remove the Emerade® and gently massage the injection site for 5 seconds.
- Note that:
  - Pens need replacing periodically (check contents are clear and colourless; check expiry date).
  - Demonstrate use with each new prescription (see above).
  - Provide a written management protocol to family, carers, school.
  - Keep spare pen at school.
  - Always carry pen.

References and resources

Emerade®. Your adrenaline pen for emergency treatment of anaphylaxis. http://www.emerade. com/adrenaline-auto-injector

EpiPen®. How to use. https://www.epipen.com/about-epipen/how-to-use-epipen

Grimshaw K, Logan K, O'Donovan S, et al. Modifying the infant's diet to prevent food allergy. Arch Dis Child 2017;102:179–86.

Jext (needs Rin a circle as per other products) then http://www.jext.co.uk/

Luyt D, Ball H, Makawana N, et al. BSACI guideline for diagnosis and management of cow's milk allergy. Clin Exp Allergy 2014;44:642–72.

National Institute for Health and Care Excellence (NICE). Food allergy in under 19s: assessment and diagnosis. London: NICE; 2011. www.nice.org.uk/guidance/CG116

Royal College of Paediatrics and Child Health. Care pathway for food allergy. 2012. http://www. rcpch.ac.uk/child-health/research-projects/care-pathways-children-allergies/food-allergy/care-pathway-food-aller

Carbohydrate intolerance

Carbohydrates in the diet *166*
Carbohydrate digestion *167*
Hypolactasia/lactose intolerance *168*
Congenital sucrase–isomaltase deficiency *168*
Glucose–galactose malabsorption *169*
Hereditary fructose intolerance *169*
Fructose malabsorption *169*
Confirmation of diagnosis of carbohydrate malabsorption *170*
References and resources *171*

Carbohydrates in the diet

Carbohydrates make up at least half the energy intake in the diet. The principal carbohydrates are the storage polysaccharides (starch, glycogen, and cellulose), the disaccharides lactose and sucrose, and the monosaccharides glucose and fructose.

- D-Glucose is the most important carbohydrate in the diet and in the intermediate metabolism of carbohydrate in humans.
- It is a hexose (a six-carbon sugar molecule), with both α- and β-stereoisomers.
- When one glucose molecule is joined to another to form a disaccharide or a polysaccharide, the link may be between the C1 of the first molecule and C4 of the second molecule (1–4 linkage) or between C1 and 6 (1–6 linkage).
- This linkage is via an oxygen bridge with either an α- or a β-glycosidic bond, depending on the stereoisomer.

Starch is made up of amylase and amylopectin. Amylose is composed of a chain of glucose units linked via a 1–4α-glycosidic bond. Amylopectin is also made up of a chain of glucose units but, in addition to the 1–4α linkages, there are 1–6α linkages at a number of branching points, approximately every 25 glucose units, along the chain.

- Lactose is made up of a molecule each of galactose and glucose, linked by a β-glycosidic bond.
- Sucrose, maltose, and isomaltose are linked by an α-glycosidic bond.
- Maltose consists of two glucose molecules linked by a 1–4 bond, whereas isomaltose (also containing two glucose molecules) is linked via a 1–6 bond.
- Sucrose (cane or beet sugar) consists of a molecule of glucose linked to a molecule of fructose via an α-linkage on the glucose side coupled to a β-linkage on the fructose side (α-glucosido-β-fructose).
- Fructose (fruit sugar) is a simple monosaccharide found in many plants where it is often linked to glucose to form the disaccharide sucrose.

Carbohydrate digestion

Salivary and pancreatic α-amylases act on starch to yield maltose, maltotriose (three glucose units), and α-limit dextrins (branched oligosaccharides with 1–6 linkages at the branching points, but otherwise 1–4 linkages containing an average of eight glucose molecules).

- Disaccharide hydrolysis occurs within the brush border of the small intestinal enterocyte.
- There is a single brush border β-galactosidase (lactase)
- There are three brush border α-glucosidases—sucrase, isomaltase (or α-dextrinase), and glucoamylase.
- Sucrase not only hydrolyses maltose and maltotriose but also splits sucrose to glucose and fructose.
- Isomaltase cleaves 1–6α as well as 1–4α links in oligosaccharides.
- After hydrolysis, the liberated monosaccharides are absorbed by active transport mechanisms.
- Glucose and galactose share the sodium-glucose-linked transporter (SGLT-1), whereas fructose has a different mechanism.

Congenital and acquired defects of disaccharidase activity have been described in children as well as congenital mutations within SGLT-1. These disorders lead to malabsorption of various sugars. Symptoms include nausea, watery diarrhoea, wind, and abdominal cramps. There is clearly overlap with cow milk protein intolerance in young children, and functional bowel disorders (e.g. irritable bowel syndrome, recurrent abdominal pain). In many patients who believe themselves to be lactose intolerant, objective testing suggests otherwise.

Hypolactasia/lactose intolerance

- Low activity of lactase in the small intestinal brush border membrane is the most common cause of carbohydrate intolerance; symptoms are provoked following ingestion of milk or lactose-containing products but the symptoms do not always occur together and the association with lactose absorption may not be obvious.
- In many populations lactase activity is normal in the first few years of life, but then declines in older children and adults; prevalence varies, being >80% in Semitics, Africans, Asians, Inuit, and American Indians, but only 10% of northern Europeans; inheritance is thought to be autosomal recessive.
- Congenital lactase deficiency is extremely rare, presenting with watery diarrhoea as soon as breast or formula feeds are introduced.
- Secondary hypolactasia commonly occurs after infective gastroenteritis but usually resolves spontaneously in a short period of time (days–2 weeks).
- Affected individuals vary in the amount of lactose they are able to tolerate so that strict exclusion of all milk products is rarely necessary (fermented dairy products such as cheese and yoghurt, for example, may not cause symptoms).
- Lactose and fructose intolerance may coexist.
- There is interest in whether lactose intolerance affects the link between dairy intake and other diseases, such as cancer, but little evidence as yet that this is the case.

Congenital sucrase–isomaltase deficiency

- Sucrase and isomaltase activity always go hand in hand (both enzymes are synthesized together, inserted into the brush border membrane as one long protein, and subsequently cleaved into two units, which remain closely associated).
- Much less common than lactase deficiency it occurs in about 0.2% of North Americans and 10% of Greenland Inuit; it is autosomal recessive in inheritance.
- Typical symptoms of carbohydrate malabsorption occur when sucrose is introduced into the diet (e.g. fruit).
- Diarrhoea may be associated with faltering growth. (NB A change to a feed containing glucose polymer as treatment for suspected cow milk protein or lactose intolerance will not resolve the problem.)
- Symptoms can be mild, and may appear clinically as 'toddler' diarrhoea.
- Mucosal biopsy analysis will show normal lactase activity and low sucrase–isomaltase.
- Dietary restriction of sucrose may help alleviate symptoms, but enzyme replacement therapy (sacrosidase/Sucraid®, Orphan Medical Inc.) is also available.
- Invertase may be an effective alternative to sacrosidase in some patients.
- Dietary management of symptoms can be very challenging as starches as well as sucrose may cause symptoms; experienced dietetic input is advised.

Glucose–galactose malabsorption

- Glucose–galactose malabsorption is the only known primary monosaccharide intolerance, exceptionally rare, and autosomal recessive in inheritance.
- Infants do not tolerate feeds containing lactose (glucose–galactose) or sucrose (glucose–fructose) and have severe diarrhoea from first feeds; they can tolerate fructose.

Hereditary fructose intolerance

- Due to deficiency of enzyme aldolase B; autosomal recessive.
- Symptoms provoked by ingestion of food containing fructose, sucrose, or sorbitol include vomiting, hypoglycaemia, jaundice (hepatomegaly; renal failure).
- May be associated with dietary aversion to fruit and other fructose-containing foods.
- Diagnosis difficult: symptoms provoked by IV fructose challenge, or measurement of aldolase B in liver biopsy (NB Cannot be diagnosed using oral challenge and breath hydrogen testing—see 'Confirmation of diagnosis of carbohydrate malabsorption', p. 170).

Fructose malabsorption

- Absorption of fructose is impaired by deficiency of fructose carriers on enterocytes.
- May cause abdominal pain, bloating, wind, diarrhoea ('IBS').
- Manage by dietary restriction.

Confirmation of diagnosis of carbohydrate malabsorption

- Samples of liquid stool will show undigested sugars on chromatography (many laboratories have stopped offering this test).
- In patients without watery diarrhoea, a sugar challenge may be given to see if symptoms are provoked and for breath hydrogen testing (if child old enough to cooperate): 2g/kg of sugar being tested given by mouth, baseline and half hourly breath hydrogen analysis for 2 h; if sugar maldigested, colonic bacteria utilize, and produce hydrogen with >20ppm in exhaled breath (positive test).
- Analysis of small-bowel mucosal disaccharidases in biopsy obtained endoscopically is the 'gold standard'.
- Clinical response to treatment (dietary modification; sacrosidase or invertase for congenital sucrase–isomaltase deficiency (CSID)).
- Gene testing now available for CSID; identifies about 75% of cases.

Case study

Sucrase–isomaltase deficiency

A male infant thrived on a standard cow milk formula but developed diarrhoea when fruit juices were given for the first time at 4 weeks of age. He was treated with oral glucose and electrolyte solution for suspected gastroenteritis and diarrhoea stopped, only to recur when a soy-based formula containing glucose polymer was introduced. He continued to be fed with this formula and was referred to a tertiary gastroenterology unit at the age of 8 months because of continuing diarrhoea and poor weight gain. Use of a modular feed with glucose polymer also caused diarrhoea, but this stopped if fructose was substituted as the carbohydrate source. Endoscopic duodenal biopsy specimens were obtained, and enzyme analysis showed normal lactase with very low sucrase–isomaltase activity. He was given a standard lactose-based cow milk formula and had prompt resolution of his symptoms. Subsequently he avoided sucrose in his diet and as symptoms were minimal did not require treatment with enzyme replacement (oral sacrosidase).

References and resources

Congenital Sucrase-Isomaltase Deficiency. Community, Advocacy, Research, Education, Support: http://www.csidcares.org

McMeans AR. Congenital sucrase-isomaltase deficiency: diet assessment and education guidelines. J Pediatr Gastroenterol Nutr 2012;55(Suppl 2):S37–9.

Newton T, Murphy S, Booth IW. Glucose polymer as a cause of protracted diarrhoea in infants with unsuspected congenital sucrase-isomaltase deficiency. J Pediatr 1996;128:753–6.

Puntis JW, Zamvar V. Congenital sucrase-isomaltase deficiency: diagnostic challenges and response to enzyme replacement therapy. Arch Dis Child 2015;100:869–71.

Treem WR, McAdams L, Stanford L, Kastoff G, Justinich C, Hyams J. Sacrosidase therapy for congenital sucrase-isomaltase deficiency. J Pediatr Gastroenterol Nutr 1999;28:137–42.

Nutritional problems in the child with neurodisability

Introduction *174*
Assessment *175*
Suggestions for optimizing oral intake *175*
Tube feeding *176*
Feeds *177*
Gastro-oesophageal reflux disease *177*
Gastrostomy placement and subsequent care *178*
Intestinal failure in patients with neurodisability *190*
References and resources *190*

Introduction

Neurological disability is common, with around 15,000–20,000 children in the UK having cerebral palsy. Of these, 50% are reported to have feeding problems, rising to 85% in more severely affected children (e.g. those with spastic quadriplegia). In an Oxford-based community study of feeding and nutritional problems in children with neurological impairment:

- 89% needed help with feeding.
- 56% experienced choking with food.
- 38% of parents considered their child to be underweight.
- 28% reported prolonged mealtimes.
- 20% reported stressful mealtimes.
- 64% reported that to their knowledge feeding and nutritional status had never been formally assessed.

Reduced energy supply as a consequence of feeding difficulties or vomiting (gastro-oesophageal reflux disease, GORD) may lead to poor growth; micronutrient deficiencies including calcium, iron, zinc, and fat-soluble vitamins are commonly encountered. Feed intolerance may be associated not only with acid reflux, but also with delayed gastric emptying, diarrhoea, or constipation.

There are many different feeding strategies including oral, partial tube, and complete tube feeding. Tube feeding can be via nasogastric, nasojejunal, gastrostomy, or gastrojejunal tube. A wide selection of feeds are available. There are many potential strategies to impact feed intolerance including changing from bolus to continuous feeds; decreasing the rate of infusion; concentrating the feed to decrease the volume; selecting an alternative feed; treating GORD, delayed gastric emptying (prokinetics), and managing constipation. Oral feeding should be promoted where possible.

Achieving and maintaining optimal nutritional status in children with disabilities helps them maximize their potential in life and is as important as it is in healthy children. Undernutrition adversely affects cognitive function and makes children apathetic and miserable. Underweight children with severe motor impairment are more likely to develop pressure sores. Overweight/ obesity will significantly impact mobility in the ambulant child, cause morbidity, and be a practical issue for carers in the non-ambulant child.

Assessment

In taking a feeding history it is important to enquire about the following:
- How long do meal times take?
- Are they enjoyable?
- What type and quantity of food is consumed?
- Is there coughing, choking, or vomiting?
- Is there a history of chest infection (?aspiration)?
- Is there a history of constipation? (delays stomach emptying, exacerbates gastro-oesophageal reflux, reduces appetite.)

Nutritional status and determinants
- Nutritional status using standard anthropometry.
- 'Height/stature' can be estimated by measuring upper arm length, lower leg length, or knee height as follows:
  - 21.8 + (4.35 × upper-arm length).
  - 30.8 + (3.26 × lower leg length).
  - 24.2 + (2.69 × knee height).
- Oromotor skills and safety of swallow are best assessed by an experienced speech and language therapist (may advise videofluoroscopy of swallowed liquid and solids).
- Occupational therapist to assess seating for mealtime, and appropriate eating aids
- Dietitian for assessment of energy needs and developmental age appropriate food; recommended daily amount (RDA) may overestimate energy needs when there is severe growth delay; energy requirements also influenced by variation in muscle tone and levels of physical activity.

Suggestions for optimizing oral intake

- Change of posture, special adaptive seating, soft cervical collar, use of wide-bore straw.
- Treatment of oral hypersensitivity (speech and language therapist).
- Thickening of foods.
- Use of energy supplements.
- Treatment of GORD, oesophagitis, slow gastric emptying, and constipation.

Tube feeding

Indications
- Severely compromised swallowing.
- Repeated aspiration pneumonia.
- Malnutrition despite 'optimizing' oral intake.
- Administration of medication.

Potential benefits
- Improved nutritional status.
- Improvement in general well-being.
- Less time spent on feeding, more on other forms of interaction.
- Oral feeding for pleasure still possible.
- Easier to give medication.
- Easier to keep well hydrated.

Long-term (>6 weeks) tube feeding is usually by percutaneous endoscopic gastrostomy (PEG). Gastrostomy requires careful discussion with family. It is not without risks and can be seen as evidence of 'failure' by some parents. The purpose is to improve quality of life for families and children; long-term follow-up is important. If energy intake exceeds energy expenditure, excessive weight gain will result. Children with impaired mobility or severe cognitive dysfunction have a relatively low energy expenditure. Resting energy expenditure is also low in children with reduced lean body mass. In severe spastic quadriplegia, around two-thirds of recommended energy intake may be adequate for growth.

Feeds

- Energy requirements are disease specific, and vary with the severity of disability and mobility.
- The best way to assess adequacy of diet is to monitor weight gain.
- Occupational and speech and language therapists can assist with oral feeding skills, correct positioning, and use of appropriate seating and utensils.
- Standard infant or paediatric casein-based formula may be used, as well as peptide-based feeds.
- Whey-based or amino acid formula empty more quickly from the stomach and are better tolerated in some children.
- If symptoms suggest cow milk protein allergy, a protein hydrolysate or amino acid feed should be given.
- Constipation may be improved by using a fibre-containing formula, although this may also cause bloating.

Blended feeds for tube-fed children

There has been recent interest in blenderized feeds, mainly driven by parents and carers who feel this approach is more 'normal' than using commercial formula feeds and may be better tolerated. There is little available research in this area; however, some children with diarrhoea or post-fundoplication may benefit. Unlike commercial formula feeds, the nutritional content of a blenderized diet is not standardized and as well as tube blockage, children may be at risk of nutritional deficiencies. From a parent's perspective, use of blenderized feeds may give them a feeling of more control over and involvement with their child's feeding and therefore have positive benefits through a sense of empowerment. Children fed in this way should remain under supervision by a dietitian.

Gastro-oesophageal reflux disease

GORD is common (15–75%) in children with neurological impairments; may relate to:
- Persistent activation of vomiting reflex.
- Generalized gastrointestinal dysmotility.
- Hiatus hernia.
- Prolonged supine position.
- Increased intra-abdominal pressure secondary to spasticity, scoliosis, or seizures.

Although PEG may sometimes exacerbate or initiate significant GORD there is no need for 'prophylactic' fundoplication. It may be in the nutritionally impaired child that a period of gastrostomy feeding will improve nutritional status and improve coexistent reflux. An initial period of NGT feeding may be useful for assessing potential need for fundoplication (i.e. if providing adequate nutritional intake provokes significant vomiting). 24-hour pH monitoring/impedance pre PEG is not generally predictive of who will need fundoplication.

Alternatives to antireflux surgery include:
- Jejunal feeding (e.g. PEG-J tube; surgical jejunostomy).
- Oesophago-gastric dissociation surgery (rarely needed).

Gastrostomy placement and subsequent care

An agreed pathway for children who need gastrostomy facilitates the process for children and their families; an example is given in Fig. 21.1.

Leaking, overgranulation, and infection of the gastrostomy site are common problems; a high standard of general care is required together with periodic tube replacement. Some practical guidance for care and maintenance of gastrostomy tubes is given in Fig. 21.2.

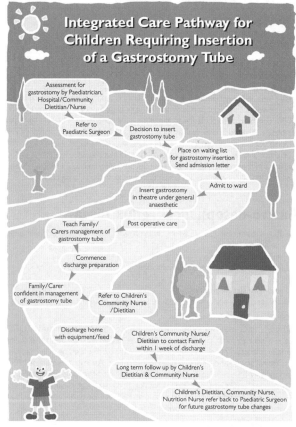

Integrated Care Pathway for Children Requiring Insertion of a Gastrostomy Tube

Assessment for gastrostomy by Paediatrician, Hospital/Community Dietitian/Nurse

Refer to Paediatric Surgeon

Decision to insert gastrostomy tube

Place on waiting list for gastrostomy insertion Send admission letter

Admit to ward

Insert gastrostomy in theatre under general anaesthetic

Post operative care

Teach Family/ Carers management of gastrostomy tube

Commence discharge preparation

Family/Carer confident in management of gastrostomy tube

Refer to Children's Community Nurse /Dietitian

Discharge home with equipment/feed

Children's Community Nurse/ Dietitian to contact Family within 1 week of discharge

Long term follow up by Children's Dietitian & Community Nurse

Children's Dietitian, Community Nurse, Nutrition Nurse refer back to Paediatric Surgeon for future gastrostomy tube changes

Fig. 21.1 Integrated care pathway for children requiring insertion of a gastrostomy tube (with grateful acknowledgement to Gill Lazonby and Cheryl Thomas, Children's Nutrition Nurse Specialists, Leeds General Infirmary).

CLEANING GASTROSTOMY STOMA SITE

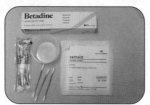

Collect equipment and wash hands thoroughly
Do not undo the fixation triangle for the first 4 days
following placement

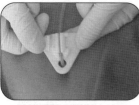

Ease the triangle up gently and clean with
soft guaze or cotton buds

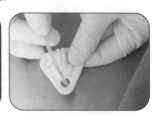

Lift tube out of fixation device and slide it down
the tube

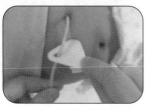

Check external length of tube

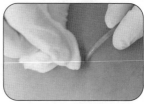

Clean around the tube with soft gauze or a
cotton bud. Use a clean piece each time, wiping
away from the gastrostomy stoma. Allow to dry
At least 4 days after placement and at
least once a week, open fixation device

Fig. 21.2 Gastrostomy tubes, buttons, and feed syringes. (a) Cleaning gastrostomy stoma site.

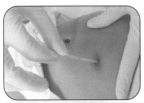 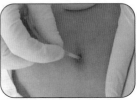

Gently push tube 1–3cm into stomach and turn the tube in a complete circle at least weekly and no more than once a day. This prevents the internal disc sticking to the stomach wall

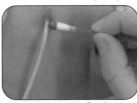 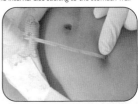

Apply antiseptic ointment (eg Betadine ointment) for the first 1–2 weeks following placement or if the gastrostomy site appears red. This reduces the risk of infection.

To check the external length of the tube, gently pull back until you feel the internal disc against the stomach wall.

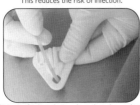 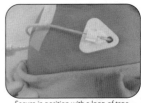

Slide the fixation device along the tube until it is close to the skin. Place your finger underneath the triangle and then press the yellow fixing clamp closed

Secure in position with a loop of tape, to prevent the tube pulling and stretching the gastrostomy stoma

Fig. 21.2 (a) (*Contd.*)

DAILY CARE OF GASTROSTOMY TUBE SITE

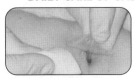

Clean around the tube with soft gauze or a cotton bud. Use a clean piece each time, wiping away from the gastrostomy site. Then clean the fixation disc

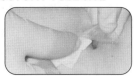

Dry around the skin and fixation disc thoroughly

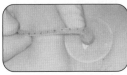

Turn the tube in a complete circle at least weekly and no more than once a day. This prevents the internal balloon sticking to the stomach wall. Gently pull back the tube and check the external length of the G tube is correct

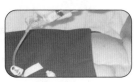

Flush the tube with cooled boiled water before and after feeds and medication and at least once a day if G tube not being used

Gastrostomy tube has migrated into stomach

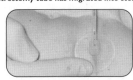

The tube appears shorter, the balloon may have migrated through the pylorus
Deflate the balloon and with drawn the tube to 6cm and then re-inflate the balloon.
Gently pull back the tube until you can feel the balloon against the stomach wall and the slide the disc to skin level

If tube continues to slip through fixation device, wrap tape around the tube above fixation device.

Aspirate tube and test for gastric acid, pH1–5, to ensure gastric placement.

Fig. 21.2 (b) Daily care of gastrostomy tube site.

**MANAGEMENT OF
OVER-GRANULATION TISSUE**

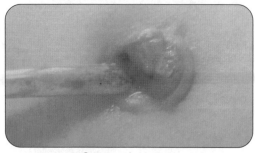

Over-granulation tissue

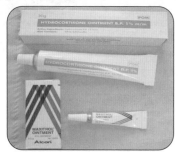

Use 1% hydrocortisone, if no improvement
after 1–2 weeks change to Maxitrol® ointment

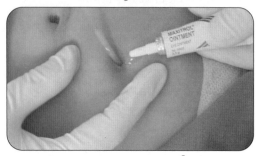

Applying hydrocortisone or Maxitrol® ointment.
Use twice a day for 10–14 days

Fig. 21.2 (c) Management of overgranulation tissue.

PERSISTENT OVER-GRANULATION TISSUE
(not responding to topical steroids/antibiotics)

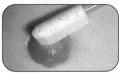

Persistent over-granulation tissue

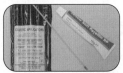

Use 75% silver nitrate applicator
and yellow soft paraffin

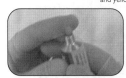

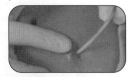

Apply soft paraffin to surrounding skin to prevent staining and damaging surrounding skin

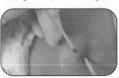

Apply silver nitrate to over-granulation
tissue, avoid touch gastrostomy tube as
this may damage the tube

Fig. 21.2 (d) Persistent overgranulation tissue.

MANAGEMENT OF A LEAKING GASTROSTOMY STOMA

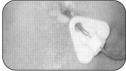

Tissue damage caused by gastric acid leakage.
Usually due to stoma being stretched by pulling or
excessive coughing/straining or a hole in the tube

Test leakage with pH paper to identify possible cause of leakage

 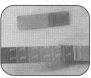

pH1–5 indicates gastric
acid leakage.

pH7–8 leakage is more likely
to be serous fluid/pus or
peritoneal fluid. This may
indicate infected gastrostomy
stoma site or misplaced tube.

 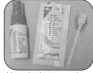

If gastric leakage is confirmed,
clean skin with cooled boiled
water or saline and allow to dry

Use a skin barrier product such as Cavilon® spray or sponge
wipe to protect surrounding skin

Fig. 21.2 (e) Management of a leaking gastrostomy stoma.

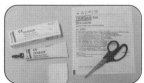

Use Orabase® paste and a key hole foam dressing to
reduce leakage and promote healing

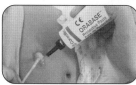

Apply Orabase® paste generously around
the tube. This creates a seal which will reduce
leakage and protects surrounding skin

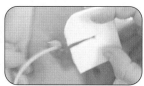

Apply key-hole foam dressing

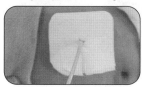

Hold in position with tape and gently
pull tube back until you can feel the
internal disc against the stomach wall

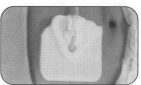

Close fixation device. Tape tube to skin
to prevent the gastrostomy stoma site
being pulled or stretched

- This treatment needs to be performed at least once a day.

- More frequent applications will be required if leakage is excessive.

- **Remember** that it will take regular applications of this treatment over
  1–2 weeks to promote healing of the stoma and gradually reduce the leakage

- **Do not** stop treatment until leakage has stopped completely for 3–5 days

Fig. 21.2 (e) (*Contd.*)

CHANGING A BALLOON GASTROSTOMY TUBE (G-TUBE)

Instil 5ml of sterile water/saline in balloon of new G tube and check balloon is a uniform shape.

Deflate the balloon on G tube in situ, using a male luer slip syringe

Lubricate the tip of the new G tube with gel. Insert G tube into stoma.

Deflate balloon and remove G tube.

Inflate the balloon with 5ml of sterile water/saline using a male luer slip syringe

Gently pull back the tube until you feel the internal balloon against the stomach wall

Attach extension set or attach catheter tip syringe directly onto the tube

Flush G tube with cooled boiled water

Test aspirate on pH paper, pH 1–5 indicates gastric placement

Check external fixation device is in correct position, use markings on the tube as a guide. The tube can be secured with tape to prevent it pulling on the stoma site. The tube can be secured with tape to prevent it pulling on the stoma site.

Fig. 21.2 (f) Changing a balloon gastrostomy tube.

CHANGING A BUTTON GASTROSTOMY
(low profile gastrostomy device LPGD)
Wash hands and collect equipment

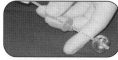

Check balloon on measuring device, if required

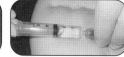

Deflate balloon on button/g-tube insitu using a male luer slip syringe

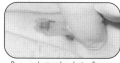

Remove button by placing fingers either side of the button. Ask patient to cough if possible.

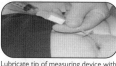

Lubricate tip of measuring device with gel, insert and inflate balloon with 5ml of water/saline

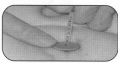

Note cm mark above the disc in both a sitting and lying position. Take an average of the two measurements to estimate shaft length

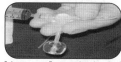

Select correct Fr size and cm length of button and check balloon for uniform shape

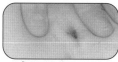

Remove measuring device

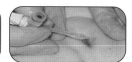

Lubricate tip with gel and insert the mini button

Fig. 21.2 (g) Changing a button gastrostomy.

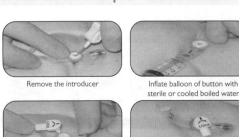

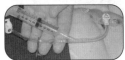

Remove the introducer

Inflate balloon of button with
sterile or cooled boiled water

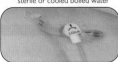

Match black mark on button and
extension and insert extension set

Turn extension to lock in position

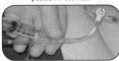

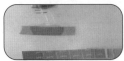

Draw back with a syringe to confirm
position in stomach

Test aspirate on pH paper,
pH 1–5 indicates gastric placement

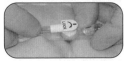

Flush with boiled cooled water

Line up black marks on button and
extension set and remove extension sets

Some buttons have an introducer which is helpful with longer shaft lengths

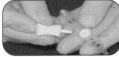

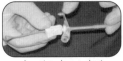

Attach clamp for the introducer
to the top of the button

Insert introducer to the tip
of the button and close the clamp

Fig. 21.2 (g) (*Contd.*)

Intestinal failure in patients with neurodisability

A small proportion of children with severe neurodisability appear to develop progressive gastrointestinal dysmotility with GORD followed by gastroparesis, then bilious reflux of small bowel contents into the stomach and abdominal pain exacerbated by enteral feeds. Under certain circumstances PN might be considered in such a child, with some returning to tolerating enteral tube feeding after a period of time. Multidisciplinary team discussions involving the family should focus on the child's best interests, and it is helpful to have a specialist in palliative care included prior to any decision to give PN.

References and resources

Allott L. Feeding children with special needs. In: Holden C, MacDonald A (eds.) Nutrition and child health. Edinburgh: Baillière Tindall; 2000, pp. 143–60.

Coad J, Toft A, Lapwood S, et al. Blended foods for tube fed children: a safe and realistic option? A rapid review of the evidence. Arch Dis Child 2017;102:274–8.

Marchand V, Motil KJ, NASPGHAN Committee on Nutrition. Nutrition support for neurologically impaired children: a clinical report of the North American Society of Pediatric Gastroenterology, Hepatology and Nutrition. J Pediatr Gastroenterol Nutr 2006;43:123–35.

Puntis JWL, Hills M. Failure and success in intestinal failure complicating neurodisability: who is at the end of the line? Arch Dis Child 2017;102:391–2.

Scope. Support for families: Food. https://www.scope.org.uk/support/families/food/A-Z-of-eating-difficulties

Obesity

Introduction *192*
Aetiology *192*
Definitions *192*
Epidemiology *193*
Prevention *193*
Evaluation *194*
Treatment *196*
Complications *198*
References and resources *200*

Introduction

Obesity is the most common nutritional disorder affecting children and adolescents in the developed world. Its importance is in its short- and long-term complications and that obese children are likely to become obese adults.

Aetiology

The reasons for a marked increase in prevalence are unclear but are linked to changes in the environment and behaviour relating to diet and activity. Energy-dense foods are now widely consumed, including high-fat fast foods and processed foods. However, there is no conclusive evidence that obese children eat more than children of normal weight. The National Food Survey showed that UK household energy intake has fallen since the 1970s, the amount of fruit purchased has increased by 75%, and the intake of full-fat milk decreased by 80%. Children's energy expenditure has undoubtedly decreased. Fewer children walk to school; transport in cars has increased; less time at school is spent doing physical activities; and children spend more time in front of small screens (video-games, mobile phones, computers, and television), rather than playing outside. Children from low socioeconomic homes are more likely to be obese; females from the lowest socioeconomic quintile are 2.5 times more likely to be overweight when compared with the highest quintile.

Definitions

Body mass index (BMI) = weight (kg)/height^2 (metres)

BMI related to reference standards for age is the most practical measure of overweight/obesity. It is objective and provides a degree of consistency with adult practice. Current British Childhood BMI charts show the 91st, 98th, and 99.6th centile lines, with a shaded area indicating healthy BMI range. The charts are also marked with the recommended International Obesity Task Force (IOTF) cut-offs for obesity and overweight in children, equating with WHO adult definitions of obesity and overweight at 18 years: BMI >30 = obese, BMI 25–30 = overweight. There is still no universally agreed definition of obesity in childhood. The National Child Measurement Programme defines overweight as BMI >85th centile, and obesity as >95th centile. For clinical use, cut offs suggested by the Scottish Intercollegiate Guideline Network and based on the 1990 Growth Cohort suggest a BMI >91st centile should be considered overweight, >98th centile as obese, and >99.6th centile as severe obesity. Clearly, use of different cut-offs may lead to some variation in estimates of overweight and obese children in different studies. Note that BMI is not a direct measure of adiposity as it cannot distinguish lean from fat mass; high waist circumference centile will provide further evidence of fatness.

Epidemiology

- In the UK, the National Child Measurement Programme measures height and weight of children in reception class at school (aged 4–5 years) and in year 6 (aged 10–11 years) to assess overweight and obesity at primary school. Among 2–5-year-olds, prevalence rates of overweight (including obesity) ranged between 19.5% (1995) and 26.0% (2007), while among 6–10-year-old boys this was between 22.6% (1994) and 33.0% (2011), and was highest among 11–15-year-olds ranging from 26.7% (1996) to 37.8% (2013). Similar findings were found for girls. Currently in the UK, one in five 5-year-olds and one in three 10-year-olds are overweight or obese.
- Obesity is an important risk factor for ischaemic heart disease (quadrupled risk in adulthood if BMI >29), hypertension, stroke, type 2 diabetes, cancers (breast, ovary, endometrium, prostate, bowel), depression, and social discrimination.
- Obesity across all ages is estimated to account for up to 7% of healthcare costs.

Prevention

There are few randomized controlled trials and most involve complex packages of interventions including decreased fat intake, increased fruit and vegetables, reduction in time spent in front of small screens, increased physical activity, and education. Of these, a reduction in time spent in front of small screens appears to be the most effective single factor.

Evaluation

When taking a history and conducting a clinical examination, assess the following:

- Family history of obesity and obesity-related illness (e.g. diabetes, cardiovascular disease).
- Family structure.
- Physical activity, diet, and eating patterns.
- Psychological effects (e.g. low self-esteem, bullying, depression).
- School attendance and attainment.
- Related morbidities (e.g. sleep apnoea, orthopaedic problems).
- Physical examination; height and weight, BMI, plotted on standard charts.
- Features of rare causes of obesity (see following paragraph), particularly short stature.
- Pubertal development; blood pressure.
- Acanthosis nigricans—a dark, velvety appearance at the neck and axillae, a sign of insulin resistance.

Consider unusual causes of obesity

Overnutrition accelerates linear growth and puberty. Obese children are therefore relatively tall and will usually be above the 50th centile for height. Therefore, if a child is obese and short, an endogenous cause, i.e. hypothyroidism and Cushing syndrome should be considered. In children who are obese with learning disabilities, or who are dysmorphic, an underlying syndrome may be present. In severely obese children under the age of 3 years, gene defects, e.g. leptin deficiency, are possible causes.

- Endocrine:
  - Hypothyroidism, e.g. in Down syndrome.
  - Cushing syndrome (truncal obesity, hypertension, hirsutism, striae).
  - Growth hormone deficiency (may have delayed puberty).
- Chromosomal abnormalities, e.g. Prader–Willi syndrome (obesity, hyperphagia, poor linear growth, developmental delay, small genitalia, dysmorphic).
- Drug related, e.g. steroid treatment.

Predisposing factors

- Spina bifida.
- Muscular dystrophy.
- Other causes of immobility.
- Polycystic ovary syndrome.

Consider further investigation if:

- Associated morbidity (e.g. apnoea, diabetes, arthritis).
- Short stature.
- Precocious (<8 year) puberty, or delayed puberty (no signs at 13 years in girls, 15 years in boys).
- Symptoms/signs of genetic or endocrine abnormality.

Treatment

Most obese children are managed in primary care. Specialist paediatric assessment is indicated in any child with complications or if an endogenous cause is suspected. The broad principles comprise management of obesity-related co-morbidities:

- Family involvement; all family members should be encouraged to eat healthily and to be physically active regardless of weight.
- A developmentally appropriate approach.
- Long-term behaviour modification.
- Dietary change.
- Increased physical activity.
- Decreased sedentary behaviours.
- A plan for longer-term weight maintenance strategies.
- In severe or complicated cases, the consideration of the use of pharmacotherapy or surgical intervention.

In the absence of evidence from randomized controlled trials, a pragmatic approach in any individual child based on consensus criteria has to be adopted. Treatment should be considered where the child is above the 98th centile for BMI and the family is willing to make the necessary difficult lifestyle changes.

Weight maintenance is a more realistic goal than weight reduction and will result in a demonstrable fall in BMI on centile chart as height increases. It can only be achieved by sustained changes in lifestyle:

- Healthier eating.
- Regular meals.
- Eating together as a family.
- Choosing nutrient rich foods that are lower in energy and glycaemic index (GI, the glycaemic index is a ranking of carbohydrate-containing foods based on the overall effect on blood glucose level; slowly absorbed foods have a low GI rating and those more rapidly absorbed a higher rating).
- Increased vegetable and fruit intake.
- Healthier snack food options.
- Decreased portion sizes.
- Drinking water as the main beverage.
- Reduction in sugary drink intake.
- Involvement of the entire family in making sustainable dietary changes.
- Physical activity can be increased by walking or cycling for transport, undertaking household chores, and playing.
- Organized exercise programmes have a role, with children and adolescents being encouraged to choose activities that they enjoy and are sustainable (e.g. football, dancing, swimming). At least 60 minutes of moderate or greater intensity physical activity is recommended each day.
- Limiting television and other small screen recreational activity to less than 2 hours per day.

Drug treatment and surgery

- Drug treatment has a part to play in children over the age of 12 who have extreme obesity (BMI >40 kg/m^2) or have a BMI >35 kg/m^2 and complications of obesity.
- It is recommended that drug treatment should only be considered after dietary, exercise and behavioural approaches have been started (NICE 2015).
- Orlistat is a lipase inhibitor, which reduces the absorption of dietary fat and thus produces steatorrhoea. It should not be used under 12 years, but may be indicated if there are co-morbidities (e.g. orthopaedic, sleep apnoea) or severe psychological disturbance.
- Bariatric surgery is generally not considered appropriate in children or young people unless they have almost achieved maturity, have very severe or extreme obesity with complications, e.g. type 2 diabetes or hypertension, and all other interventions have failed to achieve or maintain weight loss. American data would suggest that laparoscopic adjustable gastric banding is the most appropriate operation.
- Drug and surgical interventions should occur on the background of a behavioural weight management programme and be restricted to specialist centres with multidisciplinary expertise in managing severe obesity. Reducing the prevalence of obesity is a major public health challenge.
- There is recognition in the UK that there needs to be a more 'joined up' approach to obesity, with integration between health services, local government and other key partners based on the needs of the local population

Complications

Box 22.1 Complications of obesity
- Orthopaedic—slipped upper femoral epiphysis, tibia vara (bow legs), abnormal foot structure and function.
- Idiopathic intracranial hypertension (headaches, blurred optic disc margins).
- Hypoventilation syndrome (daytime somnolence; sleep apnoea; snoring; hypercapnia; heart failure).
- Non-alcoholic fatty liver disease (NAFLD).
- Gallbladder disease/gallstones.
- Polycystic ovarian syndrome.
- Type 2 diabetes mellitus.
- Hypertension.
- Abnormal blood lipids.
- Other medical sequelae, e.g. asthma, changes in left ventricular mass, increased risk of certain malignancies (endometrial, breast and colonic carcinoma).
- Psychological sequelae—low self-esteem, teasing, depression.

Metabolic syndrome
- A constellation of metabolic risk factors that appear to promote the development of atherosclerotic heart disease, including high plasma triglycerides and low high-density lipoprotein cholesterol, hypertension, insulin resistance.
- NAFLD is considered the hepatic manifestation of metabolic syndrome.

Non-alcoholic fatty liver disease
- NAFLD is thought to result from fatty infiltration of the liver due to obesity and insulin resistance, followed by inflammatory insults, possibly related to oxidative stress.
- 10% of obese adolescents in the US have elevated alanine amino transaminase.
- The most common cause of liver disease in the pre-adolescent and adolescent age groups.
- Histological changes range from simple steatosis, to steatosis with inflammation and cellular injury and fibrosis.
- Liver biopsy is the gold standard for diagnosis (applicability limited by risk and cost).
- Diagnosis usually based on elevated amino transferases and/or fatty liver on ultrasound; other causes of liver disease (hepatitis B and C, Wilson disease, α_1-antitrypsin deficiency, autoimmune hepatitis, drug-induced liver injury) should be excluded.
- Although hepatic fibrosis is common (53–100%) in children with NAFLD, the incidence of cirrhosis is unknown.
- Interventions aimed at weight reduction are currently the only therapeutic option.

Case study

Jodie was 10 years of age when referred to outpatients because of concerns about her being overweight and the possibility of a 'glandular' problem. According to her mother she was getting on well at school, but did not like taking part in physical activities. Her records show that she began to put on weight rapidly from the age of 3 years; she was tall for her age, with a BMI on the 98th centile.

The aspects of Jodie's lifestyle that predispose to obesity should be assessed, together with any emotional and behavioural difficulties. Enquiry should be made regarding what Jodie and her family eat on a normal day, and details of physical and sedentary activities. Snoring at night and lethargy in the day suggest that sleep apnoea should be considered; musculoskeletal problems are common. There may be difficulties at school, with obese children being bullied or themselves bullying; they may be depressed. Take a family history with regard to whether anyone else is overweight and whether there is a history of heart disease at a young age, or diabetes.

Nutritional obesity is very common in comparison with other causes; children with endocrine problems and overweight are usually short. Since clinical examination of Jodie was normal apart from her obesity, it was not appropriate to investigate for endocrine or genetic abnormalities. The family was given advice regarding diet options aimed at reducing energy intake, and increasing levels of exercise.

Box 22.2 Key messages for patients and parents about obesity

- Incidence of obesity in children is increasing.
- Obesity is a health concern in itself and also increases the risk of other serious health problems, such as high blood pressure, diabetes, and psychological distress.
- An obese child often becomes an obese adult.
- Obesity in children may be prevented and treated by increasing physical activity/decreasing physical inactivity (e.g. small screen time), and encouraging a well-balanced and healthy diet.
- Lifestyle changes involve making small, gradual modifications to behaviour.
- Family support is necessary for treatment to succeed.
- Generally, the aim of treatment is to help children maintain their weight at a static level (so that they can 'grow into it') rather than lose weight.
- Most children are not obese because of an underlying medical problem but as a result of their lifestyle.

Data sourced from Chapter 16 SIGN 115: Management of obesity. Scottish Intercollegiate Guidelines Network, February 2010.

References and resources

Alberti KGMM, Zimmet PZ, Shaw JE. The metabolic syndrome—a new world-wide definition from the International Diabetes Federation Consensus. Lancet 2005;366:1059–62.

Coles N, Birken C, Hamilton J. Emerging treatments for severe obesity in children and adolescents. BMJ 2016;355:30–3.

National Institute for Health and Clinical Excellence. Obesity prevention. NICE Clinical Guideline 43. London: NICE; 2015. https://www.nice.org.uk/guidance/cg43

NHS guidance on healthy eating for children and families: http://www.nhs.uk/Livewell/Goodfood/Pages/Goodfoodhome.aspx

Royal College of Paediatrics and Child Health. Tackling England's childhood obesity crisis. London: Royal College of Paediatrics and Child Health; 2015. http://www.rcpch.ac.uk/system/files/protected/news/Obesity%20Summit%20report%20FINAL.pdf

Scottish Intercollegiate Guidelines Network. Who are. http://sign.ac.uk/who-we-are.html

Scottish Intercollegiate Guidelines Network. Management of obesity. Sign Guideline 115; 2010. http://www.sign.ac.uk/sign-115-management-of-obesity.html

Wright N, Wales J. Assessment and management of severely obese children and adolescents. Arch Dis Child 2016;101:1161–7.

Gastrointestinal manifestations of cystic fibrosis

Introduction *202*
Gastrointestinal manifestations *204*
Management of gastrointestinal symptoms in children
   with cystic fibrosis *206*
References and resources *206*

Introduction

The incidence of cystic fibrosis (CF) is around 1 in 2500. Cases are diagnosed as a consequence of population screening or high-risk screening, or following presentation with clinical symptoms typical of the disorder. The basic defect is in the CFTR (cystic fibrosis transmembrane conductance regulator) protein which codes for a cyclic adenosine monophosphate-regulated chloride transporter in epithelial cells of exocrine organs. This is involved in salt and water balance across epithelial surfaces. The gene is on chromosome 7. There are multiple known mutations, the most common being ΔF508.

CF is a multisystem disorder and the primary pathology is within the respiratory system, but it can present with gastrointestinal manifestations such as meconium ileus or chronic diarrhoea. Poor weight gain is common at diagnosis. This chapter deals with the gastrointestinal manifestations relevant to the assessment of children with gut disease. Nutritional management and liver disease are covered in Chapters 24 and 25 respectively.

Gastrointestinal manifestations

Pancreatic disease

The pathophysiology of pancreatic disease is a failure of exocrine pancreatic secretion. Thickened secretions (low bicarbonate concentration) block the pancreatic ductal system; autodigestion by pancreatic enzymes follows and leads to a reduction in functional capacity.

- Pancreatic exocrine insufficiency occurs in up to 90% (80% in the first year).
- There is marked impairment of secretion of water, bicarbonate, lipase, amylase, and proteases from the pancreas into the duodenum resulting in maldigestion.
- Presentation is with chronic diarrhoea (steatorrhoea), poor weight gain, and occasionally hypoproteinaemic oedema.
- Pancreatic enzyme replacement is required and should be supervised by an experienced paediatric dietician; the dose needs to be carefully tailored to match food intake, prevent steatorrhoea, and promote weight gain.
- Energy needs are high as a consequence of the maldigestion, increased metabolic demands (primarily respiratory), and the impact of chronic disease on other body systems.
- A high-calorie diet is required but may be difficult to achieve when the child is unwell; energy-dense foods, supplements, or tube feeding are sometimes necessary.
- Fat-soluble vitamin replacement is required.
- Abnormal glucose tolerance occurs in up to 10% by the second decade and may lead to diabetes mellitus.
- Both acute and chronic pancreatitis may be seen.

Intestinal disease

Defects in CFTR lead to reduced chloride secretion with water following into the gut. This may result in meconium ileus at birth and in distal intestinal obstruction syndrome (DIOS) later in life. The basic pathophysiology results in dehydration of intestinal contents with clinical presentations as a consequence;

- 15% of children with CF have meconium ileus in the neonatal period.
- Presents with delayed passage of meconium, abdominal distension, and bile-stained vomiting.
- Management is by bowel clearance via an enterotomy using acetyl cysteine or Gastrografin®.
- Up to 30% require bowel resection.
- After bowel resection, infants will be at increased risk of bacterial overgrowth and short bowel syndrome.
- Not all children with meconium ileus have CF but it should be excluded in any child who presents in this way.
- Intussusception occurs more commonly and at a later age than in the general population.

- Rectal prolapse occurs in up to 15%; risk factors include frequent large stools, poor nutritional status, and raised intrathoracic pressure from coughing. Most cases improve with treatment of CF (NB most children with rectal prolapse do not have CF).
- DIOS (meconium ileus equivalent) results from the accumulation of thick faecal material in the terminal ileum, caecum, and ascending colon and may cause bowel obstruction. Differential diagnosis includes appendicitis, intussusception, and volvulus. Management is with IV fluids and laxatives; oral Gastrografin® or intestinal lavage is helpful in difficult cases.
- Constipation is very common; risk factors include poor fluid intake, inadequately controlled steatorrhoea, viscid intestinal secretions, energy-dense diets, dysmotility, plus all the other risk factors in the childhood population.
- Colonic strictures have been reported and are thought to be secondary to high-dose pancreatic supplementation.

Management of gastrointestinal symptoms in children with cystic fibrosis

The differential diagnosis of gastrointestinal symptoms in children with CF includes:
- CF-related complications.
- Non-CF-related bowel disease.
- Functional abdominal pain.

It is important to remember that the child with abdominal pain may have a complication of CF such as pancreatitis, non-CF-related bowel disease such as gastro-oesophageal reflux, peptic ulceration, or functional abdominal pain (recurrent abdominal pain of childhood). Gastro-oesophageal reflux is more common in children with respiratory disease, and may be exacerbated by energy-dense diets. Functional symptoms are very common in children with chronic illness, and psychosocial factors are important to take into account in the overall assessment. During adolescence, issues relating to acceptance of the underlying disease, acceptance by peers, and the gradual progression from dependence to independence are the most prominent.

References and resources

Cystic Fibrosis Trust: https://www.cysticfibrosis.org.uk/
Sathe MN, Freeman AJ. Gastrointestinal, pancreatic and hepatobiliary manifestations of cystic fibrosis. Paediatr Clin North Am 2016;63:679–98.

Chapter 24

Nutritional management of cystic fibrosis

Nutrition in cystic fibrosis 208
Pancreatic enzyme replacement therapy 212
References and resources 213

Nutrition in cystic fibrosis

There is evidence that promoting good nutritional status can slow the progression of pulmonary disease and improve long-term outcome. In 2015, the UK median predicted survival for the CF population was 45.1 years.

Risk factors for malnutrition in CF

Increased resting energy expenditure
- Chronic cough.
- Chest infections.
- Impaired lung function.

Increased nutrient losses
- Maldigestion due to pancreatic insufficiency.
- Reduced bile salt pool.
- Previous gastrointestinal surgery for meconium ileus.
- Expectoration of copious mucus can lead to losses of up to 10g protein/day, especially from *Pseudomonas aeruginosa*.
- Impaired glucose tolerance or undiagnosed/poorly controlled diabetes results in energy loss due to glycosuria.
- Vomiting following coughing, physiotherapy, or gastro-oesophageal reflux (GOR).

Poor energy intake
- Anorexia and fatigue during pulmonary infection.
- Depression.
- Behavioural feeding disorders.
- Anxiety regarding weight and weight gain, particularly in teenage group.
- Abdominal pain and GOR.

Nutritional management

- Early diagnosis by neonatal screening and early intervention assists maintenance of nutritional status.
- The Cystic Fibrosis Trust Standards of Care recommend that a specialist CF dietitian should:
  - Complete a nutritional annual review for all patients.
  - Review all inpatients at least twice a week during admission.
  - Review all patients with pancreatic insufficiency at every clinic visit.

Assessment of growth

- Weight and height should be routinely monitored at every clinic visit and hospital admission.
- BMI percentile is widely accepted as the most appropriate indicator of nutritional status and should also be monitored at every clinic visit and admission in children >2 years of age.
- Maintaining a BMI ≥50th percentile is associated with better lung function.
- A BMI <20th centile is associated with an impaired lung function and low bone mineral density.
- There is increasing concern about the rising prevalence of overweight and obesity in children with CF.
- Patients with a BMI >91st centile should therefore be given appropriate advice to reduce the rate of weight gain.
- BMI should not be used in isolation to assess nutritional status as it can mask nutritional stunting as it adjusts for height.

Assessment of requirements

- The energy needs of children with CF are estimated to be 110–200% of those estimated for healthy age and sex-matched children.
- Energy requirements should be estimated using the Scientific Advisory Committee on Nutrition (SACN) (2011) dietary reference values using estimated average requirement (EAR) for energy.
- Consider energy demands from activity levels, nutritional status, chronic and acute infection, presence of co-morbidities, pancreatic status, and control of malabsorption.
- Some children may require no more than the EAR for energy. This may be particularly evident in patients with pancreatic sufficiency.
- Regular review of growth will confirm that assessments of requirements are correct.
- Increased resting energy expenditure is associated with declining pulmonary function and subclinical infection but can be off-set by reduction in activity levels.
- There are currently no recommendations for optimal protein intakes for children with CF.
- Fibre-rich foods should be encouraged but not at the expense of energy-rich foods. Fibre can have a beneficial effect on colonic function including preventing constipation and abdominal pain.

Feeding infants and children with CF

- Normal growth can be achieved in many infants with either breastfeeding or a standard infant formula.
- Breastfeeding should be encouraged. As well as well-known benefits, breast milk also contains lipase.
- The use of a high-energy infant formula should be considered if weight gain and growth is suboptimal.
- If breast milk is unavailable, then a hydrolysed protein formula should be used in infants who have undergone surgery for meconium ileus.
- Weaning foods should be introduced between 4 and 6 months and tastes and textures progressed in the normal way.
- Full-fat cow's milk can be introduced to replace formula milk at 1 year.
- Salt-containing foods should not be restricted.
- A good variety of energy-rich, ordinary foods should be encouraged such as full-fat milk, cheese, meat, whole milk yogurt, milk puddings, cakes, and biscuits.
- Normal school meals and packed lunches are suitable for many children with CF.
- If required for growth, additional high-fat snacks between meals are helpful as long as this does not diminish the appetite for main meals.
- With increasing longevity of patients with CF, polyunsaturated and monounsaturated fats are increasingly encouraged to minimize concerns over dietary fat and blood lipid levels.
- Attention should be given to psychological, social, behavioural, and developmental aspects of feeding with encouragement of normal family mealtime routines. Psychology support may be needed if difficulties develop.

Nutrition support
- Indications for the introduction of oral nutritional supplements:
  - Weight loss or no weight gain over 2–8 weeks (<12 months),
    6–8 weeks (1–2 years), or 4–6 months (2–18 years).
  - BMI <25th centile in children over 2 years.
  - Acute disease-related reduction in appetite.
- Supplements should not replace meals.
- Prescriptions should be individually tailored based on age, preferences, and estimated nutritional requirements.
- Pancreatic enzymes should be consumed with all milk-based supplements.
- Indications for enteral feeding:
  - Sustained deviation from previous weight and/or length percentile.
  - Persisting BMI <25th centile.
  - As well as growth, enteral feeding can improve body fat, lean body mass, muscle mass, strength, and pubertal development.
- Polymeric feeds are the first choice and patients usually tolerate a 1.5kcal/mL age/size appropriate feed.
- Elemental feeds are more expensive, have a higher osmolality and lower energy density, with little evidence of greater efficacy.
- PEG is the preferred route for long-term feeding as this enables overnight feeding.
- Monitoring of enteral feeding:
  - Weight, height, and BMI—rapid weight gain is associated with an increase in fat stores.
  - Feed tolerance.
  - Glucose tolerance mid and post feeding. This should be repeated monthly at home.

Vitamin and mineral supplementation
See Table 24.1.

Table 24.1 Vitamins, their associated deficiencies, and recommended doses for children with cystic fibrosis.

Vitamin	Clinical features of deficiency	Dose			
A	Night blindness; xerophthalmia	Infants		>1 year	
		< 1500IU (0.45mg)		1500–10,000IU (0.45–3.0mg)	
D	CF-related low bone mineral density (CFRLMD); rickets	Infants		>1 year	
		400–2000IU (10–50µg)		400–5000IU (10–125µg)	
E	Haemolytic anaemia; spinocerebellar degeneration	0–12months	1–3 years	4–7 years	8–18 years
		40–80 IU	50–150IU	150–300IU	150–500IU
K	Prolonged clotting Poor bone health	<2 years		2–7 years	From 7 years
		300µg/kg/day rounded to nearest mg		5mg/day	5–10mg/day

Fat-soluble vitamins

- Malabsorption of fat-soluble vitamins is common with pancreatic exocrine insufficiency.
- Fat-soluble vitamin supplementation should be started at diagnosis in all pancreatic insufficient patients.
- Supplementation for patients with pancreatic sufficiency is indicated in the presence of evidence of deficiency.
- Levels should be checked, and adjusted where indicated, annually for all patients with CF.
- The effect of any supplemental dose changes should be assessed after 3–6 months.

Sodium

- Risk factors for sodium deficiency:
    - Infants—due to low intakes from either breast milk or standard infant formulas.
    - Infants presenting with meconium ileus, particularly those requiring a stoma.
    - Hot weather.
    - Intense physical activity.
- Suboptimal growth has been reported in infants with a low urinary sodium level following intestinal surgery.
- Infants with low urinary sodium should be prescribed additional sodium supplementation, using a sodium chloride solution that provides an additional 1–2mmol/kg/day.

Pancreatic enzyme replacement therapy

- Pancreatic status is normally determined using the faecal pancreatic elastase 1 (FPE-1) test.
- Patients with CF vary in their degree of pancreatic insufficiency and individual pancreatic enzyme replacement therapy requirements.
- Enteric-coated acid-resistant microsphere preparations are recommended.
- In the UK, Creon® is used by 95% of the CF population with pancreatic insufficiency.
- In the presence of clinical evidence of fat malabsorption, enzymes can be started prior to receipt of a FPE-1 result.
- Enzymes should be given with all meals and snacks containing fat.
- Enzymes are not required with non-fat-containing foods such as jelly, fruit, fruit juice, boiled/jelly sweets, and fizzy drinks.
- Recommended starting doses:
  - Infants: ¼–1 scoop Creon® Micro per feed.
  - Older children, 1–3 capsules per meal or snack.
- Enzyme preparations should not be crushed or chewed.
- If patients are unable to swallow the capsules whole, they should be opened and the contents mixed with a small amount of food (e.g. yoghurt, first mouthful of meal, fruit puree).
- Gradually increase dose according to clinical symptoms, appearance of stools, and weight gain.
- Meals with a very high fat content (e.g. takeaways) will likely require a higher dose.
- Enzymes are best taken at the beginning and during a meal, especially if mealtimes take >30 minutes.
- In the 1990s there were reported cases of fibrosing colonopathy (strictures of the large bowel). As a result, the Committee on the Safety of Medicines (CSM) recommended a maximum daily intake of 10,000 units of lipase/kg/day. It is now recognized that some patients require more than 10,000 units of lipase/kg/day and these patients should be closely monitored.
- Dietary fat intake should not be restricted as outlined by the CSM safety limits.
- In the event of high enzyme doses, enzyme efficacy may be improved by reducing the gastric acid secretion with H_2 receptor antagonists or proton pump inhibitors.
- Persistent problems require investigation for other disorders (e.g. coeliac disease, cow milk protein intolerance).

References and resources

Cystic Fibrosis Trust: https://www.cysticfibrosis.org.uk

Cystic Fibrosis Trust (2016). Nutritional management of cystic fibrosis. London: Cystic Fibrosis Trust.

Cystic Fibrosis Trust (2016). UK Cystic Fibrosis Registry 2015 annual data report. London: Cystic Fibrosis Trust.

Scientific Advisory Committee on Nutrition (SACN). Dietary reference values for energy. London: Public Health England; 2011. https://www.gov.uk/government/publications/sacn-dietary-reference-values-for-energy

Shaw V (ed.). Clinical paediatric dietetics, 4th edn. Oxford: Wiley; 2015.

UK Cystic Fibrosis Trust Standards of Care Working Group. Standards for the clinical care of children and adults with cystic fibrosis in the UK. London: Cystic Fibrosis Trust; 2011.

Cystic fibrosis-associated liver disease

Introduction *216*
Pathophysiology *216*
Clinical features *216*
Diagnosis *217*
Management *218*
References and resources *219*

Introduction

CF is an autosomal recessive disease resulting from mutations in the gene coding for the cystic fibrosis transmembrane conductance regulator (CFTR) (see Chapter 21). CFTR functions as a transmembrane chloride channel in the apical membrane of most secretory epithelia and the disease thus affects lungs, pancreas, exocrine glands, gut, and liver. In CF-associated liver disease, the biliary tract is most commonly involved in a spectrum from asymptomatic to biliary cirrhosis. The liver disease runs from mild and sub-clinical to severe cirrhosis and portal hypertension. Clinical disease is seen in 4–6% of cases, but there are biochemical abnormalities in 20–50%. At autopsy, fibrosis is present in 20% and steatosis in 50%.

Pathophysiology

The cause of liver disease in CF is not well understood, and is multifactorial. Reduced chloride channel function appears to result in a reduction in water and sodium movement into bile, and there are abnormalities in the composition, alkalinity, and flow of the bile. It is unclear why all CF patients have abnormal CFTR in the biliary tree, but not all develop biliary disease. In the liver parenchyma, the most common pathology is steatosis, which is present in 50%. There is no relationship between the CF genotype and the phenotype of the liver disease. Risk factors for significant liver disease include pancreatic insufficiency, possession of human leucocyte antigen (HLA)-DQ6, male sex, and presentation with meconium ileus.

Clinical features

Neonatal (uncommon)

- Conjugated jaundice.
- Fat malabsorption and faltering growth.
- Inspissated bile syndrome.

The cholestatic jaundice resolves over time, though residual fibrosis may remain. There is not thought to be an increased risk of subsequent cirrhosis.

Older children

- Asymptomatic hepatomegaly and/or splenomegaly.
- Hypersplenism.
- Complications of portal hypertension, e.g. variceal bleeding.
- Elevated transaminases, alkaline phosphatase, or gamma-glutamyl transferase.
- Malnutrition.
- Cholelithiasis.
- Sclerosing cholangitis.
- Rarely ascites and jaundice.

Diagnosis

This can be difficult as liver function tests do not always reflect the severity of the disease.

Liver function tests
- Bilirubin normal unless disease is advanced.
- Prothrombin time prolonged in severe liver disease or vitamin K deficiency.
- Gamma-glutamyl transferase raised in >30% and in severe disease.
- Intermittent rises in transaminases in 30% of patients.
- Alkaline phosphatase elevated in 50% but not specific for liver disease.

Ultrasound
- Size and consistency of liver and spleen.
- Heterogeneous liver parenchyma in steatosis.
- Portal vein flow and splenic varices.
- Cholelithiasis.

Liver biopsy
- Extent and severity of liver disease.
- Changes of giant cell hepatitis in neonates.
- Inspissated bile.
- Steatosis in older children.
- Focal biliary fibrosis.
- Cirrhosis.
- The distribution of changes in CF-associated liver disease may be patchy and therefore liver biopsy may not accurately represent the severity of the disease.

Transient elastography (FibroScan®)
Transient elastography is a non-invasive method which can be used to monitor liver stiffness which is associated with liver fibrosis. Transient elastography would not reflect liver steatosis.

Endoscopy
- Oesophageal and gastric varices.
- Portal hypertensive gastropathy.

Magnetic resonance cholangiopancreatography (MRCP)
- Sclerosing cholangitis.
- Common bile duct stricture.

Management

Management is mainly symptomatic, i.e. avoiding fat-soluble vitamin deficiency, choleretic agents to improve bile flow, endoscopic management of bleeding varices, aggressive nutritional support, and liver transplantation in a small number of patients.

Ursodeoxycholic acid

Ursodeoxycholic acid is a naturally occurring bile acid with choleretic, cytoprotective, membrane-stabilizing, antioxidant, and immunomodulatory properties. Treatment with ursodeoxycholic acid has been shown to improve biochemical and morphological parameters.

Endoscopy

Regular banding or sclerotherapy can provide good control of oesophageal varices and reduce the risk of bleeding.

Nutritional support

A dietician should be involved in the care of the patient, to give a high-energy diet with an increased proportion of fat, and protein supplements. Gastrostomy tube placement is not usually recommended in those with portal gastropathy and varices.

Liver transplantation

Most centres would consider the following complications as indications for liver transplantation in the absence of severe impairment of lung function where multiorgan transplantation should be considered:

• Deteriorating quality of life due to significant liver disease.
• Progressive chronic liver disease with increasing coagulopathy and falling albumin.
• Intractable ascites.
• Recurrent variceal bleeding not controlled with endoscopic procedures.
• Development of hepatopulmonary and portopulmonary syndrome.
• Severe malnutrition with liver disease unresponsive to aggressive nutritional interventions.
• Patients with diabetes requiring a liver transplant may be considered for a liver/pancreas transplant.
• Pulmonary and cardiac function is also assessed during the liver transplant assessment, as the patient may require a combined heart/lung/liver transplant.

References and resources

Debray D, Kelly D, Houwen R, Strandvik B, Colombo C. Best practice guidance for the diagnosis and management of cystic fibrosis-associated liver disease. J Cyst Fibros 2011;10(Suppl 2):S29–36.

Kitson MT, Kemp WW, Iser DM, Paul E, Wilson JW, Roberts SK. Utility of transient elastography in the non-invasive evaluation of cystic fibrosis liver disease. Liver Int 2013;33:698–705.

Vomiting

Introduction 222
Assessment 222
Differential diagnosis 223
Management 223

Introduction

Vomiting is a common symptom of gut disease but can also reflect disease outside the gastrointestinal tract. Vomiting refers to the forceful expulsion of gastric contents. It generally occurs as a consequence of activation of the emetic reflex.

There are three phases of vomiting:
- Nausea.
- Retching.
- Expulsion.

Nausea may manifest as irritability, pallor, excess salivation, sweating, and tachycardia. In infants, the three phases are not as easy to distinguish as in adults.

Vomiting is controlled through the emetic reflex by the vomiting centre. The vomiting centre is a functional rather than anatomical entity which responds through afferent stimuli from the cerebral cortex, cerebellum, vestibular system, and gastrointestinal tract. The vomiting centre and area postrema (previously called the chemoreceptor trigger zone) in the floor of the fourth ventricle triggers the cascade of events that results in vomiting (motor and autonomic). Endogenous (e.g. sepsis) and exogenous (e.g. drugs) factors can impact directly at the area postrema.

The threshold for vomiting may be altered by factors such as GOR, gastrointestinal dysmotility (constipation, delayed gastric emptying), lifestyle factors (e.g. high-fat diet), and gut disease.

Vomiting should be distinguished from *regurgitation*, the effortless expulsion of gastric contents which is common in healthy infants and older children who eat in excess; *rumination* is the frequent regurgitation of ingested food and is generally thought to be largely behavioural.

Assessment

The assessment and management of vomiting requires a careful history and examination considering the wide differential diagnosis listed as follows with investigation dependent on the clinical features:
- Vomiting can be acute or recurrent (chronic or cyclical).
- Acute vomiting is more likely to be infectious, surgical, or neurological.
- The differential to consider in recurrent vomiting is much wider.
- Bilious (green/yellow/brown) vomit suggests intestinal obstruction.
- Haematemesis suggests upper gastrointestinal pathology, e.g. oesophagitis, Mallory–Weiss tear.

Differential diagnosis

The differential diagnosis of vomiting is wide and almost any pathology can present with vomiting as a symptom.

- Infection, e.g. urinary tract infection, gastroenteritis.
- Intestinal obstruction, e.g. achalasia, pyloric stenosis, intestinal atresia, malrotation, volvulus.
- GOR, oesophagitis and peptic ulcer disease, Mallory–Weiss tear.
- Food allergy and intolerance, e.g. cow's milk allergy, soy allergy, coeliac disease.
- Metabolic, e.g. diabetic ketoacidosis, inborn errors of metabolism, porphyria, chronic renal failure.
- Renal, e.g. pelvi-ureteric junction obstruction, renal stone.
- Neurological, e.g. CNS tumour, epilepsy.
- Functional, e.g. functional dyspepsia/non-ulcer dyspepsia.
- Psychological, e.g. food refusal, anxiety.
- Drug induced.
- Induced illness (e.g. poisoning).

Management

The treatment is directed at the individual cause.

Indications to consider antiemetic therapy

- Motion sickness.
- Postoperative nausea and vomiting.
- Cancer chemotherapy.
- Cyclical vomiting syndrome.
- Gastrointestinal motility disorders.

Achalasia

Definition 226
Incidence 226
Presentation 226
Differential diagnosis 226
Investigation 226
Treatment 227
References and resources 227

Definition

Motility disorder characterized by failed relaxation of the lower oesophageal sphincter and disordered oesophageal peristalsis. This results in progressive dysphagia and regurgitation of ingested food/drink.

Incidence

1/10,000. Usually in older children/adults.

Presentation

Dysphagia and regurgitation, with sensation of food bolus obstruction at lower oesophagus. Initially symptoms occur with solids, but this progresses to liquid intolerance. The diagnosis is often delayed and the symptoms wrongly attributed to other causes, e.g. anorexia nervosa.

Differential diagnosis

GOR, eosinophilic oesophagitis, functional causes (anorexia nervosa, globus hystericus).

Investigation

- Upper GI series—shows typical 'bird-beak' appearance at gastro-oesophageal junction (GOJ), with dilated oesophagus.
- Endoscopy—may show oesophagitis. Passage of the endoscope through the GOJ helps to exclude reflux-associated stricture.
- Manometry—confirms the diagnosis, but may not be well tolerated in younger children. Manometry demonstrates failed relaxation of the lower oesophageal sphincter with disordered oesophageal peristalsis. Three subtypes are described in adults which may help predict outcome and response to myotomy: type I with minimal oesophageal pressurization, type II with oesophageal compression, and type III with oesophageal spasm.

Treatment

Definitive treatment is Heller's oesophago-myotomy (usually performed laparoscopically). Complications include mucosal perforation, incomplete myotomy, and recurrence.

Initial therapy to relieve symptoms may include endoscopic balloon dilatation or botulinum toxin injection, but symptoms will recur over time. There is an increased risk of oesophageal carcinoma in untreated achalasia.

References and resources

Pandolfino JE, Kwiatek MA, Nealis T, Bulsiewicz W, Post J, Kahrilas PJ. Achalasia: a new clinically relevant classification by high-resolution manometry. Gastroenterology 2008;135:1526–33.

Chapter 28

Acute gastroenteritis

Introduction *230*
Pathogenesis *230*
Aetiology *230*
Clinical features *231*
Differential diagnosis *232*
Assessment *234*
Management *236*
Prevention *238*
Complications *239*
References and resources *240*

Introduction

Gastroenteritis is one of the commonest conditions seen in childhood. Presentation to medical practitioners occurs where there is concern over inadequate intake and dehydration, and persistence of diarrhoea and vomiting.

Assessment of dehydration and consideration of the wide differential diagnosis are important factors in planning management.

Pathogenesis

Viral infections affect enterocyte function within the villi of the small intestine. Different pathogens have distinct methods of causing enterocyte damage, from toxin production to direct invasion. The damage caused leads to loss of the normal regulation of salt and fluid absorption. Inflammation can lead to a high osmotic load within the gut lumen precipitating further loss of fluid. Bacterial pathogens invade the lining of the small and large bowel and trigger inflammation.

Aetiology

In up to 50% of cases of gastroenteritis the aetiological agent is not found even when extensive investigations are undertaken. In pre-school children where an agent is looked for, the commonest cause is a viral pathogen, particularly rotavirus (see Table 28.1). Rotavirus is estimated to be responsible for up to 25% of deaths due to diarrhoeal disease worldwide. Rotavirus vaccine was introduced into the UK schedule in July 2013 with a significant reduction of reported cases. No excess morbidity or mortality was seen.

Table 28.1 Aetiology of gastroenteritis

Viruses	Bacteria	Parasites
Rotavirus[a]	Campylobacter	Giardia lambia
Norwalk-like	Salmonella	Entamoeba histolytica
Adenoviruses	Shigella	Cryptosporidium[c]
Small round virus	Escherichia coli[b]	
Astroviruses	Clostridium difficile	

[a] Rotavirus (commonest), seasonal, peaks late winter. Different pathogenicity of different strains, peak age for infection 6 months–2 years.

[b] Enteropathogenic E. coli, enterotoxigenic E. coli 0157:H7 (associated with haemolytic uraemic syndrome).

[c] Particularly in the immunocompromised host.

Clinical features

The clinical features are diarrhoea, vomiting, fever, abdominal cramps, and lethargy. A viral cause is more likely if there is a short period between ingestion of the pathogen and the development of symptoms. A bacterial pathogen should be suspected in a child with abdominal pain whose stools contain blood or mucus (colitis). Fever is more common in bacterial infection. A history of recent antibiotic administration in a febrile, systemically unwell child raises the possibility of *Clostridium difficile* infection. Foreign travel or contact with people who have been abroad widens the range of potential aetiological agents. Clinicians should also be aware of recent outbreaks of particular pathogens. The immunocompromised or malnourished child is at risk of infection with more unusual organisms, and infections are likely to be more severe with systemic sequelae.

Differential diagnosis

The differential diagnosis is wide. The symptoms of acute gastroenteritis—diarrhoea and vomiting—can be due to enteric infection or a symptom of infection elsewhere (e.g. urinary tract infection). It may also be the symptomatology of non-infective pathology in the gut (e.g. food intolerance) or another body system (e.g. diabetes mellitus, inborn error of metabolism).

> **Key differentials to consider**
> - Other infections—otitis media, tonsillitis, pneumonia, septicaemia, urinary tract infection, meningitis.
> - Surgical causes such as pyloric stenosis, intestinal obstruction (including malrotation), intussusception, appendicitis.
> - GOR.
> - Food intolerance.
> - Haemolytic uraemic syndrome.
> - Drugs—antibiotics, laxatives.

Specific pathogens

Giardia lambia
- A protozoal parasite which is infective in the cyst form.
- It also exists in the trophozoite form.
- It is found in contaminated food and water.
- Clinical manifestations vary; can be asymptomatic, acute diarrhoeal disease, chronic diarrhoea. Partial villous atrophy is occasionally seen.
- Diagnosis is by stool examination for cysts or examination of the duodenal aspirate at small-bowel biopsy.
- Treatment is with metronidazole and is often given blind in suspicious cases.

Clostridium difficile
- A Gram-positive anaerobe.
- Risk factor is disruption of the normal intestinal flora by antibiotics.
- Clinical features vary from asymptomatic carriage to life-threatening pseudomembranous colitis.
- Pathogenesis is through toxin production.
- Treatment is with vancomycin (oral) or metronidazole (iv or oral). Probiotics may have a role. *Saccharomyces boulardii* and *Lactobacillus* spp. have been used.
- Relapse rate is 15–20%.

Assessment

This is to establish the diagnosis and the degree of dehydration (Table 28.2). A careful history needs to be taken. The risk of dehydration increases portionally to the number of episodes of loose stool and vomiting, and in inverse proportionally to age, thus the frequency and duration of symptoms need to be established. A child who is extremely thirsty is likely to be dehydrated. The best measure of dehydration is documented weight change before and during illness, although this is rarely available.

The examination should help to exclude the differentials listed on p. 232 and also to exclude symptoms from systemic illness secondary to other infection such as meningitis, pneumonia, etc. The clinical assessment of degree of dehydration is difficult. There is a continuum from a child who is not dehydrated to a child in shock. Shock is apparent in a child with prolonged capillary refill (>2 seconds centrally) and tachycardia. Signs of decompensated shock include altered level of consciousness and hypotension. Shock requires urgent treatment with IV or intraosseous fluid administration according to resuscitation guidelines. Dehydration can be determined on the basis of multiple clinical parameters. The presence of a prolonged capillary refill, an abnormal skin turgor, absent tears, and abnormal respiratory pattern (deep, rapid breathing without other signs of respiratory distress suggests an acidosis) are the most reliable signs. An active, playful child with moist mucous membranes and non-sunken eyes is unlikely to be dehydrated. A normal capillary refill time (<2 seconds) makes severe dehydration very unlikely.

Risk factors for dehydration

- Age <12 months (increased surface area to volume ratio, osmotic load of an exclusive milk diet, tendency to more severe vomiting).
- Frequent stools (>5 day).
- Vomiting (>twice a day).
- Bottle rather than breastfeeding.
- Previous poor nutrition.

Hypernatraemic dehydration

- Previously common, but with more modern refined infant formulae it is fortunately now rare.
- Should be suspected in a child with a history and symptoms compatible with a considerable degree of dehydration but who has minimal clinical signs other than a doughy texture to their skin and irritability.
- Jittery movements.
- Increased muscle tone.
- Hyperreflexia.
- Convulsions.
- Drowsiness or coma.

Table 28.2 Assessment of dehydration

Dehydration %	Severity	Clinical features
3		Undetectable
3–5	Mild	Slightly dry mucous membranes
5	Moderate	Decreased skin turgor, slightly sunken eyes, depressed fontanelle, circulation preserved
10	Severe	All of above more marked, drowsiness, rapid weak pulse, cool extremities, capillary refill time >2 seconds
12–14		Moribund

Management

The vast majority of children with gastroenteritis can be managed at home.

Indications to consider hospital admission

- Age <6 months.
- Diagnosis is unclear/complications have arisen.
- Home management fails/unable to tolerate oral fluids/vomiting.
- Significant other medical condition, e.g. diabetes, immunocompromised, cyanotic congenital heart disease (risk of thrombosis with dehydration).
- Poor social circumstances.
- Difficulty to assess.
- Inability to re-assess.

Investigations

- Serum electrolytes are not helpful in establishing the degree of dehydration, but they should be performed before and during IV rehydration to ensure correct fluid administration. They are also useful to confirm a clinical suspicion of hypernatraemic dehydration.
- Stool samples are not routinely necessary, but they should be obtained where there is a history of prolonged or bloody diarrhoea or a history of recent foreign travel, and in apparent outbreaks of gastroenteritis. Stool should be cultured for bacteria and samples tested for viruses, particularly rotavirus. Basic microscopy should detect ova cysts and parasites in stool. Stool should be sent for *Clostridium difficile* toxin if infection is suspected.

Rehydration

- Enteral rehydration using oral rehydration therapy (ORT) is the recommended treatment for children with mild to moderate dehydration. This can be given by the nasogastric route if oral fluids are not tolerated. IV fluids should be reserved for children who are unable to tolerate fluids by either the oral or nasogastric route.
- Children with shock should have their fluid volume restored with appropriate boluses of normal saline. Once adequate circulation is established, further rehydration should be commenced by the enteral route.
- Water alone is not suitable for rehydration following diarrhoea and vomiting as these losses will be rich in electrolytes which also need to be replaced.
- Oral rehydration solutions (ORS) contain various quantities of electrolytes, glucose, and base. In developed countries where non-cholera-type gastroenteritis is the norm, solutions containing sodium concentrations of ~60mmol/L and carbohydrate (non-cereal) concentrations of ~90mmol/L are recommended. These solutions are slightly hypotonic to the serum osmolality of ~290mmol/L. This enables the rapid absorption of fluid. Isotonic sports drinks are not ideal for correcting dehydration secondary to gastroenteritis because the concentration of electrolytes is less than required and their major component is carbohydrate.
- In developing countries, where cholera is a major killer, the lower-osmolality ORS recommended above increase the risk of

hyponatraemia. Thus enteral rehydration is performed using ORS containing a sodium concentration of 90mmol/L. There is also evidence that using a cereal-based carbohydrate decreases the duration of diarrhoea in this population.

- Enteral rehydration is labour intensive but can be given by parents orally or by nursing staff via NGT. Oral fluid can be given by bottle or syringe, or from lollies made of frozen ORS. Most ORS needs to be consumed within 1 hour of being made, unless it is stored immediately in a fridge where it can be kept for 24 hours.
- Rapid enteral rehydration is preferred. The fluid deficit should be calculated and replaced over 4–6 hours. NICE recommend giving 50mL/kg over this time period in children with signs of clinical dehydration. Maintenance fluid requirements should be given during this time and continuing excessive losses also replaced. If there is suspicion of hypernatraemia, the fluid deficit should be corrected more slowly, over at least 12 hours, with repeated electrolyte monitoring.
- If there are continuing stool losses or vomiting these should be replaced with ORS 5mL/kg per stool or vomit, particularly if losses are large.

Feeding and gastroenteritis

Breastfed infants should continue breastfeeding even during rehydration with ORS. Formula-fed infants should restart undiluted formula after rehydration. In the older child, an age-appropriate diet should also be restarted early after rehydration. Avoid giving fruit juices and carbonated drinks until diarrhoea has stopped. These measures reduce risk of further dehydration and lead to smaller stool volumes and faster recovery.

There is no role for prolonged starvation except in some children with secondary lactose intolerance in which case feeds can be regraded one-quarter to one-half to full strength 12–24-hourly

Other treatments

- Antibiotics are of no proven benefit in cases of uncomplicated gastroenteritis, and may cause harm.
- In the case of E. coli 0157, antibiotics may precipitate haemolytic uraemic syndrome.
- Antibiotics in uncomplicated salmonella gastroenteritis may prolong salmonella excretion as well as promote resistance.
- Antibiotics are of benefit in bacterial gastroenteritis complicated by septicaemia or systemic infections. This should be done in consultation with the local microbiology/public health department.
- Antibiotics should be considered in both immunocompromised and malnourished patients. They may be used in cases of prolonged infection, e.g. giardiasis and amoebiasis.
- There is no role for antiemetics.
- There is no role for drugs to alter intestinal motility such as loperamide and opiate derivatives which have the potential to mask fluid losses by delaying gut transit.
- The role of probiotics in gastroenteritis, and the particular type of these, are yet to be established. Some evidence suggests that Lactobacillus may be of benefit in reducing duration of symptoms.

Prevention

- Most gastroenteritis is spread by faeco-oral transmission and some results from uncooked or contaminated foods. Proper sanitation and attention to food preparation and storage as well as rigorous hand hygiene can prevent infection or control the spread of disease.
- All cases of confirmed bacterial gastroenteritis should be notified to the local public health department.
- Within hospital, during an episode of gastroenteritis children should be isolated from the general ward and especially from immunocompromised patients.

Complications

- Dehydration, metabolic acidosis, and electrolyte disturbance (especially hypokalaemia, hyponatraemia, and hypernatraemia).
- Carbohydrate intolerance is relatively common after acute gastroenteritis (particularly rotavirus infection), manifested by explosive stools. This can cause significant and rapid dehydration as an osmotic effect. Most is self-limiting and, particularly if secondary to rotavirus infection, may respond to a slow regrade back on to a normal feed (see 'Feeding and gastroenteritis', p. 237). Monosaccharide intolerance (glucose malabsorption) is occasionally seen and requires a period on IV fluids. Persistent loose, frequent stool which often leads to damage to the perianal skin is usually transient. If symptoms persist, a 4–6-week trial of a lactose-free diet is advised. Topical barrier creams prevent perianal ulceration.
- Post-enteritis syndrome with enteropathy may respond to cow's milk/soya protein exclusion.
- Complications can arise from inappropriate prescription of IV fluids to correct rehydration.
- Rapid correction of hypernatraemia can lead to cerebral oedema; serum sodium should be measured regularly and a gradual reduction aimed for.
- Haemolytic uraemic syndrome occurs in 6–9% of *E. coli* 0157 infections. It is characterized by sudden onset of pallor, lethargy, and oliguria after gastroenteritis. Examination findings are of a dehydrated child, with pallor and petechiae. Anaemia and thrombocytopenia are present on the full blood count. Blood film will show fragmented red cells, burr, and helmet cells. Urinalysis often reveals mild microscopic haematuria and proteinuria.

Chronic diarrhoea

If diarrhoea persists for >2 weeks it is said to be chronic. This can reflect:
- Continued infection with the first pathogen.
- Infection with a second pathogen.
- Post-enteritis syndrome.
- Unmasking of a non-infective cause of chronic diarrhoea such as inflammatory bowel disease, food intolerance, coeliac disease, immunodeficiency, constipation with overflow, or pancreatic insufficiency.

References and resources

Guarino A, Ashkenazi S, Gendrel D, et al. European Society for Pediatric Gastroenterology, Hepatology, and Nutrition/European Society for Pediatric Infectious Diseases evidence-based guidelines for the management of acute gastroenteritis in children in Europe. Update 2014. J Pediatr Gastroenterol Nutr 2014;59:132–52. https://journals.lww.com/jpgn/fulltext/2014/07000/European_Society_for_Pediatric_Gastroenterology,.26.aspx

Murphy MS. Guidelines for managing acute gastroenteritis based on a systematic review of published research. Arch Dis Child 1998;79:279–84.

National Institute for Health and Care Excellence (NICE). Diarrhoea and vomiting caused by gastroenteritis in under 5s: diagnosis and management. Clinical Guideline CG84. London: NICE; 2009. https://www.nice.org.uk/guidance/cg84

Gastro-oesophageal reflux

Introduction 242
Reflux oesophagitis 243
Symptoms and signs of GOR 243
Approach to the management of GOR 244
Investigations 246
Management 250
Specific treatment 252
Eosinophilic oesophagitis 256
Feeding problems in cerebral palsy 257
References and resources 258

Introduction

- *Gastro-oesophageal reflux (GOR)* is the involuntary passage of the gastric contents into the oesophagus. It is a normal physiological phenomenon, particularly common in infancy. Most episodes in healthy individuals last <3 minutes, occur in the postprandial period, and cause few or no symptoms. Major factors include the high fluid volume per kilogram ingested at that age compared with older children/adults, posture, and the functional immaturity of the lower oesophageal sphincter. The natural history of GOR is generally of improvement with age, with <5% of children with vomiting or regurgitation in infancy continuing to have symptoms after the age of 14 months. This is due to a combination of growth in length of the oesophagus, a more upright posture, increased tone of the lower oesophageal sphincter, and a more solid diet.

- *Gastro-oesophageal reflux disease (GORD)* is defined as 'gastro-oesophageal reflux associated with troublesome symptoms or complications' although the authors caution that this definition is complicated by unreliable reporting of symptoms in children under 8 years of age. Gastrointestinal sequelae include oesophagitis, haematemesis, oesophageal stricture formation, and Barrett's oesophagitis. Extra-intestinal sequelae can include acute life-threatening events and apnoea, chronic otitis media, sinusitis, secondary anaemia, and chronic respiratory disease (chronic wheezing/coughing or aspiration), as well as faltering growth.

- *Regurgitation* refers to the effortless return of gastric contents into the pharynx and mouth and is distinct from vomiting which is the forceful return of gastric contents into the pharynx and mouth.

- *Adolescent rumination syndrome* is effortless regurgitation seen in older children and adolescents. The condition is benign providing complications such as weight loss do not occur. It is characterized by the presence of the following symptoms for at least 6 weeks (may not be consecutive) in the last 12 months:
  - Begins within 30 minutes of meal ingestion.
  - Is associated with either re-swallowing or expulsion of food.
  - Stops within 90 minutes of onset or when regurgitant becomes acidic.
  - Is not associated with mechanical obstruction.
  - Does not respond to standard treatment for GORD.
  - Is not associated with nocturnal symptoms.

Reflux oesophagitis

Oesophagitis implies acid- or rarely alkali-induced damage to the lower oesophagus, which can be painful. Crying and irritability may be symptoms of oesophagitis in infants, similar to the adult complaint of heartburn and chest pain. Children with oesophagitis can develop a food aversion as a consequence of experiencing pain when they eat, and food refusal can be the presenting feature. This is likely to be a significant factor in the faltering growth seen in some children with reflux. This can be difficult to diagnose and requires treatment of the oesophagitis before a feeding programme is instituted to deal with the food aversion.

Symptoms and signs of GOR

Typical

- Excessive regurgitation/vomiting.
- Nausea.
- Weight loss/faltering growth.
- Irritability with feeds, arching, colic/food refusal.
- Dysphagia.
- Chest/epigastric discomfort.
- Excessive hiccups.
- Haematemesis/anaemia—iron deficiency.
- Aspiration pneumonia.
- Oesophageal obstruction due to stricture.

Atypical

- Wheeze/intractable asthma.
- Cough/stridor.
- Cyanotic episodes.
- Generalized irritability.
- Sleep disturbance.
- Neurobehavioural symptoms—breath-holding, Sandifer syndrome, seizure-like events, dystonia.
- Worsening of pre-existing respiratory disease.
- Apnoea/apparent life-threatening events/sudden infant death syndrome (SIDS).

The association between GOR and apparent life-threatening events is somewhat controversial and probably only relevant if the infant vomits, chokes, or goes blue during or immediately after feeds.

Approach to the management of GOR

- A full assessment of infants is essential including a careful feeding history. It is important to consider the differential diagnosis (see Box 29.1). Careful attention needs to be paid to symptom severity, impact on growth, and social factors that may be relevant, e.g. parental anxiety and stress.
- Physiological reflux is common in infancy and is a clinical diagnosis. For most parents reassurance that the condition will resolve without treatment is all that is needed. It is important to consider the differential diagnosis.
- Full assessment of infants is essential, including a full feeding history to explore the possibility of overfeeding or difficulty with feeding. Careful attention needs to be paid to severity of symptoms, faltering growth, and relevant social factors, e.g. parental anxiety and stress.
- Severe cases need further assessments and investigation. These include barium study, pH study, impedance study, milk scan, oesophagoscopy, and oesophageal biopsy (see 'Oesophagoscopy and oesophageal biopsy', p. 248).
- There is a step-up approach to management.
- Difficult cases require assessment by a multidisciplinary team including dietician, speech and language therapist, paediatric gastroenterologist, and paediatric surgeon.

> **Box 29.1 Differential diagnosis of gastro-oesophageal reflux**
>
> - Infection, e.g. urinary tract infection, gastroenteritis, peptic ulcer disease.
> - Intestinal obstruction, e.g. pyloric stenosis, malrotation, intestinal atresia.
> - Food allergy and intolerances, e.g. cow's milk allergy, soy allergy.
> - Coeliac disease.
> - Eosinophilic oesophagitis.
> - Metabolic disorders, e.g. diabetes, inborn errors of metabolism.
> - Intestinal dysmotility.
> - Drug induced vomiting, e.g. cytotoxic agents.
> - Primary respiratory disease, e.g. asthma, CF.

Gastro-oesophageal reflux and respiratory disease

- Obstructive apnoea with hypoxaemia and cyanosis can be the presenting feature in GOR. There is some controversy about the causal relationship in that the obstructive apnoea may be the primary pathology with secondary GOR. The mechanism probably relates to laryngospasm and can also manifest as intermittent stridor. Upper respiratory signs such as spasmodic croup, hoarseness, or vocal cord nodules are seen in older children.
- There is a high incidence of GOR in children with chronic respiratory disease, particularly asthma. This can be primary or secondary in that the respiratory disease may be secondary to reflux or the intrinsic lung disease (asthma, CF, immunodeficiency, tracheo-oesophageal fistula) may, through excessive coughing, result in reflux.

Investigations

Barium radiology

- A barium swallow assesses the patient over only a short period. It will demonstrate reflux although is not particularly sensitive or specific. It can be diagnostic, but in less clear-cut cases may either miss pathological reflux or over diagnose physiological reflux.
- It is, however, an essential investigation in the infant with severe symptoms suggestive of reflux when it will rule out large hiatus hernia, oesophageal stricture or web, atypical pyloric stenosis, gastric web, duodenal web, malrotation, volvulus, or other anatomical cause of recurrent vomiting.
- In older children it will exclude the above-mentioned causes. It will also diagnose hiatus hernia, which functions as a reservoir for acid and increases the likelihood of reflux oesophagitis and so is relevant prognostically.

Oesophageal pH monitoring

- Acid reflux into the oesophagus occurs in all infants as a physiological phenomenon and is only significant when it occurs in excess. The pH probe is designed to measure acidity (i.e. acid reflux) in the lower oesophagus. pH monitoring measures the frequency and duration of acid reflux into the oesophagus.
- The pH probe is a microelectrode passed through the nose and down the back of the throat to sit 5cm above the lower oesophageal sphincter. A set period, usually 24 hours, is recorded A reflux episode is defined as the drop in oesophageal pH to <4.
- There are various scoring systems to quantify the degree of reflux against normal values. The normal values for all scoring systems are based on total reflux time, number of reflux periods, number of long reflux periods (> 5 minutes), and for the duration of the longest reflux period. The commonly used scores in children are
  - DeMeester score is a global measure of oesophageal acid exposure.
  - Boix-Ochoa score—best suited for children <7 years of age.
  - Vandenplas score—ideal for infants and the score takes into account the age of the patient.

Combined multiple intraluminal impedance (MII) and pH monitoring

- This uses a probe to measure oesophageal and impedance and pH to identify acid and non-acid reflux.
- Its advantages are the ability to quantify reflux over a period of time (usually 24 hours) and establish temporal relationships between reflux episodes (acid or alkali) and symptoms. It is particularly useful in children with respiratory or neurobehavioural symptoms.
- Oesophageal tracings are analysed for the typical changes caused by liquid, solid, air, or mixed bolus and can differentiate between antegrade and retrograde flow.

- The result is also affected by the clinical condition of the child on the day of the study which must, as far as possible, correlate with the normal state in terms of food intake and activity in particular.

Specific indications for pH study/combined pH/impedance
- Diagnostic uncertainty.
- Poor response to medical treatment.
- If surgery is being considered.
- Children in whom doing the test will lead to a change in management.
- Symptoms suggesting occult reflux.
- Unexplained or difficult to control respiratory disease.

There are several limitations to pH/MII studies, as follows:
- They are unable to detect anatomical abnormalities (e.g. stricture, hiatus hernia, or malrotation) or aspiration.
- The changes in environment, diet, and behaviour as a result of investigation and admission to hospital may impact the result.
- Reproducibility is poor.
- There is potential for technical difficulties.
- Provide no objective measures of inflammation, and thus are less useful than endoscopy and biopsies for the diagnosis and grading of oesophagitis.
- The severity of pathologic reflux does not correlate consistently with symptom severity or demonstrable complications.

Oesophageal manometry

- Oesophageal manometry measures intraluminal pressures and coordination of pressure activity of the muscles of the oesophagus, and is used to diagnose motility disorders of the oesophagus.
- Oesophageal manometry is indicated for the evaluation of dysphagia and primary oesophageal motility disorders (achalasia and diffuse oesophageal spasm) which can mimic GORD.
- It provides data on site, length, and resting pressure in the lower oesophageal sphincter. Data should also be collected on swallow-induced sphincter relaxation.
- Propagation pressure waves through the oesophagus are also recorded providing information on motility.

Gastro-oesophageal scintigraphy

- This uses continuous evaluation for up to an hour after a radio-labelled meal. Food or milk labelled with technetium-99m is given to the infant and stomach and oesophagus are scanned.
- Its main role is in assessment of gastric emptying times to identify the group of children with foregut dysmotility and delayed gastric emptying. It also has a limited role in diagnosis of pulmonary aspiration in patients with chronic and refractory respiratory symptoms.
- Delayed gastric emptying is especially common in children with cerebral palsy in whom vomiting may reflect an overall gut dysmotility rather than GORD.

Oesophagoscopy and oesophageal biopsy

- In children with suspected oesophagitis, upper gastrointestinal endoscopy is a useful investigation and it should be considered in all children with severe symptomatic reflux.
- Biopsies need to be taken, as a significant histological abnormality may not be obvious endoscopically.
- An eosinophilic infiltrate is characteristic of reflux oesophagitis.
- An excess of eosinophils suggests cow's milk allergic oesophagitis/ eosinophilic oesophagitis.
- The distinction between reflux oesophagitis and eosinophilic oesophagitis is somewhat controversial.

Management

- Most patients with GOR are managed in primary care by the health visitor and general practitioner.
- Simple measures are commonly used including:
  - Explanation and reassurance about the natural history, parent education.
  - Review of feeding and feeding practice, e.g. check infant is not being overfed, trial of smaller more frequent feeds, too small or too large a teat (both of which may cause air swallowing).
  - Review of feeding posture.
  - Use of feed thickeners.
  - Use of anti-regurgitation milks.

Posture

Infants have significantly less reflux when placed in the prone position than in the supine position. However, prone positioning is associated with a higher rate of SIDS. In infants from birth to 12 months of age with reflux, the risk of SIDS generally outweighs the potential benefits of prone sleeping. In children >1 year it is likely that there is a benefit to right-side positioning during sleep and elevation of the head of the bed.

Milk exclusion

Children who have persistent symptomatic reflux, and evidence of atopy (positive family history, positive skin prick test) may warrant a trial of milk exclusion. The substitute milk should be with a protein hydrolysate (peptide or amino acid-based, antigen-free) feed. Examples include Nutramigen® (Mead Johnson) and Neocate® (Nutricia). A 2-week trial is worthwhile. Solids need to be milk free. In some infants persistence to 6 weeks before making a decision about efficacy is sometimes necessary.

Soya formulae should not be used. There is significant cross reactivity between cow's milk and soya protein and because of the presence of phytoestrogens in soya milks they are not recommended in infants <6 months.

Specific treatment

The major pharmacological agents currently used for treating GORD in children are gastric acid-buffering agents, mucosal surface barriers, and gastric antisecretory agents. Acid-suppressant agents are the mainstay of treatment for all but the patient with occasional symptoms. The potential adverse effects of acid suppression, including increased risk of community-acquired pneumonias and gastrointestinal infections, need to be balanced against the benefits of therapy.

Compound alginates (e.g. Gaviscon® Infant)

Effective symptomatic treatment for GOR. Gaviscon® Infant works by reacting with gastric acid to form a viscous gel. In infants Gaviscon® Infant can be added to feed or for breastfed infants dissolved in cooled boiled water and given by spoon after a feed. Chronic use of alginates is not recommended for GORD because some have absorbable components that may have adverse effects with long-term use.

Acid suppression agents

Histamine H_2 receptor blockers

Widely used in the management of reflux. They are safe, well tolerated, and efficacious in children. Ranitidine is the most commonly used H_2 receptor blocker and has a low incidence of side effects (common side effects include fatigue, dizziness, or diarrhoea).

Proton pump inhibitors (PPIs)

PPIs such as omeprazole and lansoprazole are a group of drugs that irreversibly inactivate H^+/K^+ ATPase: the parietal cell membrane transporter. This increases the pH of gastric contents and decreases total volume of gastric secretion, thus facilitating emptying. They are metabolized by the cytochrome p450 system, and are relatively safe, with few reported side effects. PPIs are also safe in children with renal impairment, but hepatic metabolism of PPIs may be impaired.

For healing of erosive oesophagitis and relief of symptoms, PPIs are superior to histamine receptor blockers. Omeprazole is the most commonly used PPI and is known to be effective in children with GORD resistant to ranitidine. It is available as dispersible tablets or capsules given once daily. The tablet can be gently mixed or dispersed (not crushed) or the capsule broken for ease of administration in children. Liquid omeprazole can be made to order and is especially useful in children who cannot swallow tablet/capsules and where the drug needs to be administered via an enteral tube. When acid suppression is required, the smallest effective dose should be used. Most patients require only a once-daily PPI; routine use of a twice-daily dose is not indicated.

There are five PPIs approved for use in adults: omeprazole, lansoprazole, pantoprazole, rabeprazole, and esomeprazole (the pure S-isomer of omeprazole). Omeprazole is licensed in children >1 year of age in the UK, and lansoprazole is only recommended by the British National Formulary for Children when treatment with the available formulations of omeprazole is unsuitable

Prokinetic drugs

GOR is primarily a motility disorder, and the use of pharmacological agents that improve oesophageal and gastric motility are conceptually attractive as therapies. Unfortunately, the currently available prokinetic medications have only modest efficacy in relieving GORD symptoms, and the side effect profile of these agents renders them a less useful clinical practice. Examples include metoclopramide, domperidone, and erythromycin.

Domperidone is a dopamine receptor (D_2) blocker that has relatively fewer side effects but case reports of extrapyramidal side effects as well as an effect on the QT interval exist. Domperidone acts to increase lower oesophageal sphincter pressure, improve oesophageal clearance, and promote gastric emptying. It is commonly used in clinical practice either as part of empirical medical therapy of GORD or if delayed gastric emptying has been demonstrated on nuclear scintigraphy. In view of a small increased risk of cardiotoxicity, it is advisable to use domperidone in lower doses and only in cases with overt vomiting secondary to reflux. It is recommended that an ECG should be performed to rule out prolonged QT especially in children at risk (congenital cardiac disease, history, or family history of syncope, cardiac arrest or sudden cardiac death at an early age) before starting treatment.

Other agents

Buffering agents (magnesium hydroxide and aluminium hydroxide) and sucralfate are useful for occasional heart burn. Buffering agents carry significant risk of toxicity and are not recommended for long-term use. Sucralfate binds to inflamed mucosa and forms a protective layer that resists further damage from gastric acid.

Surgery

Surgery is usually fundoplication with consideration of a pyloroplasty if there is delayed gastric emptying. Most fundoplications are now done laparoscopically with good results in terms of reduced postoperative complications, reduced stay in hospital, and long-term outcome.

Indications

- Failure of optimal medical therapy.
- Extra-oesophageal manifestation (asthma, cough, chest pain, recurrent pulmonary aspiration of refluxate).
- Complication of GORD (e.g. Barrett's oesophagus or oesophageal stricture).

Children with underlying disorders predisposing to the most severe GORD such as cerebral palsy are at the highest risk for operative morbidity and postoperative failure. Before surgery it is essential to rule out non-GORD causes of symptoms and ensure that the diagnosis of chronic-relapsing GORD is firmly established. It is important to provide families with appropriate education and a realistic understanding of the potential complications of surgery, which include recurrence of reflux (10%), retching, bloating, dumping, and intestinal obstruction.

Patient groups at high risk of needing surgery

- Children with neurodisability.
- Respiratory disease with intractable reflux (e.g. oesophageal atresia, bronchopulmonary dysplasia).
- Children with complication of oesophagitis such as stricture.
- Tracheo-oesophageal fistula repair.
- Barrett's oesophagus.

Barrett's oesophagus

- This refers to the presence of metaplastic columnar epithelium in the lower oesophagus thought to be a consequence of long-standing GORD.
- There is an increased risk of adenocarcinoma of the oesophagus.
- It is rare in childhood and requires aggressive medical treatment, of the GOR and regular endoscopic surveillance.
- Surgery (fundoplication) is often considered.

Eosinophilic oesophagitis

- Eosinophilic esophagitis is a chronic, immune/antigen-mediated, oesophageal disease characterized clinically by symptoms related to oesophageal dysfunction and histologically by eosinophil-predominant inflammation (see Chapter 49).
- It is more common in older atopic boys and common presenting symptoms are dysphagia and food bolus obstruction.
- There is a symptom overlap with GOR and it should be considered in all PPI-resistant cases. Allergy testing is helpful. The pH study/impedance may be positive.
- Diagnosis is confirmed with upper gastrointestinal endoscopy and characteristic changes include oesophageal rings, thickening of mucosa with linear furrows, and rarely stricture. At least two to four biopsies should be taken from proximal as well as distal oesophagus. The main histological findings are dense eosinophilia (>15/hpf) of the oesophageal mucosa, which tends to be panoesophageal, basal zone hyperplasia, lamina propria fibrosis, and sometimes eosinophilic microabscesses.
- In symptomatic patients where histology is not diagnostic, a trial of PPIs for 8 weeks is recommended. A small group of patients with PPI-responsive oesophageal eosinophilia (PPI-REE) would improve with this treatment.
- Dietary elimination is an effective treatment and can be in the form of a targeted elimination diet or empiric elimination of common allergens (fish, wheat, dairy, soya, nuts, and eggs).
- Other treatments include use of swallowed corticosteroids for a period of 12 weeks or systemic corticosteroids in severe cases where a rapid response is required.
- There is a natural history of relapse, remission, and chronicity.
- Repeat biopsies are occasionally needed.

Feeding problems in cerebral palsy

Children with cerebral palsy commonly suffer from feeding difficulties of which GOR is a component. Assessment of the contribution of GOR requires considerable care. There are many potential causes of feeding difficulties:

- Bulbar weakness with oesophageal incoordination.
- Primary or secondary aspiration.
- Reflux oesophagitis.
- Widespread gut dysmotility.
- Mobility and posture, degree of spasticity.
- Poor nutritional state.
- Constipation.

Children require careful multidisciplinary assessment by a feeding team including dietetics, speech and language therapy, occupational therapy, and the neurodevelopmental paediatrician. An assessment of the swallow is often indicated. If present, GORD should be treated aggressively.

Attention to nutrition is of key importance and many children with feeding difficulties benefit from a feeding gastrostomy. A fundoplication is required if reflux is severe although in some cases improved nutritional status will result in improvement of the reflux.

Gut motility is a key factor in feed tolerance in children with cerebral palsy who may have delayed gastric emptying, which impacts significantly on the ability to feed particularly if nutrition is dependent on nasogastric or gastrostomy feeding. It is important to recognize this as a separate condition from reflux when the dysmotility is upper gastrointestinal only. Abdominal pain, bloating, and constipation are common feature of gut dysmotility. Therapeutic strategies include explanation and reassurance, a prokinetic agent such as domperidone, antireflux therapy, laxatives, and occasionally (if there is a need for distal gut deflation) suppositories. It may be necessary in severe cases to give feeds by continuous infusion. A milk-free diet for a trial period of 2–4 weeks can be helpful. Hydrolysed protein formula feed may be given as a milk substitute.

References and resources

Fox M, Forgacs I. Gastro-oesophageal reflux disease. BMJ 2006;332:88–93.

National Institute for Health and Care Excellence (NICE). Gastro-oesophageal reflux disease in children and young people: diagnosis and management. NICE guideline NG1. London: NICE; 2015. https://www.nice.org.uk/guidance/ng1

Papadopoulou A, Koletzko S, Heuschkel R, et al. ESPGHAN Eosinophilic Esophagitis Working Group and the Gastroenterology Committee. Management guidelines of eosinophilic esophagitis in childhood. J Pediatr Gastroenterol Nutr 2014;58:107–18.

Rudolph CD, Vandenplas Y. Paediatric gastro-oesophageal reflux clinical practice guidelines: joint recommendation of NASPGHAN and ESPGHAN. J Paed Gastro Nutr 2009;49:498–547.

Tighe M, Afzal NA, Bevan A, Hayen A, Munro A, Beattie RM. Pharmacological treatment of children with gastro-oesophageal reflux. Cochrane Database Syst Rev 2014;11:CD008550.

Helicobacter pylori infection and peptic ulceration

Helicobacter pylori 260
Other causes of antral gastritis and peptic (gastric and duodenal) ulceration 262
References and resources 262

Helicobacter pylori

- *Helicobacter pylori* is a Gram-negative organism. It is a very common infection worldwide. Infection is usually acquired in childhood, but prevalence rates are variable, being highest in developing countries. Most individuals infected with *H. pylori* do not experience symptoms or show signs.
- Persistent infection causes an antral gastritis, the most common manifestation in childhood, which may be asymptomatic.
- There is a strong relation between *H. pylori* infection and peptic ulceration in both adults and children.
- *H. pylori* is also a potential carcinogen (increased risk of gastric lymphoma, adenocarcinoma).
- There is no proven association between *H. pylori* infection and recurrent abdominal pain except in the rare cases where gastric or duodenal ulcer disease is present.
- Transmission is faeco-oral and familial clustering is common, with increased prevalence in institutions.

Investigation

- This should be considered in children with symptoms suggestive of peptic ulceration (epigastric pain, bloating, haematemesis, night pain) or proven peptic ulceration. Other causes of peptic ulceration should also be considered.
- The precise investigation (invasive or non-invasive) depends on the clinical picture, local prevalence, and tests available.
- It is not indicated in children with recurrent abdominal pain or other chronic symptoms in the absence of features which suggests peptic ulcer disease.

Investigations available

- Urea breath testing (C-13 breath test, urea labelled with carbon-13): this test has a high accuracy, sensitivity, and specificity when used in children especially >6 years of age, widely used to confirm eradication of *H. pylori* after treatment. Need to stop antibiotics, PPIs, and H_2 antagonists before the test (local protocol). The child should be given an acid drink (apple or orange juice) on an empty stomach because the urease activity of the bacteria decreases rapidly with increasing pH. After ingestion of the tracer, the drink without tracer should be provided to the child to avoid degradation of the tracer by oral flora.
- Stool antigen testing: highly sensitive and specific. Need to stop antibiotics, PPIs, and H_2 antagonists before the test (local protocol). Best used to assess success of eradication therapy; not to be used as basis for decision about endoscopy referral.
- Serology (IgG antibody): tests based on the detection of antibodies (IgG, IgA) against *H. pylori* in serum, whole blood, urine, and saliva are not reliable for use in the clinical setting. *H. pylori* infection induces an early increase of specific IgM and a later and persistent increase of specific IgA and IgG antibodies. The problem with the test is low sensitivity of 20–50% and marked interindividual variability, with a

high false-positive rate; positive serology persists for 6–12 months after infection, negative test does not exclude *H. pylori* infection. Not recommended.

- Rapid urease test (CLO test): CLO test is performed at the time of endoscopy and tissue sample is placed in a medium containing urea. A change in colour of the medium confirms the presence of urease producing *H. pylori* organisms. This test has a sensitivity of 45%, 71.2%, 81.1%, 90.1%, and 91.9% at 5, 15, 30 minutes, and 3 and 24 hours respectively.
- Endoscopy allows the detection of peptic ulcer disease, gastritis, and oesophagitis with direct visualization of the mucosa and biopsy. Lymphoid nodular hyperplasia in the gastric antrum is commonly seen. The density of *H. pylori* within the stomach may be patchy and hence, the sensitivity increases with the number of biopsies taken. Normally, the highest bacterial count is found in the antrum; however, in cases of low gastric acidity, the bacteria may be present only in the body. Therefore two biopsies each should be taken from antrum and body of stomach. The suspicion of an infection is often based on the macroscopic findings of a nodular mucosa in the antrum or bulb and/or gastric or duodenal erosions or ulcerations. Diagnosis is usually made on histology—the presence of organisms and the degree of inflammatory change. Biopsies can be sent for culture (low yield) and PCR. Rapid urease testing can be done (e.g. CLO test) on biopsies at the time of endoscopy. Ideally the child should be off antibiotics for 4 weeks and off PPIs and H_2 antagonists for 2 weeks prior to the procedure.

Treatment

- The major indication for treatment is *H. pylori* infection in the presence of peptic ulceration.
- Treatment of children diagnosed through non-invasive testing is dependent on the clinical situation and factors such as the prevalence of *H. pylori* infection in the local population and family history need to be taken into account when the decision is made. In the absence of peptic ulceration, it is unlikely that eradication therapy will resolve symptoms and this should be explained to families.
- There are various regimens. Drug resistance is common. Treatment is for 1 or 2 weeks; 2-week therapy offers the possibility of higher eradication rates although adverse effects and compliance are a problem. The most commonly used regimens include omeprazole, amoxicillin, and metronidazole or clarithromycin. Local protocols should determine which combinations are first and second line. There is no need to continue with long-term PPI therapy unless there is frank ulceration complicated by perforation or haemorrhage. The reader is referred to the current version of the British National Formulary for Children for up-to-date treatment guidelines.
- Clearance of *H. pylori* infection should be confirmed by either urea breath testing or stool antigen testing.
- Outcome after treatment is variable. Treatment failure usually indicates antibacterial resistance, reinfection within families or institutions, or poor compliance.

Other causes of antral gastritis and peptic (gastric and duodenal) ulceration

- Severe systemic illness—traumatic brain injury (Cushing ulcer), extensive burns (Curling ulcer).
- Non-steroidal anti-inflammatory drugs (NSAIDs).
- Corticosteroids.
- Inflammatory bowel disease.
- Eosinophilic gastritis.
- Autoimmune gastritis (mostly adults).
- Zollinger–Ellison syndrome.
- Coeliac disease.

Risk factors for peptic ulceration

- Genotype.
- Stress.
- Alcohol.
- Corticosteroids.
- Smoking.

Zollinger–Ellison syndrome

This results from a gastrin-producing tumour of the endocrine pancreas, presenting with gastric acid hypersecretion and resulting in fulminant, intractable peptic ulcer disease.

References and resources

Jones NL, Koletzko S, Goodman K, et al. Joint ESPGHAN/NASPGHAN Guidelines for the management of helicobacter pylori infection in children and adolescents (update 2016). J Paed Gastro Nutr 2017;64:991–1003. http://www.naspghan.org/files/Joint_ESPGHAN_NASPGHAN_Guidelines_for_the.33.pdf

Cyclical vomiting syndrome

Introduction 264
Clinical features 264
Diagnostic criteria 264
Triggers 264
Investigation 265
Management 265
Prophylaxis 266
References and resources 266

Introduction

Cyclical vomiting was first described by Samuel Gee in 1882. It refers to intense periods of vomiting with symptom-free intervals. The incidence is unknown. It occurs principally in pre-school or early school-age children and is more common in girls. Epilepsy is a risk factor. Other risk factors include a history of recurrent headache, migraine (50%), travel sickness, and irritable bowel syndrome (50%) in children and their families.

Clinical features

More than 50% of sufferers have a predictable cyclicity with a consistent pattern of attack. Symptom onset is usually during the night or first thing in the morning. Episodes last several hours to days, although rarely >72 hours. Episodes can end abruptly (suddenly better), end after sleep, or progress to severe dehydration.

There are three classical behaviours:
- Subdued but responsive.
- Writhing and moaning.
- 'Conscious coma'.

Nausea is characteristic with pallor, increased salivation, and lethargy. Epigastric discomfort occurs secondary to vomiting. Haematemesis/Mallory–Weiss tear can occur if vomiting is extreme. Autonomical features include hypertension, tachycardia, flushing. Neutrophilia and syndrome of inappropriate antidiuretic hormone secretion (SIADH) can occur. Behaviours include 'spit out' (won't swallow saliva), guzzling fluid followed by vomiting, intense thirst, irritability, inability to communicate (social withdrawal), and panic. Headache (25%), abdominal pain, fever, and loose stools are common.

Diagnostic criteria

- At least five attacks in any interval, or a minimum of three attacks during a 6-month period.
- Episodic attacks of intense nausea and vomiting lasting 1 hour–10 days and occurring at least 1 week apart.
- Stereotypical pattern and symptoms in the individual patient.
- Vomiting during attacks occurs at least four times/hour for at least 1 hour.
- Return to baseline health between episodes.

Triggers

Anxiety is a major factor. Emotional stress, life events (stressful and non-stressful, e.g. birthday), travel sickness, infections, and fatigue can trigger episodes. Often the precise trigger is unknown.

Cyclical vomiting syndrome plus refers to a subgroup of children with cyclical vomiting syndrome who develop early ketosis and have some additional neurodevelopmental problems such as neurodevelopmental delay, seizures, hypotonia, or attention deficit hyperactivity disorder. Can occur with mitochondrial disorders.

Investigation

It is important to take a full history and conduct a careful examination. Clinical examination is usually normal (apart from dehydration). Coexistent neurodevelopmental problems need to be excluded. Further investigation should be dependent on the clinical situation with a low threshold to investigate for other potential causes of vomiting, particularly if the presentation is atypical, with metabolic and neurological investigation if there are any risk factors.

Causes of intermittent vomiting with symptom-free periods include metabolic disorders (e.g. urea cycle disorders), disturbances in gut motility, congenital abnormalities of the gastrointestinal tract (e.g. malrotation, duplication cyst), renal disorders, endocrine problems (e.g. adrenal insufficiency), pancreatitis, diabetes, and CNS lesions. It is also important to consider food intolerance, GOR, peptic ulceration, constipation, and coeliac disease, all of which can present with significant vomiting.

Management

- There are no evidence-based recommendations.
- Chronic sufferers benefit from a named paediatrician and personalized management plan.

There are three phases:
- Prodrome.
- Episode.
- Recovery.

Prodrome
- This is the period between onset of symptoms and vomiting.
- Try ondansetron for nausea.
- Try lorazepam for anxiety.
- Simple analgesia for abdominal pain.

Episode
- This is characterized by intense nausea and vomiting; potential problems include dehydration (including hypovolaemic shock in extreme cases), electrolyte disturbance, haematemesis.
- Treatment needs to be initiated promptly particularly if there is a risk of dehydration.
- IV hydration with saline bolus and then maintenance fluids.
- IV ondansetron.
- Consider IV lorazepam, chlorpromazine.
- Consider other potential causes of vomiting.

Recovery
- Tend to recover rapidly, although can be prolonged.
- Consider prophylaxis and treatment plan for further episodes.

Prophylaxis

- Reduce triggers, e.g. anxiety, stress, food intolerance, prolonged fast.
- Antimigraine prophylactic agents including pizotifen, amitriptyline, and propranolol have been tried.
- The long-term outcome is generally good.

References and resources

Cyclical Vomiting Syndrome Association UK: http://www.cvsa.org.uk

Li BU, Lefevre F, Chelimsky GG, et al. North American Society for Pediatric Gastroenterology, Hepatology, and Nutrition consensus statement on the diagnosis and management of cyclic vomiting syndrome. J Pediatr Gastroenterol Nutr 2008;47:379–93.

Rome III Diagnostic Criteria for Functional Gastrointestinal Disorders. http://romecriteria.org/assets/pdf/19_RomeIII_apA_885-898.pdf

Pyloric stenosis

Pyloric stenosis 268

Pyloric stenosis

Infantile hypertrophic pyloric stenosis is a common cause of vomiting in infancy with an incidence of 2–3 per 1000 live births. Males (in particular first-born) are more commonly affected than females and there is a genetic pre-disposition.

- Aetiology is unknown—idiopathic hypertrophy of the pyloric muscle.
- Onset—peak is 4 weeks, range is a few days to 3 months.
- Presentation—non-bilious, effortless, projectile vomiting, often hungry despite regurgitation. Dehydration and weight loss result.
- The differential diagnosis includes any other cause of vomiting presenting in early infancy. In particular urinary tract infection should be excluded. GOR should be considered. The differential diagnosis of pyloric outlet/duodenal obstruction includes duodenal web, duodenal stenosis, and malrotation.
- Pylorus may be palpable ('olive') and visible gastric peristalsis present.
- Hypochloraemic, hypokalaemic metabolic alkalosis occurs as a consequence of vomiting gastric contents (rich in H^+ and Cl^-), loss of K^+ to preserve electrolyte equilibrium. Paradoxical aciduria (late) results from H^+ loss in the urine in preference to K^+ or Na^+.
- Mild unconjugated hyperbilirubinaemia may be seen and is self-limiting.
- Diagnosis—either clinical palpation of the pyloric mass or ultrasound.
- Ultrasound confirms the diagnosis demonstrating thickening of the pyloric wall. Typical sonographic diagnostic parameters are: muscle thickness >3mm, canal length >15mm. Upper gastrointestinal contrast is rarely required, unless malrotation or duodenal stenosis are suspected.
- Initial management is nasogastric decompression (size 8Fr in a term infant).
- IV fluid resuscitation is required to correct the metabolic disturbance before surgery/anaesthesia is planned.
- Initial IV fluids are 150mL/kg/day of 0.45% NaCl + 5% glucose + 10mmol KCl (per 500mL). Dehydration should be corrected if severe with a fluid bolus. Once acid–base status is corrected, continuing fluid replacement is at 100mL/kg/day.
- Definitive treatment is by Ramstedt's pyloromyotomy—never an emergency. Surgical approach is supra-umbilical incision or laparoscopic.
- Complications—incomplete myotomy, mucosal perforation (both ~1%).
- Most infants recover rapidly, and are usually discharged the following day. Continued vomiting in the first 24 hours is common and usually resolves.

Gastrointestinal endoscopy

Endoscopy *270*
Environment and equipment *271*
Indications *272*
Contraindications *274*
Bowel preparation for colonoscopy *274*
Safety/complications *275*
References and resources *276*

Endoscopy

Paediatric gastrointestinal endoscopic practice is dominated by diagnostics for non-malignant chronic intestinal disorders, to visualize mucosal lesions, and obtain biopsies.

Oesophagogastroduodenoscopy (OGD), ileocolonoscopy, and flexible sigmoidoscopy are the most common procedures.

Endoscopy also provides a minimally invasive access for therapy and imaging.

Environment and equipment

Most paediatric endoscopy is performed under general anaesthetic. The specialist endoscopy team includes nursing, recovery, and anaesthetic staff, with access to back-up support from surgical and critical care services and access to specialist paediatric pathology for biopsy interpretation.

There should be a range of age and size-appropriate flexible video endoscopes and accessories available, with image capture/storage facilities. Decontamination, reprocessing, and storage are strictly regulated to reduce the risk of infection and support safe practice.

Procedures are under general anaesthetic or deep sedation, and practice varies between units, with consideration of both safety and comfort during and after the procedure.

Indications

Diagnostic (biopsies almost always obtained)
- Chronic intestinal symptoms and/or faltering growth without clear cause.
- Anaemia with iron (and/or vitamin B_{12}) deficiency without clear cause.
- Gastrointestinal haemorrhage (see Chapter 34).
- Gastro-oesophageal reflux disease (see Chapter 29).
- Positive coeliac serology (see Chapter 38).
- Suspected inflammatory bowel disease (see Chapter 45).
- Suspected malabsorption or protein-losing enteropathy (see Chapters 20 and 37).

Surveillance/reassessment
- Inflammatory bowel disease (see Chapter 45).
- Polyposis (see Chapter 35).
- Chronic liver disease with portal hypertension (see Chapter 70).
- Eosinophilic oesophagitis (see Chapter 49).
- Barrett's oesophagus (see Chapter 29).
- Intestinal transplantation (see Chapter 16).

Therapy
- Haemostasis:
  - Injection sclerotherapy—using fibrin glue, epinephrine/saline.
  - Hemospray®—topically applied powder that solidifies on contact with moisture.
  - Clips—tamponade a bleeding lesion.
  - Diathermy probe.
  - Argon plasma coagulation.
  - Banding: application of a constricting plastic band to control or prevent bleeding.
- Polypectomy.
- Placement of feeding tubes: nasojejunal, gastro-jejunal via gastrostomy.
- PEG insertion.
- Dilatation of strictures: oesophageal (tracheo-oesophageal fistula, caustic, achalasia), Crohn's disease, anastomotic.

Imaging
- Endoscopic retrograde cholangiopancreatography.
- Endoscopic ultrasound.
- Wireless capsule endoscopy.

Foreign bodies and food bolus impaction

Ingested button batteries cause caustic burns and magnets cause compression necrosis. These require emergency removal (within 2 hours) to lessen the risk of life-threatening complications. Perforation and/or massive haemorrhage can occur after removal, even several weeks later. Symptoms from foreign body or food impaction are usually present, with pain, cough, vomiting, and/or drooling. Most foreign bodies will impact the upper oesophagus, with sternal notch pain, and are usually managed by ear, nose, and throat surgeons. Sternal area pain suggests lower impaction, either mid oesophagus or at the gastro-oesophageal junction. Radiographs will show free air in the mediastinum and/or peritoneum, and will image most foreign bodies—metal, bone, etc. Thin metal, fish bone, plastic, and wood are radiolucent. Contrast studies are best avoided, because of the risk of aspiration and affecting endoscopic views. Endoscopy is not usually required if the object is in the stomach and <2.5cm in diameter, although if >6cm long, impaction in the duodenum is more likely. Most will pass in 6–10 days. If they do not, retrieval will be required. Once perforation is excluded, endoscopy should be performed within 24–48 hours to avoid complications of mucosal injury or perforation. In the presence of perforation, surgical review is required.

Contraindications

Known or suspected intestinal perforation or toxic megacolon; recent bowel resection (within 7 days).

Colonoscopy in known acute severe colitis is very high risk—sigmoidoscopy is preferred, without bowel preparation (see Chapter 48).

Most children with uncomplicated GOR, functional abdominal pain, and irritable bowel syndrome with constipation do not require endoscopy (see Chapters 29, 42 and 43).

Bowel preparation for colonoscopy

Units vary in their practice. Most regimens use a very low-residue diet for 2 days prior to the test, with clear liquids for the 12–24 hours pre procedure. Risk: fluid/electrolyte imbalance (beware: renal disease, short gut syndrome, or cardiac disease). Children aged <2 years may not require a full preparation—clear fluids/oral rehydration solution may suffice. There are many different protocols—Table 33.1 shows the one currently used at Birmingham Children's Hospital, UK.

Table 33.1 Low-volume regimen (doses to be given the day before the procedure)

Age	Sodium picosulfate	Senna syrup (7.5mg/5mL)
12 years +	1st dose 10mg	60mL
	2nd dose 10mg	
8–12 years	1st dose 5mg	50mL
	2nd dose 5mg	
5–8 years	1st dose 2.5mg	40mL
	2nd dose 2.5mg	
2–5 years	1st dose 2.5mg	30mL
	2nd dose 2.5mg	

Safety/complications

Post-procedural pain is mild and short-lived: sore throat after laryngeal mask or endotracheal tube; abdominal cramps from air (or CO_2) used for insufflation.

Infection risk

Very low; antibiotic prophylaxis is not routinely required for diagnostic procedures, consider in immunosuppressed patients. Therapy increases risk (e.g. gastrostomy insertion): review local policy.

  Serious bleeding, requiring additional therapy and/or transfusion: very rare with diagnostic procedures. Bleeding diathesis increases risk. Seek advice for managing anticoagulation (e.g. warfarin, heparin) and antiplatelet therapies (e.g. aspirin, dipyridamole). Give platelet transfusion if platelets <50,000; give fresh frozen plasma (FFP) if PT >15 seconds.

Duodenal haematoma

1:2500–5000, probably higher in chronic liver disease. May present 1–2 days post procedure with bilious vomiting.

Perforation

Very rare in OGD (<1:10,000); rare in colonoscopy (1:1000–2000). The risk is higher in children <2 years old and in severe inflammatory bowel disease. Biopsies probably do not increase risk. Therapy increases risk (e.g. 1:200 with polypectomy). Fluoroscopic guidance and using a balloon device lessen the risk of complications after dilatation.

References and resources

Belsha D, Bremner R, Thomson M. Indications for gastrointestinal endoscopy in childhood. Arch Dis Child 2016;101:1153–60.

Thomson M, Tringali A, Dumonceau JM, et al. Paediatric Gastrointestinal Endoscopy: European Society for Paediatric Gastroenterology Hepatology and Nutrition and European Society of Gastrointestinal Endoscopy guidelines. J Pediatr Gastroenterol Nutr 2017;64:133–53.

The UK Joint Advisory Group for Endoscopy: http://www.the-jag.org.uk

Tringali A, Thomson M, Dumonceau JM, et al. Pediatric gastrointestinal endoscopy: European Society of Gastrointestinal Endoscopy (ESGE) and European Society for Paediatric Gastroenterology Hepatology and Nutrition (ESPGHAN) Guideline Executive summary. Endoscopy 2017;49:83–91.

Gastrointestinal bleeding

Introduction *278*
Definitions *279*
Initial assessment *280*
Examination *282*
Investigation *284*
Differential diagnosis *288*
Treatment *290*
References and resources *290*

Introduction

Overt gastrointestinal (GI) bleeding may occur as part of an acute illness or as a feature of chronic disease. Covert or obscure GI bleeding may be uncovered in the investigation of anaemia.

Bleeding is alarming for parents. Assessment requires a balance between urgency when necessary and reassurance when the probable cause is less serious.

The priorities in assessment are to determine the severity of bleeding, the degree of systemic upset, the site, and the cause. This allows decision-making regarding the necessity and timing of further investigation and treatment.

- In children, bright red rectal bleeding may originate from the upper or lower GI tract.
- The commonest cause of rectal bleeding in childhood is from anal fissures secondary to constipation.

Definitions

- Upper GI bleeding:
  - Haematemesis—vomiting frank blood or black material ('coffee grounds', 'soil particles'). This needs to be distinguished from haemoptysis
- Rectal bleeding:
  - Melaena—offensive black, tarry stools.
  - Haematochezia—bright red or dark red blood per rectum.
- Obscure GI bleeding is bleeding is from a presumed GI source when initial investigations, such as OGD and colonoscopy, are normal but faecal immunochemical test positivity suggests GI blood loss (FIT test has largely replaced the faecal occult blood test as it is more sensitive) or bleeding from the GI tract is presumed from the clinical assessment.

Table 34.1 Differences between haemoptysis and haematemesis

	Haemoptysis	Haematemesis
Colour	Bright red and frothy	Dark red or brown
pH	Alkaline	Acid
Consistency	Mixed with sputum	Mixed with food
Symptoms	Gurgling, coughing	Nausea, retching

Can measure the amylase in saliva (high) to clarify if saliva is mixed with blood.

Initial assessment

Resuscitation if actively bleeding

- Assess airway.
- Assess breathing.
- Assess circulation—if signs of compromise/shock:
  - Prompt IV access with large-bore cannula.
  - Group and save/cross-match blood. Inform surgeons in case urgent surgical intervention required.
  - Consider early use of 15mg/kg tranexamic acid if profound GI haemorrhage.
- Fluid resuscitate with 10mL/kg warmed 0.9% sodium chloride, consider resuscitating with blood products if available.
- Re-assess—if still shocked, further 10 mL/kg warmed 0.9% sodium chloride.
- Re-assess—if still shocked, give 5mL/kg boluses of warmed packed red cells or FFP. Aim for 1:1 ratio of red cells:FFP.
- Re-assess—if still shocked after 20mL/kg of blood products, give 10–15mL/kg platelets and 0.1mL/kg of 10% calcium chloride.

Relevant history

- Colour of blood loss.
- Amount of blood lost.
- Is it definitely blood?
- Exclude bleeding from non-GI source: haemorrhagic tonsillitis, epistaxis, dental work, haemoptysis; if breastfed, blood loss from a cracked nipple.
- Consider a bleeding disorder, thrombocytopenia.
- Ask about the presence of other GI symptoms including diarrhoea, epigastric pain, abdominal pain or cramps, constipation, vomiting, previous diagnosis of irritable bowel syndrome, weight loss, steatorrhoea.
- Consider non-GI symptoms including syncope, shortness of breath, dizziness, lethargy, palpitations, fever, rash.
- Include history appropriate to age, e.g. breast- or bottle-feeding, was infant given vitamin K?
- Ask about recent foreign travel or infectious contacts.
- Ask about history of trauma.
- Consider possibility of toxic/caustic ingestion.
- Ask about current medications, e.g. NSAIDs, warfarin, potentially hepatotoxic drugs.
- Consider pertinent past medical history including presence of liver disease, GI disorders, bleeding disorders.
- Review the family history, e.g. inflammatory bowel disease, polyposis syndromes, bleeding disorder.

Physical examination should aid in the assessment of the clinical stability of the child and may give clues as to the aetiology of the bleeding.

- It is important to look for signs of acute anaemia: pallor, tachycardia, gallop rhythm, hyper/hypotension, and chronic anaemia: pallor, poor growth, lethargy.
- Assess whether the child is hypovolaemic or has signs of cardiovascular decompensation.
- Look for signs of chronic liver disease or coagulopathy.
- In contrast to adult practice, currently there are no well-validated scoring systems to predict the need for endoscopic intervention in children. Consider use of the Sheffield scoring system to aid the decision regarding timing of diagnostic endoscopy and need for endoscopic intervention.
- The Sheffield scoring system is based on clinical history, physical examination, evidence of circulatory compromise, and anaemia requiring transfusion.

Substances that can give the stool a dark 'bloody' appearance
- Antibiotics.
- Iron.
- Liquorice.
- Chocolate.
- Blueberries.

Examination

Skin
- Pallor.
- Jaundice.
- Bruises.
- Rashes.

Ear, nose, and throat (ENT)
- Tonsillitis.
- Signs of bleeding.

Cardiovascular
- Tachycardia.
- Hypotension/postural.
- Prolonged capillary refill time.

Abdomen
- Tenderness.
- Hepatosplenomegaly.

Perianal
- Fissure.
- Excoriation or soreness/bad nappy rash.
- External haemorrhoids.
- Fistulae or previous abscess: consider Crohn's disease.

Investigation

History and physical examination should guide the appropriate investigations (Tables 34.2 and 34.3). In an acute bleeding scenario, blood results should be interpreted with caution as hypovolaemia leads to haemoconcentration and haemoglobin values can be artificially high. If a child loses half their circulating volume, the haemoglobin concentration of the remaining volume takes time to dilute down to give a true reflection of blood loss. A full blood count should be repeated after fluid resuscitation. A 'group and save' (cross-match if significant blood loss), urea and electrolytes, and liver function including coagulation screen should also be performed. Renal function is helpful to assess degree of dehydration. Urea may be elevated secondary to absorption of blood (high protein load) from the gut.

Imaging

- It can be difficult to differentiate between haematemesis and haemoptysis; in these cases a plain CXR may be helpful to look for pneumonia or a foreign body including button batteries. If there is any possibility of ingestion of a button battery, an abdominal X-ray should be requested.
- In those with swallowing difficulties or epigastric pain, an upper GI contrast study should be considered, e.g. in the diagnosis of oesophageal strictures.
- Technetium-99m pertechnetate scan (Meckel's scan) may detect functional gastric mucosa in an ectopic location, e.g. Meckel's diverticulum, duplication cyst. A negative Meckel's scan does not exclude a Meckel's diverticulum.
- In patients with hepatosplenomegaly or other signs of chronic liver disease, abdominal ultrasound should be performed with assessment of portal flow to look for evidence of portal hypertension/varices.
- Abdominal ultrasound can also be useful to look for bowel wall thickening which is suggestive of underlying inflammation.
- MRI angiography/technetium-99m labelled red cell scanning has a role if the if blood loss continues and the cause remains uncertain.
- If the source of bleeding is likely to be from the nasopharynx or the sinuses, a computed tomography (CT) scan should be considered.

Endoscopy

- Gastroscopy is indicated in children with haematemesis or melaena to establish the diagnosis and bleeding site.
- It is rarely necessary to perform diagnostic endoscopy when the child first presents. The degree of urgency depends on the likely cause of the bleeding and need to start treatment. Urgent endoscopy allows for rapid diagnosis but carries a risk of decompensation and poor visualization of the mucosa. It is carried out only if patients cannot be stabilized; surgical colleagues should be involved.

- Colonoscopy and ileoscopy with biopsies (plus or minus polypectomy) should be performed in children with per rectum blood loss who do not have evidence of infective colitis or constipation/anal fissure. It is crucial that patients have had adequate bowel preparation before colonoscopy, otherwise the information obtained is very limited.
- Push enteroscopy/laparoscopy/laparotomy should be considered if bleeding continues and the source of bleeding remains obscure.
- Wireless capsule endoscopy is useful in obscure GI bleeding, with good potential to visualize the small intestinal mucosa directly and may pick up vascular or inflammatory causes of bleeding.

Table 34.2 Upper GI bleeding: aetiology and appropriate investigation

Age	Common aetiology	Investigations that may be appropriate
Neonate/infant	Swallowed maternal blood	Apt test for maternal haemoglobin
	Oesophagitis/gastritis	
	Vitamin K deficiency	FBC, U&E, LFT, coagulation screen, gastroscopy
	Maternal NSAIDs	
	Maternal idiopathic thrombocytopenic purpura	Maternal FBC
	Pulmonary haemosiderosis	
	Factitious	CXR
Child	Mallory–Weiss tear	FBC, U&E, LFT, coagulation screen
	Haemorrhagic tonsillitis	
	Oesophagitis/gastritis/peptic ulcer disease	Gastroscopy
	Oesophageal varices/gastric varices	Abdominal ultrasound/gastroscopy ideally in a centre with experience of variceal banding in children
	Pulmonary haemosiderosis	CXR
	Factitious	
Adolescent	Mallory–Weiss tear	FBC, U&E, LFT, coagulation screen
	Haemorrhagic tonsillitis	
	Oesophagitis/gastritis/ peptic ulcer disease	Gastroscopy
	Oesophageal varices/gastric varices	Abdominal ultrasound/gastroscopy ideally in a centre with experience of variceal banding in children
	Factitious	

AXR, abdominal X-ray; CXR, chest X-ray; FBC, full blood count; LFT, liver function test; U&E, urea and electrolytes.

Table 34.3 Lower GI bleeding: aetiology and appropriate investigation

Age	Common aetiology	Appropriate investigations
Neonate/ infant	Swallowed maternal blood	Apt test for maternal haemoglobin
	Anal fissure/constipation	FBC, U&E, LFT, coagulation screen
	Allergic colitis/cow milk protein intolerance	Skin prick testing, milk RAST
	Necrotizing enterocolitis	AXR, CRP
	Hirschsprung's disease	Rectal biopsy
	Infective colitis	Stool specimen MC&S, *Clostridium difficile*
	Intussusception	Abdominal ultrasound
	Maternal ITP	Maternal FBC
	Meckel's diverticulum	Meckel's scan
	Vascular malformation	Contrast CT/MRI
	Factitious	
Child/ adolescent	Anal fissure/constipation	As above
	Threadworms	Examination of perineum
	Infectious colitis	As above
	Polyps	Endoscopy
	Inflammatory bowel disease	Endoscopy
	Coeliac disease	Coeliac screen
	Intussusception	As above
	Meckel's diverticulum	As above
	Haemolytic uraemic syndrome	Blood film, urine dipstick
	Henoch–Schönlein purpura	Endoscopy
	Vascular malformation	As above
	Factitious	

AXR, abdominal X-ray; CRP, C-reactive protein; CT, computed tomography; FBC, full blood count; ITP, immune thrombocytopenia; LFT, liver function test; MC&S, microscopy, culture and sensitivity; MRI, magnetic resonance imaging; RAST, radioallergosorbent test; U&E, urea and electrolytes

Differential diagnosis

Upper GI bleeding

(See Table 34.2, p. 285.)

Neonate and infant

- Significant haematemesis or melaena is rare in infants.
- Neonates can swallow maternal blood at delivery or amniotic fluid containing blood; breastfed babies can swallow blood from cracked, bleeding nipples.
- Critically ill neonates can develop stress ulcers in the first days of life; these can present with significant GI bleed secondary to erosive gastritis or gastric ulcers.
- Mucosal bleeding can be secondary to coagulopathy caused by: vitamin K deficiency, maternal ITP, or use of NSAIDs, haemophilia, or von Willebrand disease. It is rare for vitamin K deficiency or platelet defects to present with GI haemorrhage but relatively common for von Willebrand disease to present with mucosal bleeding.
- Significant non-GI haematemesis can occur from ENT causes. This is rare in isolation in this age group, but can occur associated with coagulopathy. Pulmonary haemosiderosis is rare but commonly presents with haemoptysis. It is caused by recurrent bleeding into alveolar spaces and interstitial lung tissue. Chest radiograph shows alveolar infiltrates, and siderophages are found on bronchoalveolar lavage.

Older child

- In the patient with preceding retching and vomiting who then develops haematemesis, a Mallory–Weiss tear with bleeding from the gastro-oesophageal junction/proximal oesophagus is a common cause.
- Infective, haemorrhagic tonsillitis can present with small-volume haematemesis (vomiting swallowed blood).
- As in infants, primary peptic ulcers are very rare but can occur secondary to multisystem disease such as head trauma or septicaemia with shock.
- Peptic ulcer disease can occur secondary to NSAID use or secondary to other medications.
- *Helicobacter pylori* gastritis or duodenal ulceration can cause acute haematemesis.
- Variceal bleeding is a rare but important cause of significant haematemesis at all ages, and signs of chronic liver impairment should be looked for.

Adolescent

- As for the older child.
- Mallory–Weiss tears can occur following vomiting caused by alcohol ingestion.
- Primary peptic ulcers more commonly present at this age.
- Higher use of NSAIDs in this age group leads to a higher presentation of gastritis as a complication.
- For all age groups, factitious/induced bleeding needs to be considered.

Mallory–Weiss syndrome refers to bleeding from tears (Mallory–Weiss tears) in the mucosa at the junction of the stomach and oesophagus, usually caused by severe retching, coughing, and vomiting.

Lower GI bleeding
(See Table 34.3, p. 286.)

Neonate/infant

- Constipation causing anal fissuring and bright red blood per rectum is probably the commonest cause of lower GI bleeding. It is not always possible to see obvious fissuring but the history is usually highly suggestive and the bleeding stops with appropriate treatment of the underlying constipation or passage of hard stools.
- Eosinophilic proctitis caused by dietary sensitivities, e.g. to cow milk protein, is a common cause of bleeding per rectum. Allergy testing and trial of an appropriate exclusion diet is usually very successful in establishing a diagnosis and stopping bleeding. This is commonly caused by non-IgE-mediated allergy to cow's milk so allergy testing is likely to be negative.
- Necrotizing enterocolitis is an important cause of bloody stools in the neonate. Clinical features and the classical radiological appearances of intramural gas or perforation usually make the diagnosis. Other causes of neonatal intestinal obstruction (e.g. volvulus) can present with blood per rectum.
- Hirschsprung's disease can present with enterocolitis.
- Infectious colitis is rare in this age group but can be a cause of bloody diarrhoea.
- Intussusception often presents with intermittent irritability, pallor, shock, and, as a late feature, 'redcurrant jelly'-like stools.
- Meckel's diverticulum is the embryological remnant of the vitellointestinal duct, and is said to be present in 2% of the population. A Meckel's diverticulum can present with large quantities of painless rectal bleeding. A Meckel's diverticulum is the likely diagnosis in children with lower GI bleeding who present with significant anaemia.
- Polyposis should be considered. Diagnosis is by endoscopy. The most likely type is a juvenile polyp. Polyps tend to produce bright red blood.

Older child/adolescent

- Children can have lower GI bleeding from many of the same causes as infants.
- In the older child with intussusception, a lead point should be looked for.
- Patients with polyposis syndromes such as familial adenomatous polyposis coli (FAP) typically present in older children. Diagnosis is by endoscopy. Management is dependent on the underlying syndrome.
- Rarely coeliac disease can present with GI bleeding.
- Inflammatory bowel disease often presents with bloody diarrhoea, particularly if there is colitis. Other causes of an inflammatory colitis should be considered.
- Infection should be considered, e.g. *Salmonella*, *Shigella*, *Escherichia coli*, *Clostridium difficile*.
- Local trauma, e.g. fissuring, prolapse, haemorrhoids, solitary rectal ulcer syndrome, sexual abuse should be considered.
- For all age groups factitious/induced bleeding should be considered.

Treatment

The management of GI bleeding requires accurate, prompt diagnosis and treatment of the underlying condition.

References and resources

Advanced Life Support Group. Advanced paediatric life support: a practical approach to emergencies, 6th edn. Oxford: Wiley; 2016.

National Institute for Health and Care Excellence (NICE). Acute upper gastrointestinal bleeding in over 16s: management. Clinical Guideline CG141. London: NICE; 2017. https://www.nice.org.uk/Guidance/CG141

Thomson MA, Leton N Belsha D. Acute upper gastrointestinal bleeding in childhood: development of the Sheffield scoring system to predict need for endoscopic therapy. J Paed Gastro Nutr 2015;60:632–6.

Tringali A, Thomson M, Dumonceau JM, et al. Pediatric gastrointestinal endoscopy: European Society of Gastrointestinal Endoscopy (ESGE) and European Society for Paediatric Gastroenterology Hepatology and Nutrition (ESPGHAN) guideline executive summary. Endoscopy 2017;49:83–91.

Chapter 35

Gastrointestinal polyposis

Introduction *292*
Hamartomas *293*
Adenomas *294*
Hyperplastic polyps *294*
Inflammatory polyps *294*

Introduction

Polyps generally present with painless rectal bleeding or through genetic screening of affected families with polyposis syndromes. There are various types, as listed in Table 35.1. Juvenile polyps (hamartomas) are the most commonly seen and generally benign.

Investigation requires full upper and lower GI endoscopy. Barium radiology or push enteroscopy is required if small-bowel polyps are suspected.

Table 35.1 Classification of polyps

Hamartomas	Juvenile polyps
	Juvenile polyposis syndrome (multiple)
	Peutz–Jeghers syndrome
	Cowden syndrome
	Bannayan–Riley–Ruvalcaba syndrome
Adenomas	Familial adenomatous polyposis
	Gardener syndrome
	Turcot syndrome
Hyperplastic	
Inflammatory	Inflammatory bowel disease
	Solitary rectal ulcer syndrome
	Post infective

Hamartomas

Juvenile polyps

- More than 90% of polyps seen in childhood are juvenile polyps. They are hamartomas and have a stalk. They are usually easily detected by colonoscopy, usually presenting between ages 2 and 6 years with painless blood per rectum.
- Most polyps are solitary and located within 30cm of the anus.
- Can regress but are seen in adults.
- Not premalignant.

Juvenile polyposis

- Juvenile polyposis (rare) refers to the presence of:
  - Presence of more than five juvenile polyps in the colon and/or rectum.
  - The presence of juvenile polyposis throughout the digestive tract, including the stomach.
  - The presence of any number of juvenile polyps in association with a family history of juvenile intestinal polyposis.
- Polyps may be present throughout the GI tract.
- Familial type is associated with autosomal dominant inheritance with variable penetrance.
- Premalignant.
- Prophylactic colectomy should be considered.

Peutz–Jeghers syndrome

- Rare: 1 in 120,000. Autosomal dominant inheritance.
- Hamartomatous polyps throughout the GI tract associated with freckling and hyperpigmentation of the buccal mucosa and lips.
- Polyps tend to be large and pedunculated.
- Small bowel polyps may present as intussusception.
- Premalignant.
- Long-term follow-up with regular endoscopic screening required.
- Increased risk of pancreatic, ovarian, breast, cervix, and testicular tumours.

Cowden syndrome

Multiple hamartoma syndrome with orocutaneous hamartomas, fibro-cystic disease of the breast, increased risk of breast carcinoma, thyroid abnormalities, and hamartomatous polyps throughout the intestine. *PTEN* gene abnormalities in >50% (the *PTEN* gene provides instructions for making a protein that is found in almost all tissues in the body and acts as a tumour suppressor).

Bannayan–Riley–Ruvalcaba syndrome

GI hamartomas, macrocephaly, speckled penis, developmental delay. *PTEN* gene abnormalities in >50%.

Adenomas

Familial adenomatous polyposis coli

- Inherited as an autosomal dominant trait. 1 in 10,000. Multiple polyps (>100) develop usually in the second decade.
- Polyps are premalignant with a lifetime risk of colonic neoplasia of 100%.
- They are often asymptomatic and a proportion present with carcinoma.
- Genetic testing is available for family screening. The gene is on the long arm of chromosome 5.
- Endoscopic surveillance should begin at age 10–12 years. Confirmation is by biopsy. Once the diagnosis is established prophylactic colectomy is advised. This is usually performed in late adolescence.
- Gastric and duodenal polyps develop in up to 50% and regular surveillance is recommended. There is an increased risk of thyroid and liver tumours.

Gardener syndrome

A variant of familial adenomatous polyposis including osteomas, skin tumours, desmoid tumours, carcinoma of the periampullary region of the duodenum and thyroid.

Turcot syndrome

The association of colonic adenomas with tumours of the CNS.

Hyperplastic polyps

Single polyps, usually in the antrum or duodenum. Can cause abdominal pain. Benign.

Inflammatory polyps

Can be multiple, common in inflammatory bowel disease, can be seen following 'other' inflammatory insults, e.g. post-infective, ischaemic.

Differential diagnosis of painless rectal bleeding

- Infectious colitis.
- Allergic colitis.
- Meckel's diverticulum.
- Vascular anomalies.
- Inflammatory bowel disease.
- Anal fissure.

Chapter 36

Intractable diarrhoea of infancy

Introduction 296
Absorption and transport of nutrients and electrolytes 297
Enterocyte differentiation and polarization 298
Enteroendocrine cell differentiation 299
Modulation of the intestinal immune response 299
References and resources 299

Introduction

Children with a congenital diarrhoeal disorder usually present in infancy in the first few weeks or months of life. Excessive watery diarrhoeal losses may be misdiagnosed as polyuria. Significant disturbances in fluid and electrolytes can lead to life-threatening hypovolaemia and commonly (but not universally) metabolic acidosis. History of consanguinity, previous miscarriage, and stillbirth is relevant as well as anomalies found on antenatal scanning and those found on careful clinical examination.

It is necessary to determine if the diarrhoea is secretory or osmotic. This can be done by catheterizing the infant to accurately differentiate urine from stool then starving the infant while providing appropriate IV fluids, and measuring the stool output. Osmotic diarrhoea occurs when non-absorbed nutrients in the GI tract produce an excessive osmotic force pulling water into the bowel lumen. It is often associated with intestinal mucosal damage most commonly seen in older children with lactose intolerance post infectious gastroenteritis. It will therefore stop if the child is fasted. Secretory diarrhoea continues in the fasted state due to alterations in electrolyte fluxes often due to active inflammation. In many cases the diarrhoea is a mixed secretory/osmotic picture. The stool osmotic gap can be calculated as follows:

$$\text{Stool osmolality} - 2\,(\text{Stool Na} + \text{K})$$

A low osmotic gap <50mOsm/kg suggests secretory diarrhoea, high >130mOsm/kg suggests osmotic diarrhoea.

Management of these children with/without a diagnosis requires meticulous attention to fluid and electrolyte losses and appropriate provision of nutrition support usually with PN in the first instance. Ongoing intestinal failure may lead to PN dependence and the need for provision for HPN.

The evolution of genetic evaluation is ever increasing our understanding of these conditions and now many of these congenital diarrhoeal disorders now have identified gene defects.

Four categories have developed based on specific defects (Canani et al. 2010). Other more common conditions such as milk allergic proctocolitis present with less severe symptoms but should be considered.

Absorption and transport of nutrients and electrolytes

Congenital chloride diarrhoea

This rare autosomal recessive condition is characterized by severe watery diarrhoea starting at birth—there is often a past history of polyhydramnios. Diarrhoea results from a failure of chloride reabsorption and bicarbonate secretion leading to loss of sodium and chloride in the stool. Secondary hyperaldosteronism promotes sodium retention in the kidney but results in loss of potassium and hydrogen ions resulting in a hypochloraemic, hypokalaemic metabolic alkalosis. Infants have a high stool chloride (>90mmol/L). Treatment is with sodium and potassium chloride supplements. Prognosis is good if diagnosis is made early.

Congenital sodium diarrhoea

This has a similar appearance to congenital chloride diarrhoea but is associated with high losses of sodium in the stool. Biochemical analysis shows high stool sodium, low urine sodium, low or normal serum sodium, and metabolic acidosis.

Glucose–galactose malabsorption

This is a rare autosomal recessively inherited condition, characterized by rapid-onset watery diarrhoea from birth. It responds to withholding glucose (stopping feeds) and relapses on reintroduction. The defect is in the sodium/glucose co-transporter encoded by the SLC5A1 gene. The diagnosis is essentially a clinical one. Sugar chromatography will be useful and small-bowel biopsy and disaccharide estimation normal. The diagnosis can be confirmed on genetic molecular analysis. Treatment is by using fructose as the main carbohydrate source. Fructose is absorbed by a different mechanism from glucose and galactose.

Abetalipoproteinaemia

This presents in early infancy with faltering growth, abdominal distension, and foul-smelling, bulky stools. Symptoms of vitamin E deficiency (ataxia, peripheral neuropathy, and retinitis pigmentosa) develop later. The pathogenesis of this autosomal recessive inherited condition is failure of chylomicron formation with impaired absorption of long-chain fats with fat retention in the enterocyte. Diagnosis is by low serum cholesterol, very low plasma triglyceride level, acanthocytes on examination of the peripheral blood film, absence of beta-lipoprotein in the plasma, low plasma vitamin E, and fat-filled enterocytes on duodenal biopsy. Treatment is with a medium-chain triglyceride-based diet. Medium-chain triglycerides are absorbed via the portal vein rather than the thoracic duct. In addition, high doses of the fat-soluble vitamins (A, D, E, and K) are required. Most of the neurological abnormalities are reversible if high doses of vitamin E are given early.

Enterocyte differentiation and polarization

Microvillus inclusion disease (congenital microvillus atrophy)

This presents as intractable diarrhoea from birth. The diarrhoea is secretory but additional osmotic diarrhoea occurs with enteral intake. The pathology is an ultrastructural abnormality at the microvillus surface. Light microscopy reveals a partial villous atrophy. Special (periodic acid–Schiff) staining is required. Electron microscopy is diagnostic. Microvilli are depleted on the apical epithelial surface and intracellular inclusions show apparently well-formed villi. Intestinal failure is profound with dependence on PN and failure to tolerate even minimal enteral intake. Fluid requirements are high as a consequence of continuing diarrhoea. Long-term nutritional support with PN is required. Liver disease is common.

Tufting enteropathy

This is rare. Presentation is similar to microvillus inclusion disease. The pathology is a primary epithelial dysplasia with the presence of 'tufts' of extruding epithelial cells on small-bowel biopsy. There is a combination of secretory and osmotic diarrhoea. Dependence on parenteral nutrition is usual, although unlike microvillus inclusion disease some gut function is present with the potential to tolerate a proportion of energy needs by the enteral route, which reduces the likelihood of liver disease.

Tricho-hepato-enteric syndrome (phenotypic diarrhoea)

Affected infants are born small for gestational age with characteristic facial dysmorphism and distinctive woolly hair that is easily removed and has non-specific abnormalities on microscopy. Biopsies from the small intestine show villous atrophy with non-diagnostic features. Liver disease can be severe. Long-term nutritional support with PN is required.

Enteroendocrine cell differentiation

Enteric anendocrinosis

This is an exceedingly rare disorder; mutations in the neurogenin 3 gene (*NEUROG3*) have been described in which affected individuals have a lack of intestinal enteroendocrine cells.

Modulation of the intestinal immune response

Autoimmune enteropathy

This refers to protracted diarrhoea presenting in infancy which usually is associated with the presence of circulating autoantibodies against intestinal epithelial cells. There is a partial villous atrophy with an inflammatory infiltrate on small-bowel histology that is similar in appearance to graft versus host disease. Treatment is with nutrition support and immunosuppression.

IPEX syndrome (immune dysregulation, polyendocrinopathy, enteropathy, X-linked)

This is a specific syndrome associated with mutations in *FOXP3*. This severe autoimmune disease presents with secretory diarrhoea associated with dermatitis, diabetes mellitus, thyroiditis, and haematological problems. Treatment is with nutrition support and immunosuppression with potential for bone marrow transplantation.

Very early-onset inflammatory bowel disease

This describes children typically aged <2 years who present usually with colitis ± perianal disease typical of inflammatory bowel disease. Many of these infants will have a single gene defect affecting proteins such as IL10 or EPCAM. Treatment is with nutrition support and immunosuppression with potential for bone marrow transplantation.

References and resources

Canani RB, Terrin G, Cardillo G, Tomaiuolo R, Castaldo G. Congenital diarrheal disorders: improved understanding of gene defects is leading to advances in intestinal physiology and clinical management. J Pediatr Gastroenterol Nutr 2010;50:360–6.

Chronic diarrhoea

Definitions 302
Assessment 303
Investigation 304
Differential diagnosis for thriving children with
    normal basic investigations 306
Other causes of Chronic Diarrhoea 308
Summary 310

Definitions

- Chronic diarrhoea refers to diarrhoea that has persisted for >2–3 weeks.
- Assessment requires a careful history, physical examination including an assessment of growth, and basic investigations.
- Visual examination of the stool is clinically valuable.

Assessment

- Is the child thriving?
- Is it true diarrhoea?
- Is the diarrhoea functional, secondary to malabsorption, or inflammatory?
- Does it stop if nil by mouth (i.e. osmotic not secretory in origin)?

The most important part of the assessment of a child with chronic diarrhoea is a careful history and clinical examination including assessment of weight gain and linear growth.

The history includes the characteristics of the stool —the Bristol Stool Chart is useful for standardizing stool description, plus other features including the appearance of grease (steatorrhoea), blood or mucous, stool frequency (e.g. night stool), presence of associated symptoms (e.g. pain, urgency, blood, weight loss), careful dietary history, assessment of general health, assessment of mental health and association of symptoms with stress or anxiety, review of risk factors (e.g. chronic disease, previous surgery, antibiotic use, foreign travel), family history (e.g. CF, coeliac disease), and social history. Height and weight (with previous measurements) need to be plotted on a growth chart and interpreted in the context of family growth data. Puberty should be assessed in older children.

A head-to-toe physical examination should be carried out. In particular, this should include evaluation of nutritional status by assessment of subcutaneous fat mass and muscle bulk. The perianal area should be visualized to exclude factors such as perianal excoriation from acid stool, rectal prolapse, soiling, or perianal signs of Crohn's disease. Rectal examination should be considered.

Investigation

The precise investigation of chronic diarrhoea is dependent on the clinical situation and outcome of the clinical assessment. A vast array of tests or no tests may be appropriate. A basic screen might include stool for infectious causes, full blood count, IgA and coeliac serology, and serum albumin.

Stool testing

In difficult cases it is essential to visualize the stool to determine what the stool actually looks like rather than relying on history alone.

Microbiological investigation

Stools should be sent for microscopy and culture, virology, ova cysts and parasites, and *Clostridium difficile* toxin if suspected.

Biochemical investigation

Some UK laboratories are no longer able to perform microscopy for fats or perform stool analysis for reducing substances.

- Sugar chromatography is performed in a few UK sites which will define the sugars present in stool.
- Stool osmotic gap—the difference between measured and calculated osmolality (can only be measured in liquid stool); stool osmolality should usually be the same as plasma osmolality:
  - Stool osmotic gap = stool osmolality − 2(stool Na + K)
  - A significant gap (>40) suggests osmotic diarrhoea with the gap reflecting the ingested, non-absorbed agent, consider possible laxative abuse.
  - No gap implies impaired electrolyte transport (secretory diarrhoea).
  - Low stool osmolality suggests contamination of the stool with water or urine or an excess of ingested hypotonic fluid.
- Stool for white cells/occult blood.
- Faecal calprotectin is a stable neutrophil protein present in stool which is a non-specific marker of bowel inflammation. High levels mean inflammatory bowel disease should be considered. However, calprotectin will be raised if the stool contains visible blood so often it isn't clinically useful in that context. Adult laboratory ranges are not applicable to children particularly those aged <4 years.
- Faecal elastase is a useful test for pancreatic insufficiency, manifest by low levels of this pancreas-specific enzyme. Low values may also be found in short gut and bacterial overgrowth. Normal levels exclude pancreatic insufficiency.
- Faecal A1-antitrypsin is a serum protein, not present in the diet with the same molecular weight as albumin. Faecal levels reflect enteric protein loss (e.g. protein-losing enteropathy).

Blood testing

- Routine blood testing should include full blood count (including blood film), basic biochemistry including inflammatory markers and albumin, serum immunoglobulins, and coeliac antibody screen.

- Fat-soluble vitamins should be checked if a fat malabsorption is suspected.
- These can range from simple, relatively benign disorders such as IgA deficiency to major life-threatening immunodeficiencies such as severe combined immune deficiency (SCID). Full immunology work-up is required if an immune deficit is suspected. The precise tests are determined by the condition considered.

Other investigations

- If laxative abuse is suspected, a urine laxative screen should be sent. Administration of an osmotic laxative will result in an increased osmotic gap on stool analysis.
- Sweat testing/CF genotype are indicated if CF is suspected.
- Hydrogen breath testing can be used to test for carbohydrate malabsorption, although there are significant false-positive and false-negative rates, and children <4 years find it difficult to cooperate. The potential offending carbohydrate is given and breath hydrogen monitored with a peak (from fermentation) suggesting malabsorption.

Endoscopy

Gastroscopy with multiple duodenal biopsies is indicated if an enteropathy (e.g. coeliac disease, cow milk protein-sensitive enteropathy, post-enteritis syndrome) is suspected. Gastroscopy and colonoscopy (plus small bowel imaging) are indicated if inflammatory bowel disease/colitis is suspected.

Chronic diarrhoea: red flags

Red flags in the history and examination for further investigation include:
- Continuous diarrhoea.
- Night stools.
- Acid stools.
- Blood and mucus in the stool.
- Faltering growth.
- Associated symptoms that suggest organic disease—fever, rash, arthritis.

Differential diagnosis for thriving children with normal basic investigations

- *Chronic constipation* is a common cause, presenting as apparent diarrhoea which is in fact overflow soiling (variable consistency, stale stool). This occurs as a consequence of faecal leakage in the presence of a megarectum/incomplete rectal evacuation. History of difficulty completely emptying bowels, spending long periods of time on the toilet, and feeling the need to void stool but not able to do so may add weight to the observer's clinical suspicion.
- *Factitious diarrhoea* needs to be considered as a potential cause. This may be loose stool that has been induced and/or created by laxative abuse or the addition of urine/water to the stool. But may also include simply reporting of 'abnormal stools or frequency' by children or carers.
- *Irritable bowel syndrome*—although this commonly has fluctuating loose stool and constipation with relief on opening bowels, some children may have a diarrhoea predominant irritable bowel syndrome. Stress and anxiety are triggers.
- *Chronic non-specific diarrhoea (toddler's diarrhoea)*—this is common, particularly in the run-up to toilet training. Children tend to pass frequent loose, often explosive stools. It can cause significant anxiety for carers. Undigested food is frequently seen in the stool and is indicative of rapid transit. There are no additional features such as pain, blood in the stool, or night stools. Incomplete rectal evacuation may also be a factor. The children are generally thriving. There are various potential factors implicated in causation—gut immaturity, dysmotility, diet (excess juice, excess fibre), and emotional stress. Fructose-containing drinks (e.g. apple juice) and excess sorbitol are common causes of chronic non-specific diarrhoea. Management is by reassurance and general advice regarding potential triggers including avoidance of excess fibre and juice (particularly excessive hyperosmolar juice).

Other causes of Chronic Diarrhoea

- Carbohydrate intolerance (see also Chapter 20) is most commonly due to lactose intolerance, and acquired. The deficient enzyme is the brush-border enzyme lactase which hydrolyses lactose into glucose and galactose. The intolerance will present with characteristic loose, explosive stools. The diagnosis is made by faecal sugar chromatography following carbohydrate ingestion. Hydrogen breath-testing can be used to confirm a peak after lactose ingestion. Treatment is with a lactose-free formula in infancy and a reduced lactose intake in later childhood. Following gastroenteritis, carbohydrate intolerance can be either to disaccharides or monosaccharides. In children with rotavirus gastroenteritis, carbohydrate intolerance is usually transient and responds to removal of the offending carbohydrate. Both mono- and disaccharide intolerance will result in positive faecal sugar chromatography.
- Sucrose–isomaltase deficiency is a defect in carbohydrate digestion; the enzyme required for hydrolysis of sucrose and alpha-limit dextrins is reduced or absent in the small intestine. Symptoms of watery diarrhoea and/or growth faltering develop after the introduction of sucrose or complex carbohydrate into the diet. Symptoms can be very mild. Sugar chromatography will make the diagnosis. Management is by removal of sucrose and complex carbohydrate from the diet.
- Post-enteritis syndrome. Acute gastroenteritis usually resolves in 7–10 days. Post-enteritis syndrome refers to diarrhoea lasting >3 weeks, particularly if associated with poor weight gain/weight loss. This is usually seen in infants. The continuing diarrhoea may be secondary to continuing infection, a further infection, carbohydrate intolerance (e.g. after rotavirus infection), enteropathy presenting as a severe malabsorptive syndrome which may reflect the 'unmasking' of another pathology (e.g. coeliac disease, cow milk protein intolerance, or CF) or secondary to the initial infection. Enteropathogenic *E. coli* (EPEC), for example, can cause a severe enteropathy.
Post-enteritis syndrome can be severe and require a period of PN. In most cases, however, treatment of the underlying condition (if unmasked) and/or a period of dietary exclusion using a cow milk free-diet using a protein hydrolysate (lactose free) as a substitute will suffice.
- Coeliac disease—see Chapter 38.
- Pancreatic insufficiency manifests as chronic diarrhoea with steatorrhoea (i.e. fat/oil in stool) secondary to fat malabsorption. Management of pancreatic insufficiency is by pancreatic enzyme replacement and nutritional support including fat-soluble vitamins; growth faltering is common. There may be evidence of fat-soluble vitamin deficiency on testing. Causes include:
  - Cystic Fibrosis (see Chapter 23).
  - Shwachman–Diamond syndrome. This is a rare autosomal recessive condition. Incidence is 1:20–200,000. The main features are pancreatic insufficiency, neutropenia, and short stature. Other features include metaphyseal dysostosis, mild hepatic dysfunction, increased frequency of infections, additional haematological abnormalities (including thrombocytopenia, increased risk of leukaemia).

- Intestinal lymphangiectasia refers to a functional obstruction of lymph flow through the thoracic duct and into the subclavian vein which leads to fat malabsorption and a protein-losing enteropathy. It can be primary (congenital disorder of the lymphatic system) or secondary to other conditions, e.g. pancreatitis, cardiac disease (pericarditis, post Fontan procedure), malignancy. Presentation is with chronic diarrhoea (steatorrhea) and oedema. Lymphopenia is common. Diagnosis is by small-bowel biopsy (multiple sites as the lesion may be patchy), which shows dilated lymphatics in the absence of other pathology or visualization by capsule endoscopy. Treatment is with nutrition support with low fat diet and formula rich in medium-chain triglycerides—absorbed directly into the portal vein.
- Inflammatory bowel disease (see Chapter 45).
- It is unusual for malignancy to present with chronic diarrhoea but it should be considered particularly in the context of significant weight loss. Lymphoma may occur particularly in patients on immunosuppression. Neuroendocrine tumours such as phaeochromocytoma or more rarely gut hormone-secreting tumours can also cause chronic diarrhoea. Primary colonic malignancy is rare but may cause a raised calprotectin in patients with a family history of bowel cancer and can occur in children with polyposis syndromes.
- Immunodeficiency—chronic diarrhoea may be an important manifestation of an immune deficiency. These can range from simple, relatively benign disorders such as IgA deficiency to major life-threatening immunodeficiencies such as SCID. A full immunological work-up is required if an immune deficit is suspected. The precise tests are determined by the condition.
- Eosinophilic enterocolitis (see Chapter 49).

Summary

Chronic diarrhoea is a common presentation to primary, secondary, and tertiary care. A careful history to determine the precise nature and frequency of stools is vital. Physical examination is necessary to look for features which may suggest underlying disease. A large range of investigations is available but each test ordered should be considered with the differential diagnosis for the specific patient in mind. Despite that, a basic level of investigations such as sending stool for microscopy and culture, virology, ova cysts and parasites ± *Clostridium difficile* toxin, and full blood count (including blood film), basic biochemistry including inflammatory markers and albumin, serum immunoglobulins, and coeliac antibody screen is worth considering in those with ongoing symptoms.

Coeliac disease

Introduction 312
Who to investigate 314
How to investigate 316
Diagnosis 318
Treatment 320
Follow-up and support 322
References and resources 322

Introduction

Coeliac disease is an immune-mediated enteropathy caused by a permanent sensitivity to gluten which is present in wheat, barley, and rye. It occurs in genetically susceptible children and adults. The classical presentation is with chronic diarrhoea, abdominal distension, and faltering growth. The widespread availability of antibody screening has considerably changed the clinical spectrum of cases seen. The testing of children with fewer classical symptoms and screening of children at high risk has brought increasing recognition of the varied presentation and increased prevalence of this now very common condition.

The prevalence of coeliac-disease based on either cross-sectional or population-based studies in developed countries is of the order of 0.3–2%, with a higher prevalence in at-risk groups. The vast majority of cases, however, remain undetected with seropositivity in apparently healthy individuals when populations are screened (asymptomatic coeliac disease). This is commonly referred to as the 'coeliac iceberg'.

The diagnosis of coeliac disease is confirmed by duodenal biopsy with classical histological features. A minority of symptomatic children with very high tissue transglutaminase (tTG) antibody can be diagnosed without a duodenal biopsy.

Who to investigate

There are three settings in which the diagnosis of coeliac disease should be considered:

- Children with frank gut symptoms.
- Children with non-GI manifestations.
- Asymptomatic individuals with conditions associated with coeliac disease.

Coeliac disease presents after 6 months, i.e. after gluten has been introduced into the diet. The classical presentation is with irritability, weight loss, pallor, and abdominal distension in infants. More often children present later with a wide range of GI symptoms including anorexia, generalized irritability, diarrhoea, abdominal pain, vomiting, constipation, anaemia, abdominal distension, and faltering growth. Recurrent abdominal pain/irritable bowel like symptoms is a common presentation and coeliac disease should be considered as part of the differential diagnosis. It is unclear what proportion of children with any combination of the above symptoms will subsequently be diagnosed with coeliac disease. However, if symptoms are significant and clinical suspicion exists then coeliac serology is indicated and it is appropriate to test all children with chronic gut symptoms. Coeliac serology should also be considered in children with non-GI manifestations of coeliac disease (see Box 38.1). Short stature is an important specific indication with a high diagnostic yield and good catch-up growth once the condition is diagnosed. Screening should be considered in children at high risk. There is considerable controversy about whether coeliac screening should be extended to the general population.

Dietary compliance is difficult to establish in children who are picked up by either high-risk group or population-based screening, particularly if the child is, and perceives themselves as, asymptomatic as this will impact on acceptance of the diagnosis and compliance.

A *coeliac crisis* is a rare complication of coeliac disease seen at presentation characterized by explosive watery diarrhoea, dehydration (with hypovolaemia and hypoalbuminaemia), abdominal distension, and electrolyte disturbance. It responds to steroid treatment.

High-risk screening

It is important to remember that children in high-risk groups who are screened (see Box 38.2) may have initially negative serology and develop positive serology later and repeat testing is indicated particularly if they develop suspicious symptoms. The British (BSPGHAN) and the European Society of Paediatric Gastroenterology, Hepatology and Nutrition (EDSPGHAN) guidelines recommend that screening should be offered to children in high-risk groups, who have been on an adequate gluten-containing diet for at least 1 year prior to testing. Screening for first-degree relatives in families with a child who has coeliac disease is also suggested. Guidance from NICE in the UK recommends screening of type 1 diabetics at diagnosis and then 3-yearly.

Box 38.1 Non-gastrointestinal manifestations of coeliac disease

- Dermatitis herpetiformis.
- Permanent dental enamel hypoplasia.
- Iron-deficient anaemia resistant to oral iron supplementation.
- Short stature.
- Delayed puberty.
- Chronic hepatitis with hypertransaminasaemia
- Arthritis.
- Osteopenia/osteoporosis.
- Epilepsy with occipital calcifications.
- Primary ataxia.
- Psychiatric disorders.
- Female infertility.
- Weakness (or muscle wasting).

Box 38.2 Conditions with an increased prevalence of coeliac disease

Children who are screened for any of these indications may have asymptomatic coeliac disease (abnormal small-bowel mucosa but no symptoms).

- Type 1 diabetes mellitus.
- Selective IgA deficiency.*
- Down syndrome.
- Turner syndrome.
- Williams syndrome.
- Autoimmune thyroiditis.
- Autoimmune liver disease.
- First-degree relatives of those with coeliac disease (one in ten).

* IgA-deficient children are at increased risk of coeliac disease. Testing based on IgA antibodies will be negative (i.e. false negative). This is a potential diagnostic pitfall.

How to investigate

Serological testing

Measurement of IgA antibody to human recombinant tTG and serum IgA is recommended for initial testing for coeliac disease. Sensitivity and specificity approach 100% although false positives are occasionally seen. IgA antibody to endomysium (EMA) is observer dependent and though very specific is not as sensitive as tTg. It is important to exclude IgA deficiency as a cause of falsely negative serology. If coeliac disease is clinically suspected in children with IgA deficiency they should be referred for a small-bowel biopsy. IgG serology may also be helpful in cases with low IgA though is not as specific or sensitive as IgA tTG.

It is crucial that children having coeliac testing are on a normal, gluten-containing diet prior to serological and histological diagnosis. Serology may be falsely negative if children are not on a normal gluten-containing diet. If children have already been started on a gluten-free diet or are eating insufficient amounts of gluten they should be referred to a paediatric dietitian and advised to recommence gluten in their diet for at least 3 months, with serial serological testing if there is a high clinical suspicion of coeliac disease and small-bowel biopsy following positive serology. After a period of gluten exclusion, it may take many months for serology to turn positive once a normal diet is re-started.

HLA testing

Susceptibility to coeliac disease is restricted to individuals possessing the major histocompatibility complex class II genes *HLA-DQA1*0501-DQB1*02* (expressing the molecule DQ2) and *HLA-DQA1*0301-DQB1*0302* (expressing the molecule DQ8). These genes have a useful negative predictive value (>99%) but are not useful for predicting who has or will get coeliac disease. HLA testing should be considered in patients with an uncertain diagnosis. It is also used to add strength to a diagnosis based on serological testing only without histological confirmation where tTg levels are greater than ten times the upper limit of normal (ULN). HLA testing may be offered to asymptomatic individuals with CD-associated conditions (group 2) to select them for further CD-specific antibody testing.

Small-bowel biopsy

Most children with positive serology will need a small-bowel biopsy. On duodenal biopsy, villous atrophy with crypt hyperplasia and increased intraepithelial lymphocytes (IELs) >30/100 epithelial cells are characteristic of coeliac disease but rarely may be found in other enteropathies.

Box 38.3 Differential diagnosis of partial villous atrophy

- Coeliac disease.
- Cow milk-sensitive enteropathy.
- Soy protein-sensitive enteropathy.
- Eosinophilic gastroenteritis.
- Gastroenteritis and post-enteritis syndrome.
- Giardiasis.
- Small-bowel bacterial overgrowth.
- Inflammatory bowel disease.
- Immunodeficiency.
- Intractable diarrhoea syndromes, e.g. autoimmune enteropathy.
- Drugs, e.g. cytotoxics.
- Radiotherapy.

IgA deficiency

IgA makes up 15% of circulating immunoglobulin. In its secretory form it is the predominant immunoglobulin at respiratory and GI surfaces. Selective IgA deficiency is a common disorder, with an incidence of 1/600. It is associated with an increased incidence of infection, atopic disease, rheumatic disorders, and coeliac disease. Immunoglobulin therapy is not worthwhile if isolated IgA deficiency is present. This is because there is only a small amount of IgA in immunoglobulin preparations and sensitization is therefore likely. If there is coexistent IgG deficiency or IgG subclass deficiency then immunoglobulin therapy may be appropriate.

Diagnosis

(See Fig. 38.1.)

- Children with symptoms suggestive of coeliac disease should have their IgA tTG tested:
    - If the level is raised but less than ten times the ULN, a duodenal biopsy is required for histological confirmation.
    - If the IgA tTG levels are greater than ten times the ULN, HLA testing and EMA should be performed which if positive confirms the diagnosis. This can be used as an alternative to biopsy in selected cases. In cases where either is negative, a biopsy should be performed.
- Asymptomatic cases identified on screening should all have a biopsy if IgA tTG levels are greater than three times the ULN. If tTG is less than three times the ULN it should be repeated in 6 months.
- The diagnosis is confirmed by complete symptom resolution on a strict gluten-free diet. Positive serology should revert to negative over time on a strict gluten-free diet. If there is no decline in anti-tTG after 6 months on a gluten-free diet, adherence with gluten exclusion should be reviewed. This may be as a consequence of inadvertent ingestion or cross contamination. A dietetic review is essential in such cases.
- It is important to remember that there are other potential causes of a small-bowel enteropathy with partial villous atrophy, including cow milk protein-sensitive enteropathy, soy protein-sensitive enteropathy, gastroenteritis, and post-enteritis syndrome, giardiasis, and autoimmune enteropathy (see Box 38.3).
- It is important to discourage gluten exclusion before diagnostic testing.

Pitfalls in the diagnosis of coeliac disease
- IgA deficiency resulting in false-negative serological testing.
- Period of gluten exclusion prior to biopsy.
- Inadequate gluten intake at the time of biopsy.
- Poor-quality biopsy specimen.

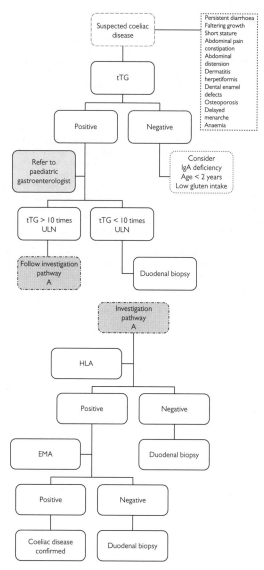

Fig. 38.1 Algorithm of investigations for suspected coeliac disease in children who are symptomatic. tTG, tissue transglutaminase.

Treatment

A gluten-free diet for life is the most effective treatment for coeliac disease (see Chapter 38). All children should be seen regularly by a paediatric dietitian to help with compliance and assess the nutritional adequacy, considering the intake both of energy and of micronutrients. There are increased risks of morbidity and mortality in those with untreated coeliac disease. Good evidence exists that adherence to a strict gluten-free diet improves growth, normalizes haematological and biochemical markers, and reduces morbidity and mortality. A gluten-free diet is nutritionally complete and there are no known complications of the gluten-free diet itself.

A small proportion of individuals who are markedly symptomatic at presentation (usually with watery diarrhoea suggestive of lactose intolerance) and who fail to settle on gluten exclusion benefit from a 6–12-week period on a lactose-free diet, although this is rarely required long term.

There is very little data on the outcome of coeliac disease in children who are asymptomatic at presentation and picked up through screening, although a pragmatic presumption that the same long-term health benefits occur as in children symptomatic at diagnosis and therefore the recommendation is that all biopsy-positive children should be treated.

Iron status should be assessed and supplements given if necessary. Calcium and multivitamin supplements may be required in some children if intake is inadequate. Dual-energy X-ray absorptiometry (DXA) scanning may be useful in children with inadequate calcium intake.

Although it has been shown that children with coeliac disease can tolerate oats, this is not recommended because oats are commonly cross-contaminated with other grains during processing.

Risks of non-adherence to a gluten-free diet

- Persistent GI symptoms.
- Impaired nutrition.
- Osteoporosis.
- Impaired growth and pubertal development.
- Reduced bone mineralization leading to osteoporosis.
- Infertility/low-birth-weight infants.
- Increased risk of GI malignancy.

Case studies

Child presents with diarrhoea and weight loss, tTG greater than ten times the ULN—what further tests are required?

Children presenting with typical symptoms where the tTg is greater than ten times the ULN, the diagnosis can be confirmed without the need for histological confirmation. A positive diagnosis in these cases would be supported by positive anti-endomysial antibodies and HLA for DQ2 or 8.

Child with positive coeliac serology, normal duodenal biopsy—what do you do?

This child is at risk (long term) of coeliac disease. The negative biopsy means that they don't fulfil the diagnostic criteria at the point it was taken. The biopsy should be reviewed by a paediatric/experienced GI histopathologist. The child should continue on a normal diet. If positive serology persists, repeat biopsy is indicated. The interval before the next biopsy depends on the clinical situation but is usually not <1 year.

Child on gluten-free diet for 3 months (gut symptoms, positive family history, no diagnostic testing)—what do you do?

This is a common situation in the clinic. The child has been started on a gluten-free diet without diagnostic testing. There may have been gut symptoms and a positive family history of coeliac disease which have prompted the carers to make this decision. In this instance the family should be encouraged to put the child back on gluten for diagnostic confirmation (gluten challenge). This doesn't need to be done urgently. The timing will depend on the clinical situation, e.g. if the child is completely well on a gluten-free diet the challenge can be deferred.

Child undergoing a gluten challenge—how long should this be for?

Gluten challenge requires the reintroduction of gluten into the diet as a powder added to foods or normal foods. This needs to be under dietetic supervision to ensure adequate amounts of gluten are ingested. The onset of symptoms after challenge is usually within 3 months but can be prolonged (months to years) and late relapse following gluten challenge is well recognized. Children should be followed with serial serology then biopsy once serology turns positive.

Case of coeliac disease on a gluten-free diet with persistent positive serology—does this matter?

The IgA-dependent coeliac serology (tTG or EMA level) should return to negative 3–6 months after starting a gluten-free diet. The failure of this to occur suggests poor compliance with gluten exclusion. In this instance, clinical and dietetic review is indicated.

Coeliac disease (index case)—what about the family members?

Family members have a lifetime increased risk of coeliac disease and family members with gut symptoms should have coeliac disease excluded. Screening of first-degree relatives should be offered but has not been universally adopted. It is important to remember that a negative screen does not exclude the possibility of coeliac disease occurring later.

Follow-up and support

Follow-up should be with a paediatrician with an interest in gastroenterology. Monitoring includes general health, growth, compliance to and adequacy of diet, haemoglobin, iron status, albumin, and calcium. Serology should become negative and can be monitored as a marker of compliance if this is in doubt. Dietetic input is crucial and the paediatric dietitian involved should liaise with the child's school. Children should be seen 3-monthly until stable, then annually or biannually if very well. Any child for whom there is a difficulty in diagnosis, investigation, or management should be referred to a paediatric gastroenterology centre.

Families should be encouraged to join a parent support group such as Coeliac UK (http://www.coeliac.co.uk).

References and resources

Hill ID, Dirks MH, Liptak GS, et al. North American Society for Pediatric Gastroenterology, Hepatology and Nutrition. Guideline for the diagnosis and treatment of celiac disease in children: recommendations of the North American Society for Pediatric Gastroenterology, Hepatology and Nutrition. J Pediatr Gastroenterol Nutr. 2005;40:1–19.

Husby S, Koletzko S, Korponay-Szabó IR, et al. European Society for Pediatric Gastroenterology, Hepatology, and Nutrition guidelines for the diagnosis of coeliac disease. J Pediatr Gastroenterol Nutr 2012;54:136–60.

Murch S, Jenkins H, Auth M, et al. Joint BSPGHAN and Coeliac UK guidelines for the diagnosis and management of coeliac disease in children. Arch Dis Child 2013;98:806–11.

National Institute for Health and Care Excellence (NICE). Coeliac disease: recognition, assessment and management. NICE Guideline NG20. London: NICE; 2015. https://www.nice.org.uk/guidance/ng20

Patient information

Coeliac UK
PO Box 220
High Wycombe
Bucks HP11 2HS
Tel.: 01494 437278
Helpline: 0870 4448804
http://www.coeliac.co.uk

Nutritional management of Coeliac disease

Introduction *324*
Gluten challenge for diagnosis *325*
Gluten-free diet *326*
Monitoring *328*
Compliance *329*

Introduction

A gluten-free diet is the primary treatment for coeliac disease. This involves the complete exclusion of wheat, rye, barley, and, in the first 6–12 months post diagnosis, oat-containing foods. If properly treated and managed, patients can eat a well-balanced, nutritionally adequate diet and therefore should be able to lead a normal, active life with no long-term complications.

Patients/parents can be daunted by the prospect of avoiding these grains that make up a large proportion of the Western diet. Avoiding many everyday foods impacts the whole family's lifestyle as well as school and social activities. It is therefore strongly advisable that families receive advice and support from a paediatric-trained dietitian at the earliest opportunity following confirmation of diagnosis. Ongoing support and review are needed particularly in the first few months after diagnosis but also at regular scheduled follow-up appointments.

Gluten challenge for diagnosis

If a patient has been excluding gluten for symptomatic relief they need to re-introduce gluten into their diet in sufficient quantity to make a valid diagnosis. A minimum of 10g of gluten in young children and 10–15g in older children is required daily for at least 6 weeks. To help ensure a sufficient minimum quantity of gluten is eaten, a 2g gluten exchange list can be helpful (Box 39.1). If gluten powder is available then 2g portions can instead be disguised in food. This is useful if gluten-containing foods are not acceptable.

Box 39.1 Food portions containing 2g gluten

- 2 rusks.
- 1 Weetabix® or Shredded Wheat®.
- 1 medium slice of bread.
- 3 chipolata sausages/2 large sausages.
- 3 fish fingers.
- 2–3 rich tea/digestive biscuits.
- 1 slice of cake (~30g).
- 30g flour.
- 4tbspns cooked or tinned spaghetti.

Gluten-free diet

- All sources of wheat, barley, and rye need to be excluded. This is a lifelong exclusion.
- Staple foods containing gluten such as bread, most breakfast cereals, pasta, biscuits, and cakes have to be avoided.
- The gluten-free diet should be based on naturally gluten-free staples such as rice, potatoes, and corn. Dietitians should take a detailed diet history and then provide suitable meal and snack ideas based around foods that are acceptable to the child keeping the diet as familiar as possible.
- Oats contain avenin, a prolamin which may have similar properties to gluten that trigger histological changes. Quantities are, however, small and studies have shown that uncontaminated oats are tolerated by most patients with gluten intolerance. It is recommended that all types of oats and oat products are withheld for 6–12 months post diagnosis until asymptomatic with normal serology having been achieved.
- At any time a patient has ongoing symptoms with abnormal serology despite reported strict adherence to a gluten-free diet, a trial of oat avoidance should be considered.
- It is essential that oats and oat products introduced are from uncontaminated sources and labelled 'Free From' as other types are likely to be contaminated with other grains during harvesting, milling and processing. Oat products are included in Coeliac UK's 'Food and Drink Directory' lists (http://www.coeliac.org.uk).
- It is advised that the risk of cross-contamination in food preparation at home is minimized by using separate chopping boards, serving utensils, butter tubs, spreads, etc. and a designated slot in the toaster used. Toaster bags are available as an alternative. Care should be taken with hand washing-up where crumbs from the water can adhere to cutlery so rinsing under the tap is advised.
- Most local authority school catering services offer a gluten-free menu choice for primary schools. Parents are encouraged to check with school that all measures are in place to prevent cross-contamination, ensure supervision of the child where necessary, and there is clear identification of the gluten-free meal. If there is doubt that mistakes are being made then a packed lunch is advised.
- A small number of children whose symptoms of diarrhoea or loose stools may persist despite good compliance with the gluten-free diet may benefit from a 6–12-week period of a lactose-free diet as small-bowel mucosa recovers and lactase enzyme function is restored. Lactose free dairy alternatives are widely available and taste matches that of normal dairy foods which helps compliance.

Food labelling

Wheat is widely used in processed foods as a filler, binding agent, thickener, or flavour carrier. Patients, parents, and carers need to be taught to read and interpret food labels in order to identify gluten and associated derivatives. All pre-packaged food is covered by food labelling legislation. Manufacturers state in **bold** if the item contains 'wheat' or 'gluten' in the list of ingredients. It is not compulsory however to list allergy information such as stating if the product is 'gluten free'.

Patients/parents are advised to be wary of packaging changes or 'new improved' products which also may include a change in the ingredients making it no longer suitable. If there is any doubt, they should refer to Coeliac UK's 'Food and Drink Directory' or manufacturers' information. If information is unobtainable, patients are encouraged to be cautious and avoid the product. If the product carries a warning such as 'may contain traces of gluten' or 'made in a factory where gluten-containing foods are made' there is a risk that the food item may contain gluten so it is advised to avoid these foods.

Coeliac UK

Coeliac UK (http://www.coeliac.org.uk) is an independent charity for adults and children with coeliac disease. Parents and patients are advised to join for support and lifestyle information. They produce the 'Food and Drink Directory' book and 'On the Move' app that contains lists of gluten-free manufactured foods and is regularly updated in line with food manufacturers' changes. Coeliac UK's website contains practical information such as recipes and suitable venues for eating out, and it produces the 'Crossed Grain' magazine for members . Members are also informed about latest campaigns and research initiatives.

Gluten-free products

An increasing amount of proprietary gluten-free foods which mimic normal gluten-containing items are available for purchase or on prescription, e.g. bread, pasta, pizza bases, biscuits, and baking mixes. These are specially manufactured foods that comply with the international gluten-free standard (WHO Codex Alimentarius 1981). Codex wheat starch can be used in gluten-free products, particularly bread, to improve the taste quality. It suggested that foods labelled 'gluten free' should contain less than 100ppm to guarantee a safe intake. Large supermarkets now stock a wide selection of these foods as well as ranges of their own label 'Free From' foods which are sold at a more competitive price. The dietitian should make families aware of these foods in order to improve variety in the diet and to supplement their prescription entitlement. Luxury gluten-free food items can be ordered and purchased through pharmacies. The use of gluten-free alternatives to previously eaten foods can help improve compliance, e.g. breads, pasta, and breakfast cereals. It should be noted that many gluten-free cakes, biscuits, and snack foods have high sugar contents and are therefore discouraged in line with healthy eating guidance.

Prescribable foods

Currently, basic gluten-free staple food items are available on prescription in the UK. There are guidelines suggesting the numbers of items prescribed for different age groups.

Better dietary compliance has been shown with the availability of gluten-free foods on prescription. Current practice is for the dietitian to guide parents and carers on the availability of prescribable food items then request an initial prescription from the patient's GP. Families should then liaise with their surgery to finalize the prescription which may be based on individual practice/local prescribing guidelines or policies.

Monitoring

Children with coeliac disease should be seen by a dietitian at diagnosis and followed up at regular intervals to assess the following:

- Height and weight recorded and plotted on growth charts.
- Faltering growth is addressed.
- Compliance with the gluten-free diet reviewed either by 24-hour recall or food diary.
- A recent history of bowel habits and GI symptoms.
- Tissue transglutaminase antibody results are reviewed to monitor compliance.
- Dietary calcium intake (meeting a minimum of the reference nutrient intake (1991) recommendation, see Table 39.1). Supplements such as Calcichew® may be required if intake is not optimal.
- Dietary iron intake assessed particularly if low on blood testing.

These reviews should be at least once a year but ideally 6-monthly. It is beneficial to offer an initial dietetic review at 3 months after diagnosis to check symptomatic improvement and that the gluten-free diet has been fully implemented.

Table 39.1 Reference nutrient intake (RNI) values for calcium

Age	RNI mmol/day	RNI mg/day
0–12 months	13.1	524
1–3 years	8.8	352
4–6 years	11.3	452
7–10 years	13.8	552
11–14 years (male)	25.0	1000
11–14years (female))	20.0	800
15–18 years (male)	25.0	1000
15–18 years (female)	20.0	800
Adults	17.5	700

Adapted from Department of Health (1991) © Crown copyright material is reproduced with the permission of the Controller of HMSO and Queen's Printer for Scotland.

Compliance

If there are problems with adherence to the gluten-free diet, patients must be seen by the dietitian and assessed at more regular intervals (3-monthly) until compliance is re-established.

If all aspects of the diet are assessed to be strictly gluten-free, consider other possible sources of ingestion:

- Any medications/supplements and advise patients/parents to seek advice from their pharmacist.
- Inhalation of wheat flour from cooking practices.
- Contamination during food preparation, e.g. utensils, toasters, surfaces, communal use of butter/margarine/jam.
- Children playing with modelling dough (alternatives can be made with a gluten-free flour).

If appropriate, consider support from psychology/mental health team/counsellor.

Risks of non-compliance

The risks of non-compliance include:
- Persistent GI symptoms, impaired nutrition.
- Osteoporosis.
- Impaired growth and pubertal development.
- Reduced bone mineralization leading to osteoporosis.
- Infertility/low birth weight infants.
- Increased risk of GI malignancy.

Bacterial overgrowth

Small intestinal bacterial overgrowth *332*

Small intestinal bacterial growth

Small intestinal bacterial overgrowth (SIBO) refers to the syndrome of stasis of the small-bowel contents leading to bacterial proliferation and excessive numbers of bacteria being present in the small bowel (normally most of the gut bacteria are in the colon). It is also known as 'blind loop syndrome' or 'stagnant loop syndrome'.

* Symptoms include abdominal pain, distension, diarrhoea (both steatorrhoea and carbohydrate malabsorption), weight loss, and anaemia.
* Repeated courses of antibiotics, prolonged used of PPIs, gut dysmotility, and previous surgery are risk factors.
* Stasis causes bacterial proliferation. The bacteria compete for nutrients, and both the bacteria and the degradation products result in damage to the small-intestinal surface and hence absorption capacity. Carbohydrate malabsorption is common.
* Deconjugation of bile salts occurs, with fat malabsorption resulting in steatorrhoea. Fat-soluble vitamin deficiency occurs.
* Vitamin B$_{12}$ deficiency is common.
* Diagnosis is by a high index of suspicion—particularly in patients with risk factors, e.g. multiple courses of antibiotics, previous gastrointestinal surgery (particularly involving loss of the ileocaecal valve, which normally prevents the reflux of colonic contents into the small bowel), strictures, short-bowel syndrome, small-bowel dysmotility, pseudo-obstruction, use of PPIs to block gastric acid secretion.
* Any condition that reduces small-bowel motility is a risk factor.
* Culture of duodenal juice is helpful to isolate specific pathogens and inform treatment regimens. There is the potential for the emergence of resistant strains. Duodenal juice can be taken at endoscopy if performed.
* Hydrogen breath testing may be useful with an early hydrogen peak 30 minutes after ingestion of a carbohydrate load secondary to hydrogen production from the small-bowel bacteria (NB the hydrogen peak occurs when bacteria metabolize the ingested carbohydrate, usually in the colon at 2 hours).
* Small-bowel imaging should be performed if obstruction is suspected.
* D-lactic acidosis is a complication of SIBO which presents as neuroencephalopathy (irritability, confusion, aggressive behaviour, and depressed consciousness), increased anion gap metabolic acidosis, and hyperchloraemia. It is a by-product of bacterial digestion of carbohydrate and most commonly produced by Gram-positive bacteria including *Lactobacillus*. The brain is unable to metabolize d-lactate and convert it to pyruvate as it lacks D-2-hydroxyacid dehydrogenase. This leads to accumulation in the brain and neurological manifestations.
* Levels of D-lactate can be measured in blood and it can be prevented by controlling SIBO with use of antibiotics.
* Treatment involves appropriate management of the underlying cause.

- Correction of any nutritional deficit, with supplementation of nutrients and fat-soluble and B$_{12}$ vitamins if indicated. Lactose exclusion may be beneficial in the short term.
- Metronidazole, which is effective orally and intravenously, is the antibiotic of first choice to normalize the gut flora. It may require use in combination or cyclically, e.g. in children with short-bowel syndrome. Local microbiological advice should be sought in difficult cases. Alternative antibiotics include gentamicin (the IV preparation given orally) and rifaximin. Prolonged courses are often required.
- Probiotics can be used.

Acute abdominal pain

Introduction *336*
Appendicitis *337*
Intussusception *338*
Miscellaneous conditions *338*

Introduction

The commonest surgical diagnosis in children who present to hospital with acute abdominal pain is appendicitis. The differential diagnosis is wide, however (see Box 41.1), and in >50% of admissions no specific cause is found.

Box 41.1 Differential diagnosis of acute abdominal pain

This is very wide, with abdominal pain being a common presenting symptom of pathology both within and outside the gastrointestinal tract.

- Appendicitis.
- Intussusception.
- Urinary tract infection.
- Mesenteric adenitis.
- Constipation.
- Peptic ulceration.
- Meckel's diverticulum.
- Pancreatitis.
- Gastroenteritis.
- Ovarian pathology, e.g. torsion/cyst.
- Primary peritonitis.
- Henoch–Schönlein purpura.
- Hernia.
- Testicular torsion.
- Cholecystitis.
- Renal colic.
- Metabolic, e.g. acute porphyria.
- Trauma.
- Inflammatory bowel disease.
- Pelvic inflammatory disease.
- Sickle cell crisis.
- Non-abdominal causes, e.g. pneumonia.

The approach to assessment is through a detailed history and careful physical examination considering the wide differential diagnosis. Further investigations should be dictated by the clinical presentation. Age is a factor in the differential diagnosis. Other important factors in the assessment of the pain include the site, type, duration, time of day, associations, and the presence of associated symptoms including nausea, vomiting, urinary tract symptoms, or changes in bowel habit. Physical signs to assess include fever, pallor, abdominal tenderness and rigidity, presence of bowel sounds, faecal loading, and organomegaly. In boys, a testicular examination is mandatory.

The urgent priority is to establish whether there is a surgical cause that requires intervention or a medical cause that requires urgent treatment. Initial investigations to consider include a basic blood screen including full blood count, inflammatory markers, serum amylase, and urine microscopy and culture. Plain abdominal radiograph is only indicated if bowel obstruction is suspected, chest radiograph if there are any chest signs; abdominal ultrasound should be considered.

Appendicitis

- Appendicitis can occur at any age. Presentation can be as simple appendicitis, perforated appendicitis, or an appendix mass.
- The classical symptomatology is initial colicky central abdominal pain progressing to persistent localized pain in the right lower quadrant. Fever, anorexia, nausea, and vomiting are usual. Loose stool or urinary symptoms may be an associated feature. The abdomen will be tender and there may be guarding in the right lower quadrant—'Mc Burney's point' (two-thirds of the way along a line from the umbilicus to the anterior superior iliac spine). A pelvic appendicitis may not manifest with the classical abdominal signs. Rectal examination is rarely required and should only be performed if pelvic appendicitis is suspected, and undertaken once by an experienced doctor.
- White cell count is rarely helpful. A normal CRP at >24 hours is very much against the diagnosis of appendicitis (99% cases). Other investigation (urine, amylase) are to exclude differential diagnosis.
- Ultrasound is increasingly used as an acute investigation which can be diagnostic although even in experienced hands there is a false-negative rate particularly if the appendix cannot be seen or is retrocaecal. However, the absence of secondary signs of appendicitis if the appendix is not visualized is also very much against the diagnosis of appendicitis. CT is rarely required.
- Management is by appendectomy unless there is an appendix mass in which case a period on IV antibiotics with or without an interval elective appendectomy is preferred. Laparoscopic techniques are widely used.

Intussusception

- The peak incidence is at age 6–9 months although it can present later, with a male-to-female ratio of 4:1.
- Presentation is with spasmodic pain, pallor, irritability, and inconsolable crying. Vomiting is an early feature and rapidly progresses to being bile stained. Passage of blood-stained 'redcurrant jelly' stools often occurs (late) and a 'sausage-shaped' mass is frequently palpable. The presentation is often atypical, however, and requires a high index of suspicion in children who present with acute abdominal pain.
- The intussusception is usually ileocaecal, the origin being either the ileocaecal valve or the terminal ileum.
- An identifiable cause is commoner in those who present later, particularly children who present aged >2 years—Meckel's diverticulum, small-bowel polyp, cystic fibrosis, duplication cyst, lymphosarcoma, and Henoch–Schönlein purpura being examples. Preceding viral infection is a common trigger.
- Diagnosis is confirmed by ultrasound.
- Resuscitation with IV fluid is always required (usually 40mL/kg).
- Treatment is either with air-enema reduction (if the history is short, <24 hours) or surgically at laparotomy, if air enema fails or there is peritonism.
- Contraindications to air enema include peritonitis and signs of perforation.
- Recurrent intussusception occurs in ~10%.

Miscellaneous conditions

Henoch–Schönlein purpura

This is a vasculitis that affects the skin, gut, joints, and kidneys. Gastrointestinal manifestations include abdominal pain, gastrointestinal bleeding, and intussusception. Pain can be severe and corticosteroids can be used. Abdominal pain occurs secondary to the vasculitis. If intussusception occurs it tends to be in the proximal small bowel and is difficult to treat, with PN required for difficult cases. Ultrasound is the best initial investigation.

Acute porphyria

Porphyrias are rare inherited or acquired disorders of the enzymes of haem biosynthesis, and can manifest with skin (erythropoietic) or neurological (hepatic) problems or both. Acute porphyria primarily affects the nervous system resulting acute abdominal pain, vomiting, neuropathy, seizures, and mental disturbance. Abdominal pain can be severe and chronic. Constipation is common. Diagnosis is by estimation of urinary porphyrins which should be raised during an acute attack. Treatment is with a high carbohydrate load or dextrose infusion if severe.

Recurrent abdominal pain

Introduction *340*
Classification *342*
Personality type and family factors *344*
Therapeutic options *346*
Recommended clinical approach *348*
References and resources *354*

Introduction

- Recurrent abdominal pain occurs in 10–15% of school-aged children and is a frequent presenting complaint in general practice and general paediatric and paediatric gastroenterology clinics. Patients often have vague symptoms and investigation usually results in a low yield of organic disease. Treatment strategies are varied and often subjective with limited evidence upon which to base them.
- Apley described the syndrome of recurrent abdominal pain in childhood as three episodes of abdominal pain occurring during a period of 3 months, which were severe enough to affect daily activities.
- The symptom of abdominal pain in childhood is so common that it is unusual for a child to go through school years without experiencing it at some stage and up to half of all children with recurrent abdominal pain do not present to the doctor although their pain is often as severe as in those who do. Therefore, this symptom is often considered trivial by the patient or family, presumably because of mild severity or transient nature. Usually, it is only when the pain impacts the functioning of the child or family that medical help is sought.
- The differential diagnosis is wide and one of the early priorities in the assessment of children with recurrent abdominal pain is the exclusion of serious underlying organic pathology. The various significant organic disorders are dealt with in the relevant chapters of this handbook. In most patients the aetiology is functional or unclear.
- Multiple factors have been implicated in the aetiology of childhood abdominal pain, including psychological stress, visceral hypersensitivity, previously undiagnosed organic disorders, infection with *Helicobacter pylori*, gastrointestinal motility disorders, abdominal migraine, food intolerances, and constipation.
- The psychological environment within the family may be relevant in the aetiology. The biophysical model proposes that recurrent abdominal pain is the child's response to biological factors, governed by an interaction between the child's temperament and the family and school environments.
- Acceptance by parents and child of a biopsychosocial model of illness is an important factor for the resolution of symptoms.
- Many cases of childhood recurrent abdominal pain respond to acknowledgement of the symptoms and reassurance regarding the lack of serious underlying organic disease.
- Recent evidence points to a slightly increased future relative risk of inflammatory bowel disease in those with functional symptoms; referral of those who develop new red flag symptoms is recommended.

Classification

It is useful in the clinical assessment to classify cases by subtype (see Table 42.1):

- Functional abdominal pain.
- Functional dyspepsia.
- Irritable bowel syndrome (IBS).
- Abdominal migraine.

However, not all children can be easily classified into one group.

- Children with functional dyspepsia require consideration of organic disease such as GOR, peptic ulceration, or *H. pylori* infection. Night pain should prompt referral for endoscopy. Constipation should be excluded, as severe constipation with loading can present as epigastric discomfort/bloating. Dyspeptic symptoms may follow a viral illness.
- It is estimated that 10–20% of adolescents have symptoms suggestive of IBS. The diagnosis of IBS is supported by abnormal stool frequency (frequent, infrequent), abnormal stool type (loose, hard, mixed), abnormal stool passage (pain, incomplete rectal evacuation), passage of mucus, and bloating/distension. There are many physical and psychosocial factors that can impact symptoms, with functional and family factors being relevant.
- It is likely that abdominal migraine, cyclical vomiting syndrome, and migraine headache are different manifestations of the same disorder along a symptom spectrum. The diagnosis of abdominal migraine is supported by a positive family history of migraine headache. Many patients have a history of travel sickness. Dietary triggers include caffeine and foods containing nitrites or amines.
- Children with functional abdominal pain are often the most difficult to manage.
- Stress is often a major factor. It is important, however, to remember that stress can be either physical or psychological or a combination of the two, and reflects the response to external factors of the inherent personality type.
- Parents often associate pain severity and persistence with increased likelihood of disease; identifying absence of red flag symptoms (including the absence of symptoms when asleep) is a key part of reassurance.

Table 42.1 Classification of recurrent abdominal pain according to the Rome IV criteria

Functional dyspepsia	*Criteria must be fulfilled for at least 2 months before diagnosis and must include all of the following:* One or more of the following features for ≥4 days/ month: 1) Persistent or recurrent epigastric pain or burning not relieved by defecation or change in bowel pattern (i.e. not IBS) 2) Early satiety 3) Postprandial fullness After appropriate medical evaluation, the symptoms cannot be attributed to another medical condition
Irritable bowel syndrome	*Criteria must be fulfilled for at least 2 months before diagnosis and must include all of the following:* Abdominal discomfort or pain for ≥4 days/month that has two out of three features: 1) Related to defecation 2) Pain with change in frequency and/or form of stool 3) In children with constipation, pain persists despite constipation resolution 4) After appropriate evaluation, the symptoms cannot be attributed to another medical condition
Functional abdominal pain	*Criteria must be fulfilled for at least 2 months before diagnosis and must include all of the following:* ● Episodic/continuous abdominal pain for ≥4 days/ month ● Pain unrelated to physiological events (e.g. eating) ● Loss of daily functioning. The pain is not feigned ● Insufficient criteria for other functional gastrointestinal disorders that would explain the abdominal pain
Abdominal migraine	*Criteria fulfilled two or more times in the preceding 6 months and must include:* ● Paroxysmal episodes of intense, acute periumbilical pain that lasts ≥1 hour ● Intervening periods of normal health ● Pain is incapacitating and impacts on functioning Two of the following features: ● Anorexia ● Nausea ● Vomiting ● Headache ● Photophobia ● Pallor After appropriate evaluation, the symptoms cannot be fully explained by another medical condition.

Adapted from Hyams JS et al. Childhood Functional Gastrointestinal Disorders: Child/ Adolescent: Gastroenterology 2016;150:1456–1468 with permission from the AGA Institute and Elsevier.

Personality type and family factors

Children with functional symptoms tend to be rather timid, nervous, anxious characters. They are often perfectionists—overachievers with an increased number of stresses, who are more likely to internalize problems than other children. School absence is common. There may be a degree of school refusal or separation anxiety in the younger child. There may be specific issues of importance in the school environment.

There may be significant stresses within the family environment, such as marital discord, separation, divorce, excessive arguing, and extreme parenting (over-submissive or excessive punishment). Factors such as a family history of alcoholism, antisocial or conduct disorders, or the presence of somatization disorders within the wider family setting may be relevant.

Children with recurrent abdominal pain that becomes chronic often come from families with a high frequency of medical complaints, particularly recurrent abdominal pain, nervous breakdown, migraine, or maternal depression.

Common stresses in children with recurrent abdominal pain

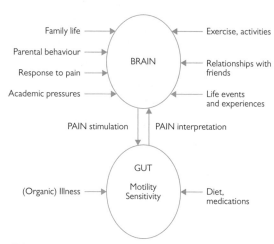

Fig. 42.1 A biopsychosocial model of pain: for use with parents and patients.

Physical stresses
- Recent physical illness.
- Postviral infection which can present as a postviral gastroparesis.
- Food intolerance—poor diet, wheat, carbohydrate intolerance, excess sorbitol.
- Different and/or multiple medications, e.g. NSAIDs, antispasmodics.
- Constipation.
- Lack of exercise/obesity.
- Chronic illness.

Psychosocial stresses
- Death of a family member.
- Separation of a family member—divorce, child going to college.
- Illness in parents or sibling including functional illnesses.
- School problem.
- Altered peer relationships.
- Poverty.
- Geographical move.

Therapeutic options

The evidence base for therapeutic interventions is poor, probably reflecting the wide spectrum of different aetiologies and considerable differences in clinical phenotypes and triggering factors. This means management that tends to be subjective and based largely on the experience of individuals working in the field

Standard medical care/reassurance

This is the cornerstone of effective medical management. Many cases will respond to acknowledgement of the symptoms and reassurance regarding the lack of serious underlying organic disease, including comparison with the high proportion of adults with IBS and its significant functional impact.

Psychological intervention

The aims of psychological therapy are to modify thoughts, beliefs, and behavioural responses to symptoms and the effects of illness. Therapeutic modalities include biofeedback, relaxation therapy, behavioural therapy, cognitive therapy, coping skills training, hypnosis or self-hypnosis, and family therapy. Explanation of the role of these strategies to families, and the evidence base, helps the psychological intervention, and often contributes a detailed evaluation of the psychological stressors.

Lifestyle and dietary management

There is a lack of published evidence, but it seems sensible to recommend healthy eating including plenty of fruit and vegetables, regular sensible meals, and plenty of fluids. Food that can potentially aggravate symptoms (e.g. fatty food, spicy food, fizzy drinks) should be avoided. Dietary triggers should be avoided in abdominal migraine. Dietary strategies should go hand in hand with a daily routine which includes exercise and is not unduly sedentary. An extended part of this strategy is to promote school attendance if that is an issue.

Pharmacological therapy

Many pharmacological interventions have been tried in treatment of recurrent abdominal pain but few have been tested in clinical trials. Managing parental expectations given the limitations of prescriptions for functional symptoms is important:

- Medication that can aggravate symptoms should be avoided, e.g. NSAIDs in functional dyspepsia.
- Commonly prescribed agents include simple analgesics and antispasmodics.
- Pizotifen is probably of use in abdominal migraine (see Table 42.1).
- There is a role for a trial of H_2 antagonists and probably PPIs in children with functional dyspepsia, and should be continued only if effective. Prokinetics such as domperidone should not routinely be used (note Medicines and Healthcare products Regulatory Agency alert).
- Peppermint oil is useful in children with IBS.
- Laxatives are helpful when constipation or incomplete rectal evacuation is felt to contribute to recurrent abdominal pain. This can be a feature in children with functional dyspepsia secondary to faecal loading or IBS.

Outcome

Recurrent abdominal pain may be the antecedent of IBS in adults, but there have been few long-term studies. Retrospective data suggest an increased incidence of psychiatric disorders in adulthood, particularly anxiety disorders.

The acceptance of the biopsychosocial model by the patients and their families is an important factor in the response to therapy

Recommended clinical approach

Exclude organic disease

The history and examination should be carefully scrutinized for features suggestive of organic pathology, bearing in mind the wide-ranging differential diagnosis of organic disorders that may present with recurrent abdominal pain.

- It is important to recognize that diet, lifestyle, and constipation may be significant factors in the child with recurrent abdominal pain.
- In the absence of likely underlying organic disease, it is often useful to elicit clinical features known to be associated with recurrent abdominal pain, such as psychological stress and anxiety. Many of these will become apparent while taking a detailed social history. Typical adverse social factors leading to psychological stress include bereavement, altered peer relationships, school problems, and illness of a family member. High achievers are at risk, particularly those who have excessive out-of-school activities. It is important not just to ask about illnesses in the family but also to ask about how those illnesses impact the family. In some families there is an 'illness model' and this puts the child at increased risk of functional symptoms. This part of the assessment may also reveal a family history of anxiety disorders, or an anxious temperament in the child.

Box 42.1 Important organic causes

- GOR/oesophagitis.
- Peptic ulcer disease.
- *Helicobacter pylori* infection.
- Food intolerance.
- Coeliac disease.
- Inflammatory bowel disease.
- Constipation.
- Urinary tract disorders.
- Dysmenorrhoea.
- Pancreatitis.
- Hepatobiliary disease.
- Anatomical abnormalities, e.g. Meckel's diverticulum/malrotation.

Box 42.2 Symptoms suggestive of organic disease

- Age <5 years.
- Constitutional problems:
  - Fever.
  - Weight loss.
  - Delayed growth.
  - Skin rashes.
  - Arthralgia.
- Vomiting—particularly if bilious.
- Nocturnal pain that wakes the child.
- Pain away from the umbilicus.
- Urinary symptoms.
- Family history:
  - Inflammatory bowel disease.
  - Coeliac disease.
  - Peptic ulcer disease.
- Perianal disease.
- Bloody stool (gross or occult).

Classify by symptomatology

The next key step is to attempt to classify the abdominal pain according to symptom subtypes, as documented in the Rome criteria (see Table 42.1). Establishing a diagnostic label helps give families certainty and move families towards rehabilitation. Although these criteria are not strictly validated, they do allow the clinician to target further investigation and management.

Targeted investigations

The mainstay of management of these patients is reassurance. Nevertheless, the symptoms may impact the child's and family's functioning enough to warrant further investigation. For such cases, suggested initial investigations are listed in Box 42.3. Overall, in the absence of red flag symptoms, <5% of patients have identifiable disease, and investigations should be rationalized accordingly and potential risks (e.g. from endoscopy) explained to families.

The role of initial investigations is to help identify organic disease. However, secondary investigations may be indicated if there are suggestive symptoms and signs, initial investigations are suggestive of organic disease symptoms, or symptoms are atypical. It is logical to use a targeted approach to further investigation according to symptom subtype. If initial investigations are normal, and based on the clinical assessment organic

---

Box 42.3 Suggested initial investigations

- Full blood count/erythrocyte sedimentation rate/CRP.
- Renal and liver function.
- Coeliac antibody testing (tTG IgA and total IgA).
- Urine microscopy and culture.
- Faecal calprotectin.

---

pathology is felt to be unlikely, it is important to avoid doing more tests and emphasize the normal results.

Second-line investigations that might be appropriate include ultrasound of the abdomen, renal tract and pelvis, barium radiology, and endoscopy. *H. pylori* testing may be appropriate in functional dyspepsia.

Explanation

Finding the right way of explaining how functional conditions can cause pain is key to helping parents accept your diagnosis and implement your management plan. Using understandable language appropriate for the family is vital, and different models can be used.

Helping parents know that increased pain doesn't mean increased likelihood of disease in the absence of red flags:

At the easier conceptual end:

> 'You know many children have "butterflies" before a stressful situation, e.g. an exam or a roller-coaster ride. Your child's on the severe end of this and her "butterflies" cause her pain, but aren't a disease.'

One can also discuss visceral hypersensitivity (substance P and other nociceptive transmitters increased by physical/psychological stressors causing normal bowel activity such as peristalsis to be perceived as pain—see Fig. 42.2).

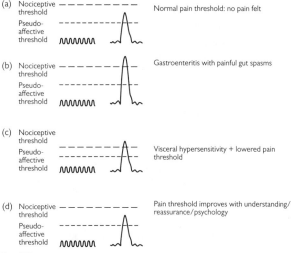

Fig. 42.2 Modifiable pain thresholds in recurrent abdominal pain. Adapted from Sarna SK. (2010) Colonic Motility: From Bench Side to Bedside, In: Colloquium Series on Integrated Systems Physiology, ed. Granger DN and Granger JP. https://doi.org/10.4199/C00020ED1V01Y201011ISP011. Used with permission from Morgan & Claypool Life Sciences.

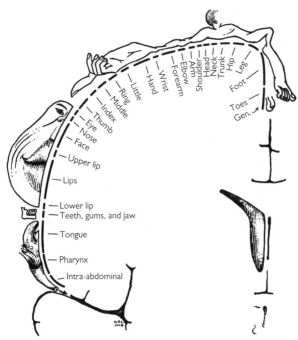

Fig. 42.3 Sensory homunculus (postcentral gyrus). Reprinted from The Hermunculus: What Is Known about the Representation of the Female Body in the Brain? Cereb Cortex. 2012;23(5):1005–1013. doi:10.1093/cercor/bhs005 Cereb Cortex © The Author 2012. Published by Oxford University Press. All rights reserved.

Many children appreciate the concept of the sensory homunculus (Fig. 42.3) and that children can easily develop a persistent 'pain feedback loop' within the brain, even when the gut has recovered and that reassurance and distraction helps reduce or break this loop.

Treatment/therapeutic approach

- The mainstay of treatment is reassurance, and the emphasis being on rehabilitation. Therefore, the first step is to acknowledge to the family and child that the pain is a real symptom.
- It is then necessary to recognize and treat any underlying or contributing factors. This may include a tendency to constipation.
- Avoid excessive medications such as NSAIDs.

- Promote a healthy diet and lifestyle. Assessment by a dietitian may be helpful. It is worthwhile identifying dietary triggers, and suggesting alternatives.
- If the patient has an anxious temperament or is missing an excessive amount of school, consider psychology/mental health assessment.
- Parents who adopt a strategy of distraction and normalization for their children markedly improve their children's self-reported pain and anxiety scores over time, however parents who worry and get distressed by their children's symptoms are more likely to see their child's pain scores remain high or worsen over time. Many families are looking for an explanation for the symptoms and need to have discussed with them the inseparability of physical and psychological causes of symptoms, e.g. stress following viral illness, 'sick with worry', anxiety (with 'butterflies') prior to exams.
- Graded rehabilitation with a goal-based approach, setting simple targets such as optimizing school attendance, graded exercise programme, and reducing NSAIDs.
- Most children can be discharged once the diagnosis has been made. The more severe and long-standing cases in whom, for example, school attendance is poor may benefit from psychological support and require follow-up until symptoms resolve and to give an opportunity for any psychiatric co-morbidity to emerge.

References and resources

Berger YM, Gieteling MJ, Benninga MA. Chronic abdominal pain in children. BMJ 2007;334:997–1002.

Brown LK, Beattie RM, Tighe MP. Practical management of functional abdominal pain in children. Arch Dis Child 2016;101:677–83.

Hyams JS, Di Lorenzo C, Saps M, Shulman RJ, Staiano A, van Tilburg M. Childhood functional gastrointestinal disorders: child/adolescent. Gastroenterology 2016;150:1456–68.

Spiller R, Aziz Q, Creed F, et al. Guidelines on the irritable bowel syndrome: mechanisms and practical management. Gut 2007;56:177–98. Available from http://www.bsg.org.uk

Tighe MP, Beattie RM. Functional abdominal pain and other functional gastrointestinal disorders. In: Guandalini S, Dhawan A, Branski D (eds.), Textbook of pediatric gastroenterology, hepatology and nutrition. Cham: Springer; 2016, pp. 215–31.

Chronic constipation

Introduction 356
Pathogenesis 358
Clinical assessment 359
Investigation 360
Practical management 362
Outcome 368
Indications to refer for specialist advice 'red flags' 369
Case studies 369
References and resources 370

Introduction

Chronic functional constipation is a common problem in childhood. Without early treatment, the condition is likely to impact all aspects of the child's life, including education and psychological well-being as well as physical growth and development.

The key to successful management is early diagnosis and prompt treatment with an emphasis on practical management strategies with multidisciplinary support where needed. Conventional treatment relies on patient education, behavioural modification, and drugs.

- Constipation is defined as a delay in the passage of stool leading to distress and may include other symptoms such as pain, discomfort, anorexia, soiling, or encopresis.
- Soiling refers to the leakage of stool in the context of a megarectum.
- Encopresis (inconsistently defined in the medical literature) refers to the passage of normal stool at an inappropriate time/in an inappropriate place in the absence of constipation.
- The Paris Consensus on Childhood Constipation Terminology (PACCT) Group's recommended terminology is shown in Table 43.1.
- The mean stool frequency in the first week of life is around 4 a day, although some breastfed normal infants may not pass a stool for several days.
- In general, the trend throughout childhood is a decreasing stool frequency up to the age of 4 years, at which time stool frequency is the same as in adult life with most schoolchildren in the range between three a day and one every 2 days.

The prevalence of constipation in childhood varies with age. The peak incidence of occurs around toilet training (age 2–4) although prevalence remains high throughout childhood and into adult life.

Table 43.1 Paris Consensus on Childhood Constipation Terminology (PACCT) group's recommended terminology

Suggested terminology	PACCT group definition
Chronic constipation	The occurrence of two or more of the following characteristics, during the last 8 weeks:
	Frequency of bowel movements <3/week
	>1 episode of faecal incontinence per week
	Large stools in the rectum or palpable on abdominal examination
	Passing of stools so large that they may obstruct the toilet
	Display of retentive posturing and withholding behaviours
	Painful defecation
Faecal incontinence	Passage of stools in an inappropriate place
Organic faecal incontinence	Faecal incontinence resulting from organic disease (e.g. neurological damage or sphincter abnormalities)
Functional faecal incontinence	Non-organic disease which can be subdivided into:
	Constipation-associated faecal incontinence
	Non-retentive (non-constipation-associated) faecal incontinence

Reprinted from Benninga M, Candy DC, Catto-Smith AG, et al. The Paris Consensus on Childhood Constipation Terminology (PACCT) Group. J Pediatr Gastroenterol Nutr 2005;40(3):273–275 with permission from Wolters Kluwer.

Pathogenesis

The physiology of normal defecation depends on the interplay of multiple factors:

- Stool is moved through the distal colon by peristaltic contractions of the bowel wall.
- This movement is influenced by colonic tone, which in turn is influenced by diurnal variation and the gastrocolonic reflex (altered colonic tone in response to a meal).
- Once the stool enters the rectosigmoid junction, distension of the rectal wall results in reflex rectal contraction with concomitant relaxation of the internal anal sphincter.
- Stool is therefore presented to the anal canal and enters the so-called firing position.
- Stool is perceived in the anal canal, and a decision to expel or withhold the faeces is made.
- Interruptions at any stage during this process may lead to constipation.

The commonest interruption is a painful stimulus perceived during defaecation at around the time of toilet training (e.g. anal fissure secondary to the passage of hard stool). Once the painful stimulus has occurred, the child may learn that voluntary withholding of stool prevents recurrence of the stimulus. This may lead to a stool-withholding cycle, which may ultimately lead to faecal impaction and overflow faecal incontinence. Prolonged faecal impaction can lead to chronic rectal distension and eventual loss of normal rectal sensation. This can lead to further impaction of stool and megarectum. This is known as functional constipation—i.e. constipation in the absence of underlying organic disease. It is the cause of childhood constipation in ~95% of cases.

Chronic functional constipation may coexist with other functional disorders. One example of this is irritable bowel syndrome (IBS), which may exist in a 'constipation-predominant' form. The symptom of incomplete rectal evacuation is likely to be a factor and although there is no good quality evidence that IBS may improve with laxatives in children, there is some evidence from adults.

Differential diagnosis of chronic constipation

- Hirschsprung disease.
- Anorectal anomalies (e.g. anal stenosis).
- Neuronal intestinal dysplasia.
- Spina bifida.
- Neuromuscular disease.
- Hypothyroidism.
- Hypercalcaemia.
- Coeliac disease.
- Food allergy/intolerance.
- Cystic fibrosis.
- Perianal group A streptococcal infection.
- Anal fissure.
- Pelvic/spinal tumours.
- Child sexual abuse.
- Drugs.

Clinical assessment

Key features in the history

- Delay in passage of meconium: the vast majority of infants will pass meconium within 48 hours of birth; delayed passage of meconium raises the possibility of Hirschsprung disease.
- Age at onset of symptoms: typical age of onset for functional constipation is 2–4 years, around the age of toilet training.
- Consistency/nature of stool: infrequent, very large stool (large enough to block the toilet) is common in chronic functional constipation.
- Painful or bloody stools: the differential diagnosis should include anal fissure, perianal group A streptococcal infection, or, rarely, sexual abuse.
- Abdominal pain: a very common symptom in childhood, and is a feature of many organic and functional disorders. Many constipated children have recurrent abdominal pain, which may be relieved by the periodic passage of large stool.
- Stool-withholding behaviour: voluntary stool withholding may manifest as unusual behaviour, which may be mistaken for straining.
- Soiling: occurs as a result of involuntary passage of liquid stool around faecal impaction in the rectum. It is almost always associated with psychological distress in the child or family.
- Diet: children with chronic constipation may have a history of anorexia, poor energy intake, and poor fluid intake. Low fibre intake is common. Cow's milk allergy may be a factor in some children, particularly if other atopic features are present.
- Urinary symptoms: urinary tract infections, urinary frequency, and nocturnal enuresis are common in chronically constipated children.
- Family history of constipation/IBS.

Key points in examination

- General health, nutritional status, and growth.
- Abdominal palpation: this will reveal a faecal mass in at least half of all chronically constipated children. The size of the mass reflects the extent of rectal/colonic involvement. Usually the mass is palpable in the suprapubic area, but in severe cases may extend above the umbilicus. If the child is obese or if the stool is soft (e.g. after laxatives have been introduced) palpation can be difficult.
- Perianal inspection: the perianal area should be carefully inspected for signs of soiling, inflammation (which may be due to streptococcal infection), anal fissure, or congenital abnormalities such as anterior anus. In rare cases there may be signs of sexual abuse.
- Rectal examination: if the clinical features are typical of functional chronic constipation, the digital rectal examination is unlikely to add further useful information. Furthermore, a rectal examination is invasive and may compound the underlying fear of anal pain and toileting. However, if there are clinical features suggestive of underlying organic pathology (e.g. Hirschsprung disease, anal stenosis particularly in infancy) a single rectal examination be indicated to assess anal tone, calibre, position, and the presence of stool in the rectum. It should only be done by a healthcare professional competent to interpret findings including anatomical abnormalities.
- Neurological assessment including inspection of the lumbar-sacral spine and examination of the lower limbs is essential.

Investigation

If the history and examination are typical of chronic functional constipation, further investigations are not generally indicated. The following lists some of the investigations that can be considered but should not be routine:

- Abdominal radiograph: useful to demonstrate underlying spinal abnormalities and to delineate the extent of faecal loading. Only indicated in rare cases, where there is a strong suspicion of neural tube defect, or the abdominal examination is not conclusive. This should not be routine as there is a high radiation dose.
- Bowel transit studies: segmental colonic transit time may be assessed by measuring the position of swallowed radio-opaque markers on plain abdominal radiographs. This is a specialist investigation and its diagnostic use is questionable, since up to 50% of chronically constipated children may be shown to have normal colon transit time, although severely delayed transit is associated with a poor prognosis.
- Anorectal manometry: this is an invasive investigation not indicated as first line, the main purpose being to demonstrate the normal relaxation of the internal anal sphincter in response to rectal distension.
- Full thickness rectal biopsy: diagnostic of Hirschsprung disease and indicated only if there is a strong clinical suspicion.
- Coeliac antibody screen: coeliac disease is common and constipation can be the presenting feature.
- Electrolytes, micronutrients, endocrine assessment: iron deficiency is common in childhood constipation. Electrolyte (e.g. hypercalcaemia) and endocrine abnormalities (e.g. hypothyroidism) should be considered if the history and examination are suggestive.
- Allergy: in children with atopic features (rhinitis, dermatitis, or bronchospasm) and evidence of proctitis or perianal erythema, investigation for cow's milk allergy/allergic colitis should be considered.

Practical management

The practical management of chronic constipation is not just about laxatives. Patients and their families need a full clinical assessment as outlined previously in this chapter, emphasizing in particular family and social factors that may impact the condition and its management. If, for example, there is a coexistent behavioural or emotional problem then the management of that will be relevant to the management of the constipation. The successful management of the constipation, particularly when soiling is a major factor, may impact the behavioural problem.

Emphasis on the many factors relevant in the aetiology of chronic constipation is fundamental from the outset.

There are seven general principles of management, of which drug therapy plays a major role. Unless the first six principles are considered, drug therapy is rarely effective.

1. Explanation of normal bowel function

Careful explanation of this process to the parents (and child if appropriate) helps the family understand the disorder and aids compliance with therapy. A basic understanding of the pathophysiology may also relieve tensions in the family associated with blame and guilt.

2. Diet/fluids and exercise

A high-fibre diet is recommended, along with adequate fluid. Dietary fibre/bulking agents help retain water in the gut lumen by osmosis, and stimulate peristalsis by adding bulk to the stool. Regular exercise promotes intestinal peristalsis and helps with bowel transit.

3. Behavioural advice

Gaining a child's trust is important. Time needs to be spent reassuring children about their condition and the treatment. The psychological principle of ignoring failure and rewarding success is important. Anything that helps relax the child will help with the defecation problem, whether it is fear of pain or persistent soiling. Conflict should be avoided. It is vital that the child wants to get better.

4. Toilet training advice

Regular toileting is a crucial part of the management. Children need to be encouraged to sit on the toilet on waking, after all meals, and before bed. It is important the child has a comfortable position, e.g. toilet seat with foot support. It must be stressed to the parents that this is the most important part of the child's management. It is important that the child sits on the toilet for long enough.

5. Simple reward schemes

Reward schemes can be highly effective in the behavioural management. The star chart can be used but any attractive variation of this can be used to appeal to each particular child (e.g. sticker charts, computer game time). Rewards can be given for compliance at first (e.g. sitting on toilet twice a day after breakfast and tea), and later rewards are given for success (e.g. bowels opened into the toilet).

6. Reassurance and encouragement

Parents ought to be reassured that constipation is common and that the prognosis is generally good.

7. Ongoing support

The child and family need ongoing support from specialist healthcare professionals/school nurses/specialist nurses.

Drug therapy

There is no right strategy for pharmacological intervention, and there is wide variation between different units in the regimens used. The evidence base is poor. There is no best fit for all patients and many cases require individual treatment plans. Open discussions are needed from the outset about compliance. Parents and the child need to be aware that any laxative regimen may in the short-term increase soiling particularly if the toileting regimen is not being adhered to. Frequent support and follow-up is required during the initial phases with encouragement not to give up as soon as the stools become loose. Many medications are available (see Table 43.2).

Table 43.2 Pharmaceutical agents used in the treatment of constipation: mode of action

Class of drug:	Mode of action/properties	Example drugs
Osmotic agents	Increase quantity of water in large bowel by osmosis	Lactulose, Macrogols, e.g. polyethylene glycol Magnesium sulfate Phosphate enema
Stimulant laxatives	Increase intestinal motility	Anthraquinones, e.g. Senna, Bisacodyl, Docusate, Picosulfate
Lubricants/softeners	Lubricate/soften impacted stool	Mineral oil, e.g. arachis oil, liquid paraffin, Docusate
Bulking agent	Increase faecal mass and therefore stimulate peristalsis	Fibre, Bran, Isphagula Methylcellulose Erythromycin
Other agents	Prokinetics	

Reprinted from Plunkett A, Phillips CP, Beattie RM. Management of chronic constipation in childhood. Pediatr Drugs 2007;9(1):33–45 with permission from Springer.

Disimpaction

The basic principle is to first disimpact if there is a megarectum in order to facilitate normal defecation dynamics and then give a sufficiently high laxative dose to ensure regular emptying.

Local therapy (manual evacuation, enemas, suppositories) can be used although can exacerbate the stool withholding and/or exacerbate toilet-phobic behaviour, which is usually present in children with chronic constipation, so oral therapy is often preferred. Options include polyethylene glycol, senna, sodium picosulfate elixir, bisacodyl, liquid paraffin, sodium docusate,

Picolax,® or local therapy (e.g. Micralax® enema, phosphate enema) if the above options fail.

It is essential that high doses are used and that mechanisms are put in place to monitor the child and ensure compliance. Increased soiling is often seen during the early phase of disimpaction.

Senna can be used as a sole agent given in the evening in stepwise increasing doses, increased by 5mL (7.5mg) at a time until at least daily evacuation is achieved. This can be usually done as an outpatient. Doses of 15–30mL, as syrup or tablets, are generally required. It is important to make patients aware that senna takes 10–12 hours to work and therefore an adequate evening dose should result in a bowel motion the next morning. It is important to stress that the child needs to sit on the toilet regularly for this to occur. The peak stimulant effect is in the morning and after breakfast there will be an enhanced gastrocolonic reflex.

Polyethylene glycol can be used similarly as a sole agent in increasing doses until effective bowel emptying is achieved. It is best given in a twice-daily regimen. High doses are generally required particularly if there is significant loading.

In children in whom impaction is severe, other agents may be needed including sodium picosulfate, as the elixir (5–10mL) or Picolax® sachets (half to one) given daily or polyethylene glycol sachets at higher dose. All three are options and the regimen needs to be tailored to the needs of the individual child.

Regimens may take several days to take effect. Sodium picosulfate in particular has a significant osmotic effect and requires a high fluid intake.

Maintenance

Laxatives are often required for a prolonged period. The laxative regimen used needs to be consistent and given regularly, with weaning only after a sustained period of normal stooling with no soiling. The choice of laxative is probably less important than the compliance of the child and parent with the treatment regimen.

There is considerable debate about which laxative to use long term; long-term stimulant laxatives (other than as rescue) are not advocated in North America but they are widely used in the UK.

Many centres use polyethylene glycol as first line.

Senna given in the evening can be effective. Children with long-standing, severe constipation will often require high doses. The aim is to produce a formed or semi-formed stool regularly (hopefully daily), although some children on senna will always produce an unformed stool. It may take a few weeks to find the correct dose for an individual child; maintenance dose is usually 10–20mL senna nocte. The maximum dose is usually not more than 30mL.

Alternative laxatives can be used when senna fails.

Weaning from high-dose laxatives

Treatment may be needed for many months, or even years in very severe cases. Eventually almost all children will require progressively less and wean off over time. The weaning regimen should be cautious, tailored to the individual child, and regularly reviewed. Early weaning will invariably result in relapse of the constipation.

Notes on commonly used laxatives

- *Lactulose* is a non-absorbable disaccharide of the sugars D-galactose and D-fructose. It is not absorbed from the small intestine because it is resistant to hydrolysis by digestive enzymes. It is fermented by colonic bacteria in the colon. The by-products of this process exert a local osmotic effect, resulting in an increased faecal bulk and stimulation of peristalsis. The side effects of treatment are predominantly secondary to intraluminal fermentation and gas production. This may lead to flatulence, bloating, and cramping abdominal pains. Lactulose may exacerbate soiling in the presence of faecal impaction. It is often the first-line choice of drug prescribed for acute/mild constipation in children.

- *Polyethylene glycol* has been used for some time in high dose for bowel lavage prior to gastrointestinal procedures. Recently, a lower-dose form (PEG 3350, Movicol,® Movicol Paediatric Plain®) has become available and been used successfully as an alternative treatment for acute and chronic constipation being effective in both the disimpaction and maintenance phases. Its large molecular size renders it unabsorbed in the intestinal tract. It therefore produces a local osmotic effect, preventing the absorption of water from the faeces. Unlike lactulose it does not result in the production of gas secondary to bacterial fermentation and consequently has fewer side effects (such as bloating and flatus).

- *Stimulant laxatives* include *senna, bisacodyl, sodium docusate* (also a softener), and *sodium picosulfate*. These agents work by increasing intestinal motility. A common side effect is, therefore, colicky abdominal pain particularly in the presence of retained stool. Stimulant laxatives are widely used in the management of chronic functional constipation—in both the disimpaction and the maintenance phase. They are both safe and effective. Despite the ubiquitous nature of the use of drugs such as senna, docusate, and sodium picosulfate, there is very little empirical data to support their use. A recent Cochrane review of the use of stimulant laxatives for the treatment of constipation and soiling in children found no randomized controlled trials that met the selection criteria for analysis. The authors concluded that there is insufficient evidence to guide the use of stimulant laxatives and more research is needed. Nevertheless, in the UK, senna in particular is commonly used in the maintenance phase of treatment. Its longer mode of action compared with other agents such as lactulose make it more applicable to the school-aged child, where an evening dose may precipitate a bowel motion the following morning.

- *Liquid paraffin (or mineral oil)* is a petroleum derivative. Historically it has been a popular choice of drug for the treatment of constipation and faecal impaction. Its main effect is thought to be as a stool lubricant (although the conversion of the oil to fatty acids also exerts an osmotic effect). Although widely used in North America, it is not commonly used in the UK.

- *Enema therapy* is occasionally required in acute faecal impaction or oral medication fails. Children find this treatment unpleasant and it can exacerbate stool-withholding behaviour. There have been numerous reports about toxicity of phosphate enemas secondary to absorption, leading to profound metabolic changes.

Key points in management
- Chronic functional constipation is a common problem in childhood with soiling a significant issue. The morbidity is high and treatment complex.
- There is a very poor evidence base for the drug treatments used and considerable differences in practice in different units.
- The key to successful management is early diagnosis and prompt treatment with multidisciplinary support where needed.

Outcome

Children with chronic constipation require follow-up until full recovery and then benefit from a consolidation period. There is a high frequency of relapse. It is usual practice therefore to offer long-term follow-up. The length of follow-up depends on time to full recovery and the likelihood of relapse.

Early identification and effective treatment will improve the outcome.

Indications to refer for specialist advice 'red flags'

- Children in whom aggressive bowel clearance, e.g. picosulfate, needs to be considered.
- Children in whom significant behaviour/psychosocial problems are impacting the management of their constipation.
- Failure to respond to high doses of laxatives.
- Persistent soiling despite laxatives.
- Structural/physical cause cannot be excluded.
- Concern regarding nutrition/poor growth.
- Anal fissure or rectal prolapse if there is failure to be cured by a reasonable course (3 months) of laxatives.

Case studies

Case study 1

A 3-year-old boy (previously toilet trained) presents with constipation. He has just recovered from an acute gastrointestinal illness. He is off his food, irritable, and stooling only once every 3 days passing hard stools with pain and fresh blood per rectum. He is rather pale. Growth is normal. He has palpable stools and perianal soreness. Basic investigations are normal including urine culture, perianal skin swab, and coeliac antibody screen. He is in a stool-withholding cycle whereby it is painful to pass stool so he doesn't, but resisting the urge to pass stool compounds the problem. This is managed with laxatives (at reasonable doses), regular toileting, and explanation and reassurance.

Case study 2

A 10-year-old boy presents with soiling. He is a rather picky eater and doesn't eat breakfast. His fluid intake is poor. He has had recurrent urinary tract infections and wets at night. He has behavioural problems although is in mainstream education. He is constantly teased. He was born preterm. His brother has attention deficit disorder. Clinical examination is unremarkable apart from palpable faecal loading and old stool around the anal margin. Basic investigations are unremarkable. His faecal loading suggests that the soiling is secondary to overflow. The normal defecation dynamics have been lost as a consequence of his permanently distended rectum. Management is with high-dose laxatives (disimpaction then maintenance) with attention to diet, fluids, and regular toileting particularly after meals. He is clean within a few days, but laxative dependent for several months. He continues with his early morning routine of breakfast (with a drink), then toileting. He gradually becomes dry at night. His confidence and behaviour improve.

References and resources

BMJ Best Practice. Constipation in children 2017, http://bestpractice.bmj.com/best-practice/monograph/784.html

Education and Resources for Improving Childhood Continence: http://www.eric.org.uk

National Institute for Health and Care Excellence (NICE). Constipation in children and young people: diagnosis and management. Clinical Guideline CG99. London: NICE; 2017. http://www.nice.org.uk/Guidance/CG99

Tabbers MM, DiLorenzo C, Berger MY, et al. Evaluation and treatment of functional constipation in infants and children: evidence based recommendations from ESPGHAN and NASPGHAN. J Pediatr Gastroenterol Nutr 2014;58:258–74. http://www.espghan.org/fileadmin/user_upload/guidelines_pdf/IBD/Evaluation_and_Treatment_of_Functional.24.pdf

Perianal disorders

Examination *372*
Anal fissure *372*
Perianal streptococcal infection, 'soggy bottom' *373*
Threadworm infestations *373*
Rectal prolapse *373*
Solitary rectal ulcer syndrome *374*
Inflammatory bowel disease *374*

Examination

The perianal examination is one of the most important parts of the examination of the gastrointestinal tract. This is best done by inspection with the patient lying in the left lateral position. The perianal region can be inspected by gently parting the buttocks.

Perianal redness is most commonly seen.

Differential diagnosis of perianal redness

- Poor perineal hygiene.
- Soiling/encopresis.
- Perianal streptococcal infection.
- Threadworm infestation.
- Lactose intolerance (acidic stool).
- Anal fissure.
- Inflammatory bowel disease.
- Cow's milk protein allergy.
- Sexual abuse (rare).

Anal fissure

- Commonly seen, often caused by the passage of a hard stool and results in 'stool-withholding' cycle exacerbating constipation if present.
- Presents with pain and bright red blood either on the surface of the stool or post defecation.
- Usually anterior or posterior and if lateral more suggestive of inflammatory pathology.
- May be a skin tag at the site of a healed fissure.
- Treat underlying cause (e.g. constipation).
- Local treatment rarely indicated.
- Most settle conservatively.
- Inflammatory bowel disease should be considered if fissures are atypical or resistant to medical treatment.
- Child sexual abuse should be considered if fissures are atypical or resistant to treatment.

Perianal streptococcal infection, 'soggy bottom'

- Common cause of perianal redness.
- Can present as constipation or perianal pain or both.
- Characterized by erythematous, well-demarcated, tender perianal margin.
- Secondary to group A beta-haemolytic *Streptococcus* infection.
- Perianal skin swab should be sent for diagnostic confirmation.
- Treatment is with penicillin for 7–10 days. Children who do not respond to penicillin should be treated with either co-amoxiclav or clarithromycin.
- There may be a need for a period on laxative therapy as there is a risk even after treatment of the child developing stool-withholding behaviour secondary to perianal discomfort.
- Infection can recur and require a more prolonged course of antibiotics. Choice of antibiotics should where possible be determined by sensitivities.

Threadworm infestation

- This is very common secondary to *Enterobius vermicularis* (pinworm).
- Common cause of perianal redness and itch.
- Transmission is faeco-oral.
- The life cycle is 6 weeks.
- Eggs are laid on perianal skin.
- Commonest symptom is itch, results in scratching; eggs on fingers are then swallowed, which perpetuates the infective cycle.
- Diagnosis is mostly clinical based on the presenting symptoms and signs.
- Can do a Sellotape slide test whereby the tape is placed on the skin around the perianal margin and then taped onto a slide and sent for microscopy to look for eggs.
- Treat with mebendazole (single dose) or piperazine (two doses, 2 weeks apart). Re-infection is common. The whole family needs to be treated and bedding changed to try to reduce this.

Rectal prolapse

- This is the abnormal protrusion of the rectal mucosa through the anal margin.
- Usually spontaneously reduces.
- Aetiology includes chronic straining secondary to constipation, chronic diarrhoea, malnutrition, polyps, cystic fibrosis as a manifestation of chronic diarrhoea (15%).
- Medical treatment of the underlying cause is appropriate.
- Surgical management (either through a perineal or abdominal approach) is rarely indicated.

Solitary rectal ulcer syndrome

- This rare condition is poorly understood.
- Occurs usually in adults but can occur in children with chronic constipation (particularly those who strain) and may be due to injury to the rectum.
- Usually manifests as a single ulcer (or occasionally multiple/polypoid mass) in the rectum.
- Symptoms include rectal bleeding, straining during bowel movements, constipation, soiling (particularly mucous), and a feeling of incomplete evacuation.
- Treatments include regular toileting, attention to diet and fluid intake, laxatives. In resistant cases, biofeedback or surgical intervention can be considered as an option. If surgery is contemplated, the advice of a colorectal surgeon should be sought.

Inflammatory bowel disease

- The presence of perianal abscess, persistent fissuring (usually lateral), skin tags, and fistula should raise the possibility of perianal Crohn's disease.
- Fissures are resistant to treatment and at atypical sites, e.g. lateral.
- Skin tags are generally large and 'fleshy'. Although minor skin tags are seen in up to 10% of the normal population, (particularly at the site of healed fissures), larger tags are strongly suggestive of inflammatory bowel disease. Need careful histological examination with multiple layers looking for granulomas if resected. Pathologist needs to be told that Crohn's disease is suspected.
- Fistula with discharge may be present.
- There is often surprisingly little discomfort in the presence of extensive perianal Crohn's disease (in the absence of perianal abscess formation).
- Management is complex, with anti-inflammatories and immunosuppressive agents. MRI is useful. Surgery should be minimal (abscess drainage, seton placement, diversion).

Inflammatory bowel disease: introduction

Introduction *376*
Differential diagnosis of inflammatory bowel disease *378*

Introduction

- 25% of inflammatory bowel disease (IBD) presents in childhood, usually as Crohn's disease or ulcerative colitis. The UK incidence is 5.2/100,000 children <16 years of age. Crohn's disease is the more common. Family history of IBD is common and both diseases can occur in the same family.
- *Crohn's disease* is a chronic inflammatory disease that can affect any part of the bowel, from mouth to anus. The most common sites are terminal ileum, ileocolon, and colon. The typical pathological features are transmural inflammation and granuloma formation, which may be patchy.
- *Ulcerative colitis* is an inflammatory disease limited to the colonic and rectal mucosa. The characteristic histology is mucosal and submucosal inflammation with goblet cell depletion, cryptitis, and crypt abscesses but no granulomas. The inflammatory change is usually diffuse rather than patchy.
- 10–15% of children with IBD have *indeterminate colitis or inflammatory bowel disease unclassified*, which means the histology is consistent with IBD but not characteristic of Crohn's disease or ulcerative colitis.
- Colitis is inflammation of the colon. Characteristic features include abdominal pain, tenesmus, bloody diarrhoea, and blood and mucus per rectum. Children with IBD who have colitis can have either ulcerative colitis or Crohn's disease.
- The precise aetiology of IBD is unknown and reflects a complex interaction between genetic predisposition, immune dysfunction, and environmental triggers. Smoking is a risk factor for Crohn's disease.
- The differential diagnosis of IBD is wide and should be considered in the diagnostic work-up.
- IBD runs a chronic relapsing course, with a significant morbidity particularly during the adolescent growth spurt.
- Growth and nutrition are key issues in the management with the aim of treatment being to induce and then maintain disease remission with minimal side effects.
- Diagnosis is by upper and lower endoscopy and small-bowel imaging with MRI, barium radiology, or ultrasound.
- Management is by careful clinical assessment and multidisciplinary management as part of an IBD service led by a physician with expertise in the condition.

Differential diagnosis of inflammatory bowel disease

Infective
- *Salmonella.*
- *Shigella.*
- *Campylobacter pylori.*
- *Escherichia coli* 0157 (and other strains of *E. coli*).
- *Yersinia enterocolitica.*
- *Amoebiasis*
- *Giardia lambia.*
- Tuberculosis.
- Cytomegalovirus.
- *Entamoeba histolytica.*
- Pseudomembranous enterocolitis (*Clostridium difficile* infection).

Non-infective
- Eosinophilic gastrointestinal disorders including eosinophilic gastroenteritis, eosinophilic colitis, eosinophilic proctitis.
- Vasculitis and autoimmune conditions, e.g. Henoch–Schönlein purpura, haemolytic uraemic syndrome.
- Polyposis syndromes.
- Immunodeficiency states (e.g. chronic granulomatous disease).
- Coeliac disease.
- Intestinal lymphoma.
- Ischaemic colitis.
- Hirschsprung enterocolitis.
- Necrotizing enterocolitis (newborn).
- Behçet disease.
- Solitary rectal ulcer syndrome.
- Carbohydrate intolerance.
- Laxative abuse.
- NSAID-induced enterocolitis.
- Lymphoid nodular hyperplasia.

Chronic granulomatous disease

- Can present with granulomatous inflammation in the gastrointestinal tract (Crohn's like).
- Mostly X-linked.
- Defect of neutrophil killing.
- Presents with recurrent bacterial infections, abscesses, osteomyelitis usually in the first year of life.
- Diagnosis is by detection of the impaired neutrophil respiratory burst using the nitroblue tetrazolium test (NBT).
- Treatment is with prophylactic antibiotics, anti-inflammatories, and corticosteroids if there is significant gut inflammation.
- Bone marrow transplant offers the potential for cure.

Behçet syndrome

- Orogenital ulceration with/without non-erosive arthritis, thrombophlebitis, vascular thromboses, or CNS abnormalities including meningoencephalitis.
- Treatment of orogenital ulceration is often unsatisfactory, however local/systemic steroids may be used acutely.
- Other drugs that have been used in prophylaxis include azathioprine and thalidomide.

Abdominal tuberculosis

- Tuberculosis can involve any part of the gastrointestinal tract and the bacteria reach the gastrointestinal tract via haematogenous spread, ingestion of infected sputum, or direct spread from infected contiguous lymph nodes.
- The most common site of involvement of gastrointestinal tuberculosis is the ileocaecal region.
- It is characterized by ulceration, fibrosis, thickening and stricturing of the bowel wall, with caseating granulomas seen on histology.
- Management is with conventional anti-tubercular therapy for at least 6 months.

Crohn's disease

Introduction *382*
Clinical features *382*
Investigation *384*
Clinical course *386*
Management *388*
Anti-tumour necrosis factor therapy *392*
References and resources *396*

Introduction

Crohn's disease is a chronic inflammatory disease that can affect any part of the bowel, from mouth to anus. Family history is common. 25% of patients present in childhood (age <18 years), most commonly during the adolescence.

- The diagnosis should be considered in children who present with abdominal pain, diarrhoea, weight loss, unexplained growth failure, and pubertal delay.
- The clinical course is one of recurrent relapses.
- Particularly in adolescence, the disease significantly impacts growth and development.
- Assessment includes upper and lower GI endoscopy and small-bowel imaging (MRI, barium radiology or ultrasound).
- Medical management is complex, requiring multidisciplinary input and a major emphasis on nutrition.
- Surgery is sometimes required in resistant Crohn's disease but the relapse rate is high and continued medical therapy is usually required.

Clinical features

The disease may be florid at presentation or insidious in onset. The diagnosis may therefore be delayed, sometimes for many months or even years. Most cases are underweight and up to 50% have significant growth failure, usually associated with delay in pubertal development. Growth failure can be the presenting feature.

The commonest presenting symptoms are abdominal pain, diarrhoea, and weight loss. In the British Paediatric Surveillance Unit (BPSU) survey, this triad was seen in only 25% of children. Abdominal pain was the commonest symptom occurring in 75%, nearly 60% had weight loss preceding diagnosis, 56% of children had diarrhoea, while only 45% reported both diarrhoea and weight loss. Abdominal pain is, however, common in children. The presence of additional features such as vomiting, diarrhoea, blood per rectum, weight loss, joint pains, and/or systemic upset, particularly if growth failure is present, should always prompt consideration of Crohn's disease and further evaluation and/or investigations if appropriate.

- The perianal examination is crucial in the assessment of such children as perianal skin tags, fistulae, and resistant fissures make Crohn's disease likely.
- Large, fleshy skin tags are strongly suggestive of Crohn's disease.

Nutritional status is frequently compromised at diagnosis. This is multifactorial:

- There is decreased food intake because of anorexia and abdominal pain following food which reduces the desire to eat.
- There may be reduced absorption in the presence of bowel mucosal inflammation.
- Particularly, there may be excessive losses through diarrhoea.

Investigation

- Basic investigation includes a full blood count, basic biochemistry, liver function tests, and inflammatory markers.
- Most (not all) children with active Crohn's disease will have raised inflammatory markers at presentation.
- Inflammatory markers are less likely to be raised in ulcerative colitis, particularly if not florid.
- Infective colitis should be excluded by stool culture (including ova, cysts, and parasites), Stool should be sent for *Clostridium difficile* toxin.
- Faecal calprotectin (FC) has high negative predictive value, i.e. can reliably rule out IBD when normal.
- *Endoscopy is indicated in all cases in order to get a tissue diagnosis and assess disease extent.*
- Endoscopy should include upper GI endoscopy and ileocolonoscopy.
- A positive family history should lower the threshold for investigation.

Most children in the UK have endoscopy under general anaesthetic, although some centres will investigate children using controlled sedation. Adequate bowel preparation is essential, as a good mucosal view will only be obtained if the bowel is clear. Ileocolonoscopy and upper GI endoscopy with biopsy provide information about disease severity and extent (in conjunction with small bowel imaging) as well as a tissue diagnosis in most cases. The disease extent will influence the choice of treatment and follow-up. It is essential to take biopsies as there may be no endoscopic abnormality but significant histological change.

- Small-bowel disease is best assessed by MRI, barium meal, and follow-through or small-bowel enema. Ultrasound will assess bowel wall thickening and is specific but less sensitive.
- MRI pelvis is useful in the assessment of difficult perianal disease.
- Histology is indeterminate in a significant number of children with colitis (indeterminate colitis, IBD-unclassified) and in these cases serological markers may help in the assessment (perinuclear antineutrophil cytoplasmic antibody (pANCA) positive in 70% of ulcerative colitis, perinuclear anti-*Saccharomyces cerevisiae* antibody (pASCA) positive in >50% of Crohn's disease).

Faecal calprotectin (FC)

- FC is a simple, cheap and non-invasive test with high sensitivity which can be useful in identifying children with IBD.
- The high negative predictive value of a normal FC (levels <50mcg/g) can be utilized in risk stratification and screening of children with suspected IBD.
- High levels of FC are also seen in a number of other conditions associated with mucosal inflammation, such as GI infections and coeliac disease.

FC correlates well with bowel inflammation and is not influenced by sex, age, IBD type, or disease location.

Growth failure

Occurs as a consequence of:
- Nutritional impairment.
- The systemic consequences of gut inflammation.
- Disturbances of the growth hormone/insulin-like growth factor axis.
- The side effects of corticosteroids when used.

Extraintestinal manifestations of Crohn's disease

- Joint disease in 10%.
- Skin rashes—erythema nodosum, erythema multiforme, pyoderma gangrenosum, cutaneous Crohn's disease.
- Liver disease—sclerosing cholangitis, autoimmune liver disease.
- Iritis/uveitis.
- Osteoporosis.

Complications of Crohn's disease

- Growth failure with delayed puberty.
- Emotional disturbance—difficulty with friendships, impact of a chronic disease with chronic symptoms, impact of pubertal delay.
- Treatment toxicity, e.g. corticosteroids.
- Osteoporosis.
- Long-term cancer risk.

Diagnostic work-up in children with suspected inflammatory bowel disease

- Full blood work-up including inflammatory markers.
- Stool culture.
- Gastroscopy.
- Ileocolonoscopy.
- MRI abdomen or barium meal and follow-through.

Clinical course

Crohn's disease runs a chronic relapsing and remitting course. A single episode of active disease followed by a sustained clinical remission is rare. The chronic nature of the inflammatory process (and frequent need for steroids) leads to ongoing growth failure, usually with delayed onset of puberty. Many children will miss periods of schooling, and their illness may disrupt their social and psychological well-being. They often look younger than their peers and are treated accordingly. Children who are chronically ill and who lag behind physically, educationally, and socially may struggle during their adolescent years and into adulthood.

Management

A multidisciplinary approach is important. Key professionals include paediatric gastroenterologist, general paediatrician, paediatric surgeon, radiologist, histopathologist, paediatric dietician, nurse specialist, and psychologist. Close liaison with education is essential. Appropriate strategies need to be in place for transition to adult services. Guidelines and recommendations for management of Crohn' disease have been published by BSPGHAN and European Crohn's and Colitis Organisation (ECCO).

- The aim is to induce remission and to normalize growth and development, minimizing treatment impact and complications.
- The initial treatment will be determined by the clinical state of the child and the disease extent.
- In most children exclusive enteral nutrition is appropriate as first-line treatment.
- Corticosteroids are indicated in severe colitis.
- Additional therapies are often required, however, because of the frequently relapsing nature of the disease and surgical input required in up to 50% of cases.
- Basic anthropometry, including height and weight together with pubertal status, is an essential part of the initial clinical and follow-up assessment.
- Multidisciplinary care with attention to disease control and social, family, and educational issues is a fundamental part of management.

Exclusive enteral nutrition

The use of liquid dietary therapy as a substitute for normal diet for a period (6–8 weeks) will induce disease remission in 70–80% of children if cases are selected appropriately and compliance is good. Large volumes are required, with individualized volume and feed concentration to achieve weight gain and to prevent hunger. The volume of feed is increased over 5–7 days depending on tolerance. Often children require 120% or more of their predicted calorific requirements. Most children tolerate their feed orally, divided evenly through the day. The formula can be flavoured to improve compliance. Nasogastric feeding is an option, and is most useful in children who cannot tolerate a volume large enough to meet their calorific needs by mouth.

Modulen® IBD (Nestlé) and Alicalm® (Nutricia) are polymeric feeds specifically designed for use in IBD. Elemental O28® (Nutricia), an elemental feed, is an effective alternative but less palatable. There have been no published controlled trials comparing the types of feed. Both induce improvement in symptoms. Often an improvement in well-being is felt in a matter of days. Weight gain is frequently established in the first week when the feed is well tolerated. Inflammatory markers almost universally improve within 2 weeks of treatment in children who are going to do well.

Motivation (patient, family, and healthcare professionals) is key, and ongoing support is needed to maintain compliance. Food reintroduction after a period of enteral nutrition is staged and begins with low-residue foods, new food groups being added every few days over a period of 2–3 weeks. Enteral nutrition is weaned slowly during this period in order to ensure nutritional requirements are met during the weaning period. Having returned to a normal diet, a reduced volume of the enteral feed or an alternative oral nutritional supplement may be recommended to further restore nutritional status and growth.

Corticosteroids

Oral corticosteroids are recommended for inducing remission in children with severe active luminal disease if enteral nutrition is not an option or those who fail to respond to it. They are an effective treatment for Crohn's disease with a similar efficacy to enteral nutrition although can impact growth, at least in the short term. Steroids are usually given as prednisolone 1–2mg/kg (maximum dose 40–60mg). When oral corticosteroids have failed, IV corticosteroids may prove efficacious in some patients. High-dose prednisolone is continued until remission is achieved, and then the dose is weaned by reducing the daily dose by 5mg each week. Enteric-coated preparations should not be used because of the risk of poor absorption. Calcium and vitamin D supplements such as Calcichew D3 forte® should be given to children at risk of deficiency, particularly during the adolescent growth spurt. DXA scanning of bone mineral density is useful although needs to be interpreted in the context of height, weight, and pubertal status. An antacid preparation may be required in children with gastritis.

Budesonide (which has a high first-pass metabolism and therefore less toxicity) has been used with good effect in ileocaecal (right-sided) disease.

Side effects of steroid therapy
- Immunosuppression with increased susceptibility to infection.
- Cushingoid facies (moon face).
- Inappropriate weight gain (central obesity) and fluid retention.
- Acne, hirsutism, and striae.
- Osteopenia/osteoporosis/aseptic necrosis.
- Hypertension.
- Glucose intolerance.
- Pancreatitis.
- Hyperlipidaemia.
- Depressed mood.
- Growth suppression, adrenal suppression, delayed puberty.
- Cataract.

Maintaining remission
- 50–90% of people diagnosed with Crohn's disease will relapse within the first 12 months.
- Maintaining remission is therefore a major challenge.
- 5-aminosalicylic acid (ASA) derivatives are widely used but of little proven benefit; however, they are useful to control continuing active disease or for the management of acute flare-ups. High doses are generally used. Sulfasalazine in syrup form is most appropriate for the younger children, with mesalazine given as either controlled- or delayed-release preparations in older children. Controlled release preparations

(e.g. Pentasa®) work better proximally and delayed-release preparations work better distally (e.g. Asacol®).

- Continued emphasis on good nutrition is essential with a number of children electing to remain long term on nutritional supplements. Most children require higher than normal requirements, particularly when well.
- Children with long-term nutritional needs may benefit from gastrostomy placement for supplementary feeding.
- Repeated courses of exclusive enteral nutrition and/or steroids can be given.
- Corticosteroids are not effective as maintenance therapy.

Further management

Azathioprine

Azathioprine (or 6-mercaptopurine, a metabolite of azathioprine) is a steroid-sparing agent that is effective in 60–80% of cases inducing a sustained remission and growth spurt in many cases. Azathioprine is used more commonly in the UK. More than 50% of children with Crohn's disease are likely to need azathioprine. The usual indication is to give after two or three relapses, particularly if over a short period. Growth failure is a factor in the decision to treat, particularly if steroid requirements are high. Azathioprine is increasingly being used at diagnosis in severe cases. It can take 3–6 months to take effect. There is significant potential toxicity, with flu-like symptoms, GI symptoms, leucopenia, hepatitis, pancreatitis, rash, and infection. Side effects result in stopping treatment in up to 18% of children. The dose of azathioprine is 2–2.5 mg/kg per day and for 6-mercaptopurine 1–1.5 mg/kg per day, given as a single daily dose. Thiopurine methyl transferase (TPMT) is important in the metabolism of thiopurine derivatives. Genetic polymorphisms for this enzyme will increase the risk of toxicity and consideration should be given to checking this before starting. There is small increase in the risk of lymphoma with long-term use of thiopurine derivatives. Frequent blood monitoring is required. There are various suggested regimens. The British National Formulary for Children recommends a weekly full blood count for 4 weeks, then 3-monthly. Parents/children should be told to report any symptoms or signs of bone marrow suppression (bruising, bleeding, and infection) acutely. Measurement of active metabolite 6- thioguanine nucleotide (6-TGN) and 6-methylmercaptopurine (6-MMP) concentrations in plasma can be used in children failing to respond to assess compliance and risk of developing toxicity. A significantly greater therapeutic effect can be achieved in paediatric IBD patients with level of the thiopurine metabolite 6-TGN >235pmol/8 $\times$ 10^8 erythrocytes while hepatotoxicity correlates with elevated 6-methyl mercaptopurine (MMP) levels (>5700pmol/ 8 $\times$ 10^8 erythrocytes).

Methotrexate

Methotrexate is an antimetabolite, which exerts an immunomodulator effect by inhibiting purine synthesis. It can be used as primary maintenance therapy or in children who are intolerant to or fail to respond to thiopurine derivatives. It can be used orally or subcutaneously. Treatment is usually initiated as parenteral as bioavailability of oral methotrexate is variable. It is prescribed at a dose of 15mg/m^2 once a week to a maximum dose of 25mg, with oral folate 5mg once weekly or 1mg once daily for 5 days per week. The main side effects include nausea/vomiting, flu-like symptoms, hepatocellular liver disease, and myelosuppression. Among these, nausea and vomiting are very common and severe enough to limit the use. Monitoring of liver functions, full blood count, and kidney functions is advised fortnightly for 4 weeks and 1–3-monthly from there on.

Anti-tumour necrosis factor therapy

Tumour necrosis factor (TNF)-α is a proinflammatory cytokine produced in lymphocytes and macrophages that has been implicated in the pathogenesis of Crohn's disease. There are several therapeutic modalities that antagonize its effects. Infliximab and adalimumab are the commonly used anti-TNF agents in management of paediatric Crohn's disease.

The indications for using anti-TNF treatments are:
- Inducing remission in children with steroid-refractory disease.
- Primary therapy in children with perianal, fistulating, or stricturing disease.
- Inducing and maintaining remission in children with chronically active luminal Crohn's disease.

Prior to commencing anti-TNF therapy, patients have to be screened for tuberculosis and hepatitis B to prevent reactivation. Varicella immunity should also be established and in seronegative cases, varicella zoster immunization should be considered before treatment.

They both have comparable efficacy and adverse event profile though most paediatric centres would use infliximab as the first agent. Infliximab is administered at the dose of 5mg/kg with three induction doses over 6 weeks (week 0–2–6) followed by maintenance therapy of 5mg/kg every 8 weeks.

Adalimumab is administered as induction therapy at 2.4mg/kg (maximum 160mg) at baseline, 1.2mg/kg (maximum 80mg) at week 2, followed by 0.6mg/kg (maximum of 40mg) every other week. Alternatively, for patients under 40kg, dosing regimens of 80–40–20mg were proposed, and for patients over 40kg dosing regimens of 160–80–40mg.

Side effects of treatment include acute infusion reactions, delayed hypersensitivity reactions, serious infections, risk of opportunistic infections (e.g. invasive fungal infections, reactivation of latent tuberculosis), and potential risk of malignancy (e.g. lymphoma, skin cancers).

Infliximab treatment failure can be primary, i.e. lack of response despite three doses, or can be due to loss of response in children who had previously responded. Loss of response can be due to:
- Decrease in viable drug level due to clearance or development of antibodies.
- Complications of disease, e.g. stricture.
- Superimposed infection.

In cases with loss of response to infliximab trough and antibody levels should be checked and drug levels can be improved by either increasing dose to 10mg/kg or reducing interval to 6-weekly.

Use of combination therapy with thiopurines or methotrexate reduces the risk of antibody formation and is used as standard treatment in children.

Biosimilars are subsequent versions of innovator biopharmaceutical products made by a different sponsor following patent expiry on the innovator product. The lower cost of biosimilars is anticipated to increase access for many more patients to effective biologic therapies.

Surgery

Surgery is indicated in children with chronically active disease resistant to medical therapy and is especially useful in children with refractory short segment ileal disease. It is also indicated for complications such as stricture or perianal disease unresponsive to anti-inflammatories. Emergency surgery may be needed in the child who presents with acute toxic colitis and colonic dilatation. Elective or semi-elective surgery is indicated in children with chronic disease resistant to the medical therapy, particularly if there is chronic symptomatology, chronic steroid use, and/or growth failure. Surgical options range from removal of isolated disease segments or strictures to extensive panproctocolectomy and the possibility of permanent stoma formation. Surgical resection of active disease can lead to rapid increases in growth and a prolonged period of disease remission, therefore timing of surgery relative to the pubertal growth spurt is crucial.

Specific situations

Oesophagitis

Most children with oesophageal involvement present with disease elsewhere in the bowel. Treatment of symptomatic oesophagitis or gastritis with a PPI is helpful, particularly if corticosteroids are being given.

Oral disease

Oral manifestations of Crohn's disease may occur as recurrent aphthous ulceration, as orofacial granulomatosis (swelling of the lips and cheeks), or as a manifestation of panenteric disease. Orofacial granulomatosis implies oral disease in isolation without disease elsewhere in the GI tract. Management can be local or systemic. Oral disease may also respond to enteral nutrition.

Cinnamon and benzoate free-diets have been used. Systemic antibiotics, corticosteroids, and thiopurines are required in difficult cases. Intralesional corticosteroids can reduce swelling and improve cosmesis.

Perianal Crohn's disease

Active perianal disease can occur in isolation, although it is usually associated with active Crohn's disease in other locations. Treatment of the active disease will often result in improvement of perianal disease and/or closure of fistulae. Specific therapeutic strategies used include 5-ASA derivatives; local and systemic corticosteroids and other immunosuppression including azathioprine; and antibiotics, particularly metronidazole. Tacrolimus may be administered topically, although systemic treatment can be used if the conventional treatments fail. Infliximab is effective in difficult cases with reasonable efficacy. Surgical management is by abscess drainage, Seton placement to encourage fistula drainage, and diversion in the most resistant cases.

Case study

A 15-year-old boy presents with a 6-month history of abdominal discomfort, loose stools, and weight loss and has a reduced height velocity (<4cm/year) over the last 12 months. He has not yet entered puberty. He has missed >50% of school. He looks pale and unwell. Basic investigations show a mild normochromic anaemia, thrombocytosis, raised CRP, and a low serum albumin. Crohn's disease is suspected—further investigation including upper GI endoscopy, ileocolonoscopy, and barium radiology confirm ileocaecal Crohn's disease.

Management priorities include getting him well, establishing weight gain, promoting growth and the onset of puberty, and getting him back into school.

He is treated with enteral nutrition given as sole therapy for 8 weeks, which induces a clinical remission. He is then well for >6 months with good weight gain. He does unfortunately relapse and requires a further course of enteral nutrition. Steroids are avoided because of the potential toxicity (on growth in particular) and azathioprine introduced as steroid-sparing therapy. He then has a more sustained remission with improved liner growth and the onset of puberty. His final adult height is normal.

Medical therapy will suffice in most cases of ileocaecal Crohn's disease particularly with the early introduction of azathioprine as steroid-sparing medication. Monoclonal antibody therapy, e.g. infliximab, can be used. If the disease proves resistant to medical management, particularly if there are persistent symptoms or stricturing disease and/or persistent growth failure, then ileocaecal resection is appropriate which will affect a remission, although recurrent disease is common.

References and resources

Beattie RM, Croft NM, Fell JM, Afzal NA, Heuschkel RB. Inflammatory bowel disease. Arch Dis Child 2006;91:426–32.

Kammermeier J, Morris M, Garrick V, et al. Management of Crohn's disease. Arch Dis Child 2016;101:475–80.

Levine A, Koletzko S, Turner D, et al. ESPGHAN revised porto criteria for the diagnosis of inflammatory bowel disease in children and adolescents. European Society of Pediatric Gastroenterology, Hepatology, and Nutrition. J Pediatr Gastroenterol Nutr 2014;58:795–806.

Mowat C, Cole A, Windsor A, et al Guidelines for the management of inflammatory bowel disease in adults. Gut 2011;60:571–607.

National Institute for Health and Care Excellence (NICE).Crohn's disease: management. Clinical Guideline CG152. London: NICE; 2012. https://www.nice.org.uk/guidance/CG152

National Institute of Clinical Excellence (NICE). Guidance for the use of infliximab. Technology Appraisal Guidance TA187. London: NICE; 2010. https://www.nice.org.uk/guidance/ta187

Ruemmele FM, Veres G, Kolho KL, et al. Consensus guidelines of ECCO/ESPGHAN on the medical management of pediatric Crohn's disease. J Crohns Colitis 2014;8:1179–207.

Sawczenko A, Sandhu BK, Logan RF, et al. Prospective survey of childhood inflammatory bowel disease in the British Isles. Lancet 2001;357:1093–4.

Patient support groups

Crohn's and Colitis UK: https://www.crohnsandcolitis.org.uk

Crohn's in Childhood Research Association (CICRA). Pat Shaw House, 13–19 Ventnor Road, Sutton, Surrey, SM2 6AQ. http://www.cicra.org

Nutritional management of Crohn's disease

Introduction *398*
Nutritional status *398*
Nutritional requirements *399*
Treatment *400*
Refeeding *402*
Monitoring *402*
Food reintroduction *403*
Continued nutritional support *404*
References and resources *404*

Introduction

Crohn's disease in childhood can have a significant effect on nutritional status and growth. Exclusive enteral nutrition (EEN) as a treatment for Crohn's disease was first introduced in the 1970s and is used as a primary therapy in children because of its proven efficacy, lack of side effects, and positive impact on growth. The aim is to induce remission while promoting weight gain with subsequent height gain and pubertal development.

EEN can induce remission in 70–80% of children. The enteral feed replaces a normal diet for a 6–8-week period followed by gradual reintroduction of a normal diet as the feed volume is weaned.

Nutritional status

In active Crohn's disease, nutritional status is compromised by:
- Malabsorption due to mucosal inflammation.
- Pro-inflammatory cytokine action leading to tissue catabolism.
- Nausea, anorexia, abdominal pain resulting in decreased nutrient intake.
- Increased gut losses of protein and micronutrients.

These factors can lead to significant malnutrition, weight loss, and growth failure with delayed onset of puberty. Growth failure is seen in up to 50% of children. A low serum albumin and iron deficiency are common as well as micronutrient deficiencies, most commonly zinc and selenium. Fat-soluble vitamins A, D, and E stores may be low.

In clinical practice, nutritional status is assessed by the following measures (indicating possible refeeding risk):
- Anthropometry (height, weight, and mid-arm circumference).
- Weight, height, and BMI.
- Diet history including normal diet and recent changes to intake.
- Approximate weight loss.
- Appetite status.

Nutritional requirements

There are several methods of assessing energy requirements. Schofield equations are commonly used in clinical practice although estimated average requirement (EAR) (see 'References and resources') provides a similar result. Exclusive enteral nutrition should be commenced at 50–75% EAR to avoid the risk of refeeding and increased according to appetite. Dietary intakes during EEN can reach 120% EAR particularly if there is a need for catch up growth. A nutritionally complete formula, i.e. macro- and micronutrient sufficient, should be provided. Fluid requirements should be based on current body weight. Assessment of normal activity levels/sport involvement should be considered in assessment of energy requirements.

Treatment

EEN should be given exclusively over a 6–8-week period with no other foods or drinks (other than water or no-added sugar squash type drinks). Disease-specific feeds are:

- Polymeric (whole protein, lactose-free) feeds:
  - Modulen® IBD (Nestlé).
  - Alicalm® (Nutricia).
- Elemental feed:
  - Elemental O28® (Nutricia).

Polymeric feeds have been found in numerous studies to be as effective as elemental feeds. They are also cheaper and more palatable. A multidisciplinary approach to treatment is essential. An initial 2–4-day inpatient admission to assess tolerance, establish feed volume, and regimen may improve subsequent compliance. Access to members of the multidisciplinary team and experienced nursing staff can address the following:

- Spending time with the family promoting the benefits of enteral nutrition.
- Building up feed volumes as tolerated to meet requirements.
- Addressing practical issues such as school, holidays, and special occasions.
- Involve psychologist/psychiatrist input for emotional support if needed.
- Parents/carers can observe the method of feed preparation.
- Arrange prescription for enteral feeds through contact with the GP and community pharmacist.
- Nursing support and encouragement.
- Adjustment of the feed recipe if necessary to optimize nutritional content within a manageable volume.
- Consider and establish exclusive or partial nasogastric feeding if the patient fails to take it orally.
- Assess tolerance and monitor refeeding bloods.

In order to meet requirements large volumes are needed but the recipe can be individualized. The advantage of using powdered feeds is that if high energy requirements are to be met within an acceptable volume, the feed may be concentrated. This also improves compliance if the prescribed volume is more acceptable to the patient and some find a slightly thicker consistency more palatable. The standard concentration of Modulen® IBD is 20% (1kcal/mL) but in practice concentrations up to 30% (1.5kcal/mL) are tolerated. Standard concentration should be given for at least the first 3–5 days. At higher concentrations, if symptoms of abdominal discomfort, loose stools, or diarrhoea are reported, then the concentration should be reduced by 1–2% until tolerance is regained. In severe disease, an isocaloric standard concentration feed should be given as a hyperosmolar concentrated feed may aggravate the inflamed gut mucosa.

Preferably feeds should be taken orally with the total volume divided into a minimum of six to eight drinks per day given at regular intervals to simulate meal and snack times. Initially, if there are issues with nausea or vomiting then drinks can be of a smaller volume taken 2-hourly. Feeds can be taken unflavoured or flavoured with commercially available milkshake flavourings but with attention to oral hygiene and regular, thorough teeth brushing. Elemental 028® Extra powder, if required for milk-intolerant patients, is available in ready-to-feed flavoured cartons as well as in powdered form. Of note, a larger volume of this feed would be required in order to meet energy and protein requirements. Feeds taken from a beaker with a lid and straw or a sports bottle prevent the patient being put-off by the smell of the drink. Most patients prefer the feeds to be taken chilled from the fridge although they can be warmed (not boiled) if preferred. Arrangements for transporting and storing feed at school should be discussed.

Nasogastric feeding is an option if, despite input from the multidisciplinary team, there are difficulties with volumes and dislike of taste. Feeds are given as boluses that are gravity fed unless there is a risk of refeeding syndrome or severe malnutrition warrants a continuous feeding regimen using a pump. Avoiding use of the pump allows easier and earlier discharge home with minimal equipment and training needs.

Once full volumes of feed are established, patients are allowed to take sugar-free chewing gum, sugar-free boiled sweets, and no-added sugar squash-type drinks if desired. It is advised that sugar-free boiled sweets are limited to four to five sweets per day because they contain polyol sweeteners which is a fermentable carbohydrate and has a laxative effect if taken in excess.

Refeeding

'Refeeding' is defined as 'the occurrence of severe fluid and electrolyte shifts with associated complications in malnourished patients undergoing enteral/parenteral nutrition' and is a risk in children with Crohn's disease who present with a poor nutritional intake, unintentional weight loss >10%, and low phosphate, potassium, and magnesium blood levels prior to feeding. Careful questioning is essential to establish recent dietary intake, amount of weight lost, and over what period of time. If the patient is deemed 'at risk', enteral feeds can be introduced at as low as 10–20kcal/kg current body weight/50% of requirements (up to a maximum of 1000kcal) for the first 48 hours to avoid rapid shifts in electrolytes. It may be prudent for those patients 'at very high risk' to have 25% of requirements from feed for the first 48 hours. Feeding too quickly can result in severe drops in phosphate, potassium, and magnesium which can lead to disturbances in body systems including cardiac arrhythmias. Refeeding bloods, i.e. serum phosphate, potassium, and magnesium, should be checked 24 hours after feeds commence. Careful monitoring of serum electrolytes is required, with supplementation if necessary, and feeds increased cautiously over 5–7 days to meet requirements.

Monitoring

It is assumed that as energy levels return and patients resume normal activities that energy requirements will increase and therefore weekly contact by telephone over the 6–8-week period of EEN ensures that appetite is being met and nutritional status optimized by adjustment of the feed recipe. Appetite is used as a primary indicator to increase quantity either as volume or concentration of feed. If a patient is getting hungry on the prescribed volume, compliance is more likely to be compromised.

Children who are particularly active and regularly participate in sport should be given an additional extra drink recipe, i.e. 250–300mL to allow for extra nutritional demands.

Failure to respond clinically may be due to poor compliance, presence of a stricture, or disease that is unresponsive to EEN treatment. Insufficient follow-up and monitoring can result in poor compliance and failure to gain expected weight if feed quantity is not being adapted to needs and appetite.

Patients are usually reviewed in clinic in the first few weeks of EEN treatment and then towards the end to introduce the food reintroduction programme.

Food reintroduction

This involves a 2–3-week period of gradually reintroducing food. There is no consensus or standardized protocol, however it is widely accepted that food should not be introduced too rapidly. During this period, nutritional support needs to be maintained by a gradual weaning of EEN. Table 47.1 is an example of a food reintroduction programme that has proven to be acceptable to patients based on variety of foods in the initial stages and the length of time taken to return to a normal diet.

If any symptoms are experienced at any stage then it is advised to pro-long the stage before moving on to the next or move back to a stage that is well tolerated. If there are ongoing bowel symptoms it is worth considering whether a reduction in lactose or other fermentable carbohydrates such as fructose can give symptomatic improvement.

Table 47.1 Example food reintroduction programme

Stage 1	Introduce 'bland' foods that are wheat/gluten free, milk and dairy free, low fat and fibre, non-spicy over 5 days
Stage 2	Introduce wheat and gluten containing foods over 5 days
Stage 3	Introduce milk and dairy foods over 5 days
Stage 4	Introduce high-fibre, higher-fat, spicy foods over 10 days

Continued nutritional support

Children who have severe growth failure and malnutrition will require nutritional monitoring once in remission and off EEN to continue repletion and achieve catch-up growth. Optimizing nutritional intake in the period following EEN and in remission can be assisted with the use of various nutritional supplements. It may be that maintenance enteral nutrition in this form can prolong length of remission. Many patients prefer to continue to take 300–600mL of the enteral feed used during EEN as maintenance enteral nutrition. Nutritionally complete alternatives are Fortini® (Nutricia), Paediasure® (Abbott), Fortisip Compact® (Nutricia), Fortijuce® (Nutricia), Ensure Plus® (Abbott). Higher calorie supplements made up with cow's milk such as Scandishake® (Nutricia) or Calshake® (Fresenius) are well accepted by children as long as cow's milk is well tolerated. Calogen® (Nutricia), Pro-cal® Shots (Vitapro), and Calogen® Extra Shots (Nutricia) can be used as calorie supplements if other drink-style supplements are refused.

An age-appropriate multivitamin and mineral supplementation is recommended for all patients, e.g. Sanatogen® A to Z Complete, Centrum® A to Z, Wellkid® Smart Chewable (Vitabiotics), Wellteen® (Vitabiotics), and supermarket own-brand A to Z-type versions.

References and resources

Scientific Advisory Committee on Nutrition. Dietary reference values for energy. London: TSO; 2011.
Schofield WN. Predicting basal metabolic rate, new standards and review of previous work. Hum Nutr Clin Nutr 1985;39(Suppl 1):5–41.

Ulcerative colitis

Introduction *406*
Clinical presentations *406*
Investigation *407*
Clinical course *407*
Management *408*
References and resources *414*

Introduction

25% of IBD presents in childhood, one-third as ulcerative colitis. Presentation can occur at any age and ulcerative colitis is the commonest cause of IBD in the younger child. A family history of Crohn's disease or ulcerative colitis is common in index cases.

Clinical presentations

- Acute toxic colitis.
- Pancolitis—mild, moderate, or severe.
- Left-sided disease/distal colitis.

Pancolitis is the most common presentation in children. Characteristic symptoms are abdominal pain, diarrhoea, and blood per rectum although atypical presentations can occur. There may be significant pain before or during bowel movement, relieved by the passage of stool (tenesmus). Night stools are common. A history of foreign travel should be excluded. Systemic disturbance can accompany more severe disease including tachycardia, fever, weight loss, anaemia, hypoalbuminaemia, leucocytosis, and raised inflammatory markers. The presentation can be more indolent with occult blood loss or non-specific abdominal pain. Constipation can be a feature, particularly in distal colitis.

- Extraintestinal manifestations include:
  - Arthropathy (10%), usually knees, ankles.
  - Ankylosing spondylitis (rare in childhood).
  - Liver disease (sclerosing cholangitis, autoimmune liver disease).
  - Erythema nodosum.
  - Iritis and uveitis.
- Disease associations include:
  - Pyoderma gangrenosum.
  - Ankylosing spondylitis and sacroileitis.
- Complications include:
  - Toxic megacolon.
  - Osteoporosis.
  - Growth failure.
  - Colorectal cancer.
- There is an increased thrombotic tendency in severe disease.
- It is common to develop an 'irritable bowel type syndrome' as the colitis enters remission.
- Proximal constipation is common in distal colitis.

Investigation

Clinical presentation is generally with abdominal pain and bloody diarrhoea. It is important to give careful consideration to the differential diagnosis. Investigation is by careful history and examination with basic blood testing including blood count, differential, inflammatory markers including CRP and erythrocyte sedimentation rate, and liver function. Bloods tests can be normal. It is essential to culture the stool to exclude an infective cause. Further investigation is with upper and lower GI endoscopy including ileoscopy with biopsies. This will help differentiate between ulcerative colitis and Crohn's disease. In children with indeterminate changes (not diagnostic of Crohn's disease or ulcerative colitis) on histology, pANCA status may be useful. pANCA is positive in 70% of ulcerative colitis and <10% of patients with Crohn's disease or controls.

If liver function is abnormal, then a more detailed autoantibody screen and liver ultrasound should be performed with consideration of MRCP/liver biopsy. A family history of IBD should lower the threshold for investigation.

Endoscopy is indicated in all cases in order to get a tissue diagnosis and assess disease extent unless disease is so severe (e.g. toxic megacolon) and empirical treatment required, in which case it can be deferred.

Clinical course

Ulcerative colitis runs a chronic relapsing and remitting course. A single episode of active disease followed by a sustained clinical remission is rare. Growth failure can be a feature, particularly when high doses of corticosteroids are used or disease becomes steroid dependent. Many children will miss periods of schooling, and their illness may disrupt their social and psychological well-being. Major anxieties can occur about school toilets, for example. These are important issues that need to be addressed by the multidisciplinary team responsible for the management of this chronic condition.

Management

General principles

- The general principles are similar to those for Crohn's disease (Chapter 46) and involve careful assessment, follow-up, and input from the multidisciplinary team. Psychological factors are of particular importance.
- The aim of treatment is to induce and maintain a disease remission avoiding either disease or treatment-related complications. The choice of treatment is influenced by disease severity and extent (Fig. 48.1 and Table 48.1). Comprehensive guidelines and recommendations of treatment have been published by BSPGHAN and ECCO. Many of the therapies used have significant toxicity and the reader is referred to these guidelines and the paediatric British National Formulary (https://www.evidence.nhs.uk/formulary/bnfc/current) for a fuller account of these including the specific monitoring regimens.
- The lifelong nature of the condition means that appropriate arrangements need to be put in place for transition to adult care.
- It is important to pay attention to general factors including the importance of good nutrition, educational strategies (e.g. access to the toilet in school, recognition of the impact of a chronic disease on learning), and management of psychological problems including anxiety.
- Many patients claim benefit from fish oil supplements and probiotics.

Acute severe colitis

This implies that in addition to colitic symptoms (pain, diarrhoea, and blood per rectum) the child has systemic upset with pyrexia, tachycardia, and abdominal tenderness/distension. *Toxic megacolon* (colonic dilation on plain abdominal radiograph) is a life-threatening complication of this, although fortunately rare in childhood. It is important to obtain multiple stool cultures to exclude infection which can be a trigger either for disease presentation or for disease flare-up, and is important in the differential diagnosis. It is important to specifically request testing for *Clostridium difficile* toxin, which can precipitate an acute exacerbation.

- It is important to remember that Crohn's disease can occasionally present as acute toxic colitis.
- Children with acute toxic colitis are best managed in specialist centres by paediatric gastroenterologists in conjunction with paediatric/adult surgeons.

Pancolitis

Pancolitis—mild, moderate, severe but not toxic—is the more usual presentation in childhood.

Prednisolone and 5-ASA derivatives (sulfasalazine, mesalazine) should be started in most cases. In very mild disease, 5-ASA derivatives can be used as sole therapy. Prednisolone is given as 1–2mg/kg (maximum 40mg) for 2–4 weeks weaned once remission is achieved over the subsequent 6–8 weeks. Calcium and vitamin D supplements should be given to children at risk of deficiency, particularly during the adolescent growth spurt. DEXA scanning of bone mineral density is useful, though needs to be interpreted in the context of height, weight, and pubertal status. Mesalazine

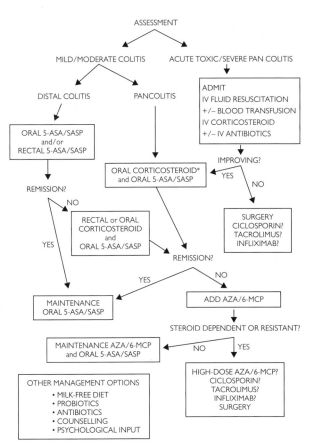

Fig. 48.1 Algorithm for the treatment of UC in children. 5-ASA, 5-aminosalicylates; AZA, azathioprine; 6-MCP, 6-mercaptopurine; SASP, sulfasalazine.

*Consider initial 2–5 days of IV therapy in moderate to severe pancolitis.

preparations are generally given at high dose and can be given once daily if tolerated. Sulfasalazine, which is available as syrup, can be given to younger children. Higher doses of prednisolone are occasionally used. IV steroids may be useful for 2–5 days in severe disease. It is sometimes necessary to use an antacid preparation in children with gastritis on upper GI endoscopy. Exclusive enteral nutrition has no role. Dietetic input is useful, as most children with colitis will be in energy deficit with high calorific needs. Ongoing dietetic input is essential.

Table 48.1 Disease severity in ulcerative colitis—Paediatric Ulcerative Colitis Activity Index (PUCAI)

Item	Points
1. Abdominal pain	
No pain	0
Pain can be ignored	5
Pain cannot be ignored	10
2. Rectal bleeding	
None	0
Small amount only, in <50% of stools	10
Small amount with most stools	20
Large amount (>50% of the stool content)	30
3. Stool consistency of most stools	
Formed	0
Partially formed	5
Completely unformed	10
4. Number of stools per 24h	
0–2	0
3–5	5
6–8	10
>8	15
5. Nocturnal stools (any episode causing wakening)	
No	0
Yes	10
6. Activity level	
No limitation of activity	0
Occasional limitation of activity	5
Severe restricted activity	10
Sum of PUCAI (0–85)	
Score <10, remission; 10–34, mild; 35–64, moderate; ≥65, severe.	

Reproduced from Turner D. et al. (2007) Development, validation, and evaluation of a pediatric ulcerative colitis activity index: a prospective multicentre study, Gastroenterology 133(2):423–432 with permission from Elsevier.

The 5-ASA derivative should be continued long term and will reduce the risk of relapse and of colorectal carcinoma. Toxic effects include headache, nausea, vomiting, and diarrhoea. Rare side effects include Stevens–Johnson syndrome, pancreatitis, renal failure, and agranulocytosis. Mesalazine preparations are generally better tolerated than sulfasalazine.

There is no role for long-term steroids and these should be avoided where possible.

Practical management of acute toxic colitis

- *Fluid resuscitation* with saline bolus if required for reduced peripheral perfusion.
- *Blood transfusion* if Hb <8g/dL.
- *IV fluids*—initially 0.9% saline/dextrose with 20mmol KCl per 500mL modified depending on fluid balance and electrolyte results.
- *Intravenous steroids.* Methylprednisolone at a dosage of 1–1.5mg/kg/day (up to a maximum of 60mg/day) given in one or two divided daily doses Or hydrocortisone 10mg/kg in four divided doses—maximum 100mg four times daily.
- *Sequential PUCAI scores* can be useful in identifying cases not responding to treatment and needing second-line therapy.
- *Second-line therapy* should be started in cases not responding to treatment with steroids. This can be in form of infliximab or IV ciclosporin. Both treatments are used to induce remission and as bridge to establishing therapy with thiopurines.
- *Plain abdominal radiograph* should be performed if toxic megacolon is suspected. Dilatation of the transverse colon >56mm (>40mm in children <10 years) is diagnostic.
- Abdominal ultrasound to look at bowel wall thickening.
- *Surgical review* (at presentation) as up to 50% with toxic megacolon will require colectomy, although most with an acute toxic colitis (not megacolon) will settle.
- *Subcutaneous heparin* for prophylaxis of venous thrombosis if the illness is prolonged.

Distal colitis

In children, rectal treatments are not well tolerated and most will require systemic treatment. In older children, local therapy should be considered, particularly if disease is distal involving sigmoid colon and rectum only. 5-ASA derivatives tend to be more effective than corticosteroids. Mesalazine preparations can be given as an enema (usually in 100mL) or suppository. Steroid preparations include Predfoam,® Predsol® (prednisolone), and Colifoam® (hydrocortisone).

It is important that children and families are adequately supported in the administration technique and positioning required. This will improve adherence and acceptability. Enemas are best given with the patient lying on their left side with the foot of the bed elevated and ample time given for the enema to act locally, i.e. 30–45 minutes before getting up and going to the toilet. Suppositories and small-volume enemas are easier to apply but are only effective for rectal disease. Proximal constipation is common in distal disease and should be treated with laxatives if present.

Local therapy should also be considered in children who fail to respond to systemic treatment (as additional treatment).

Thiopurine derivatives (azathioprine, 6-mercaptopurine)

- The main indication for azathioprine in ulcerative colitis, like Crohn's disease, is for steroid-sensitive, frequently relapsing disease (two or more flare-ups in 12 months), steroid-dependent disease (early relapse on weaning or discontinuation of steroids), and steroid-resistant disease (failure to respond to steroids).

- The aim of thiopurine therapy in children is to improve clinical well-being and reduce steroid requirements. There is an increasing tendency to give it at diagnosis in severe disease, particularly to those who don't respond rapidly to treatment. It can take 3–6 months to take effect. There is significant potential toxicity, with flu-like symptoms, GI symptoms, leucopenia, hepatitis, pancreatitis, rash, and infection.
- Thiopurine methyl transferase (TPMT) is important in the metabolism of thiopurine derivatives. Genetic polymorphisms for this will increase the risk of toxicity and this should be checked before starting.
- There is a small increase in the risk of lymphoma with long-term use of thiopurine derivatives.
- Frequent blood monitoring is required. There are various suggested regimens. The British National Formulary for Children recommends a weekly full blood count for 4 weeks then 3-monthly. Parents/children should be told to report any symptoms or signs of bone marrow suppression (bruising, bleeding, infection) acutely.
- 6-mercaptopurine is effective in a number of children either intolerant to or resistant to azathioprine.
- Dose of azathioprine is 2–2.5mg/kg per day and 6-mercaptopurine 1–1.5mg/kg per day given as a single daily dose.
- There is no evidence base for the use of methotrexate in paediatric ulcerative colitis.
- Measurement of active metabolite 6-TGN (thioguanine nucleotide) and 6-MMP (methyl mercaptopurine) concentration in plasma can be used in children failing therapy to assess compliance and risk of toxicity. A significantly greater therapeutic effect can be achieved in paediatric IBD patients with level of the thiopurine metabolite 6-TGN >235pmol/8 $\times$ 10^8 erythrocytes while hepatotoxicity correlates with elevated 6-methyl mercaptopurine (MMP) levels (>5700pmol/ 8 $\times$ 10^8 erythrocytes).

Anti-TNF

Infliximab should be considered for treatment of children with acute toxic colitis in whom there is a failure to respond (see earlier), steroid-refractory acute severe disease, or steroid-dependent persistent disease. It is given in three doses over 6 weeks (0, 2, and 6) at 5mg/kg; this can be followed by maintenance treatment every 6–8 weeks. Side effects include acute infusion reaction, delayed hypersensitivity reactions, serious infections, risk of opportunistic infections, and potential risk of malignancy. In children on moncolonal antibody therapy in whom there is no response/loss of response/toxicity, other treatments such as adalimumab can be tried.

Surgical management

Surgery will be required in at least 15% within 5 years of diagnosis and 25% by 10 years. Subtotal colectomy and temporary ileostomy is the most commonly performed operation. This can be performed as an emergency (acute toxic colitis with failure to respond to medical treatment) or electively, leaving a rectal stump as short as is practical. Indications for elective colectomy include disease resistant to medical treatment with morbidity either from the disease or complications of treatment, e.g. growth failure, high-grade dysplasia. Reconstruction is usually timed after puberty to coincide with the holidays after school exams (aged 16+). This is usually done laparoscopically to reduce the risk of complications such as infertility in conjunction with the adult colorectal team.

Colectomy is curative from the point of view of the colitis. Following reconstruction, bowel frequency will be 10–12/day initially, reducing to 3–4/day by 1 year. However, there may be major long-term morbidity from faecal incontinence, defecation at night, adhesion obstruction, or problems with the rectal stump. Pouchitis affects at least 33% of all pouches, though antibiotics (metronidazole) may be helpful if given intermittently. Infertility can be a problem in women.

20% of patients prefer a permanent ileostomy combined with excision of the rectal stump, especially if there have been multiple complications following reconstruction.

Stoma management

This needs to be discussed before surgery where possible with the support of a stoma nurse who will advise about the practical management. Careful attention needs to be paid to stoma losses. The colon normally functions to reabsorb salt and water. Salt supplements may be required. Sodium status can be monitored by urine electrolytes, with low urinary sodium being suggestive of sodium depletion. If stoma losses increase significantly, e.g. during infection, there is a high risk of dehydration and IV fluid replacement may be required.

Cancer surveillance

Patient with colitis for >10 years, particularly if active, are at increased risk of colorectal cancer. Regular colonoscopic surveillance is indicated every 2–3 years. This is an issue for the paediatrician in children who have presented with disease at a young age. Risk factors for malignancy include young age at onset, longer duration of disease, and extent of colonic involvement. Colectomy is recommended if there is high-grade dysplasia or malignancy.

Case study

A 10-year-old girl presents with abdominal discomfort associated with frequent loose stools containing blood and mucus. Investigations show anaemia with thrombocytosis. Stool cultures are negative. Colonoscopy shows severe pancolitis with no normal mucosa. Histology is consistent with ulcerative colitis and she is treated with IV steroids. Despite some initial improvement she does not respond to treatment by day 5. Second-line therapy with infliximab is started following CXR to rule out tuberculosis. She completes a 6-week induction course and remains on maintenance treatment with azathioprine and infliximab. She does well initially, but her disease relapses three times in the first year necessitating further courses of steroids. Repeat colonoscopy shows a featureless 'hosepipe' colon. After appropriate preoperative counselling she undergoes a subtotal colectomy with ileostomy and mucus fistula formation and does well with a symptom-free adolescence. She will be a good candidate for future reconstructive surgery after she has completed her schooling.

References and resources

British National Formulary for Children: https://www.evidence.nhs.uk/formulary/bnfc/current

Carter MJ, Lobo AJ, Travis SP, IBD Section, British Society of Gastroenterology. Guidelines for the management of inflammatory bowel disease in adults. Gut 2004;53(Suppl 5):V1–16.

Fell JM, Muhammed R, Spray C, et al. Management of ulcerative colitis. Arch Dis Child 2016;101:469–74.

National Institute for Health and Care Excellence (NICE). Ulcerative colitis: management. Clinical Guideline CG166. London: NICE; 2013. https://www.nice.org.uk/guidance/cg166

Mowat C, Cole A, Windsor A, et al. Guidelines for the management of inflammatory bowel disease in adults. Gut 2011;60:571–607.

Turner D, Levine A, Escher JC, et al. Management of pediatric ulcerative colitis: joint ECCO and ESPGHAN evidence-based consensus guidelines. J Pediatr Gastroenterol Nutr 2012;55:340–61.

Eosinophilic disorders

Introduction *416*
Eosinophilic proctocolitis of infancy (dietary protein-induced
    proctocolitis of infancy) *418*
Eosinophilic enterocolitis of infancy (dietary protein-induced
    enterocolitis of infancy) *420*
Eosinophilic enterocolitis in the older child *421*
Eosinophilic oesophagitis *422*
Features suggestive of food allergy as a cause of gastrointestinal
    disease *423*
References and resources *424*

Introduction

This chapter discusses the wide spectrum of eosinophilic (allergic) disorders of the gut. They are generally not IgE mediated and because of this, standard allergy testing using a skin prick test of specific IgE may not elucidate the cause. Presentation is with the full spectrum of GI symptoms and signs. Outside infancy, the disorders may only become apparent on investigation of chronic gut symptoms by endoscopy to exclude oesophagitis, peptic ulceration, enteropathy, or colitis. Important disorders to consider are:

- Eosinophilic proctocolitis of infancy (dietary protein-induced proctocolitis of infancy).
- Eosinophilic enterocolitis of infancy (dietary protein-induced enterocolitis of infancy).
- Eosinophilic enterocolitis in the older child.
- Eosinophilic oesophagitis.

Eosinophilic proctocolitis of infancy (dietary protein-induced proctocolitis of infancy)

- This is a common disorder and generally benign with a good prognosis.
- Most infants present having been exposed to cow's milk formula although the condition can occur while being breastfed secondary to transmission of cow's milk protein in breast milk.
- Mean age at diagnosis of 2 months.
- Infants are generally healthy with visible specks or streaks of blood mixed with mucus in the stool. Blood loss is usually minimal, and anaemia is rare. The infants are generally thriving.
- It is often associated with other non-IgE-mediated symptoms including vomiting and gastro-oesophageal reflux.
- Differential diagnosis includes infection, constipation, and anal fissures. Bleeding associated with vitamin K deficiency should be excluded.
- Cow's milk protein is the most common implicated antigen.
- Symptoms occur as a result of maternally ingested proteins excreted in breast milk or whole dairy protein-based feeds.
- Endoscopic examination is usually deferred but if indicated will show a predominantly distal colitis with an eosinophilic infiltrate on biopsy.
- Endoscopic examination is indicated in infants in whom there is doubt about the initial diagnosis or a poor response to treatment.
- Blood investigations are usually unremarkable. Mild anaemia, thrombocytosis, and a low serum albumin may be seen. Peripheral eosinophilia is occasionally seen. Serum IgA may be low. IgE antibody skin prick testing and specific IgE (formerly RAST) testing are often negative.
- Diagnosis is secured by response to dietary elimination of the causal antigen. For breastfed infants, strict maternal avoidance of cow's milk is required. This requires dietetic advice. For cow's milk formula-fed infants substitution with an extensively protein hydrolysate formula (e.g. Nutramigen®, Mead Johnson; Simillac Ailmentum®, Abbott Nutrition; SMA® Althera, Nestlé) generally leads to cessation of bleeding. An amino acid-based formula (e.g. Neocate®, Nutricia; Pure Amino®, Mead Johnson; SMA® Alfamino, Nestlé) may be needed in those who have prolonged bleeding or persistence of other symptoms, e.g. GOR, vomiting, while taking an extensive hydrolysate formula. Bleeding is expected to resolve within 72 hours of dietary exclusion. Continued bleeding may be an indication for referral for more invasive testing (i.e. endoscopic biopsy).
- It is usual to challenge within 3 months of exclusion diet to confirm the diagnosis. With the following proviso, this can be conducted at home with careful medical or dietetic follow-up.
- The disorder is not usually IgE antibody mediated, but infants with severe eczema who have excluded cow's milk for >6 weeks should have skin prick testing or specific IgE before the re-introduction of milk. Some infants will switch from non-IgE to IgE-mediated disease, and will

experience immediate urticaria, angio-oedema, and even anaphylaxis on reintroduction of cow's milk protein. Therefore infants with evidence of raised IgE to milk should have reintroduction as a food challenge under hospital supervision.

- The condition generally resolves completely by age 1–2 years, and the causal food protein can be gradually added back to the diet at that time with monitoring. If there are no extenuating factors (see next bullet point) then this could be done from 12 months of age as tolerated.
- Delayed weaning until 6 months should be encouraged, with dairy free solids in the first instance.

Eosinophilic enterocolitis of infancy (dietary protein-induced enterocolitis of infancy)

- This is part of a disease spectrum. Enterocolitis implies involvement of the small and large bowel and therefore the more severe end of the spectrum of eosinophilic proctocolitis of infancy.
- It can present with severe diarrhoea, dehydration, lethargy, and acidosis with raised inflammatory markers and hypoalbuminaemia.
- Infants may require resuscitation if fluid losses are severe.
- Wide differential diagnosis.
- Cow's milk is the most common implicated antigen. Infants with severe eczema may also have multiple food allergens.
- Upper and lower GI endoscopy is indicated.
- Biopsy may show an enteropathy and/or a colitis, both of which can be severe. A dense inflammatory infiltrate with eosinophilic degranulation is characteristic.
- Treatment is by removal of the offending antigen. Amino acid-based formulas are generally required. Weaning should be delayed until 6 months and dairy/soya/wheat/egg free in the first instance.
- Cases should be managed jointly between paediatric gastroenterologists and specialists in paediatric allergy.
- Challenge can result in severe reactions (acute and delayed), so should be done in hospital.
- A proportion of the most severe cases may require a period of bowel rest on total PN, anti-inflammatories/steroids, and/or other immunosuppression.
- Most infants outgrow the allergy by the age of 3 years.
- The disorder is not IgE antibody mediated but may be associated with severe atopy and multiple food allergies.

Eosinophilic enterocolitis in the older child

- This is a spectrum of disorders which have in common eosinophilic inflammation of the gut.
- Different subtypes:
  - Eosinophilic oesophagitis
  - Eosinophilic gastritis
  - Eosinophilic enterocolitis
  - Eosinophilic colitis.
- These conditions present with a full spectrum of GI symptoms and presentations including nausea, dysphagia, pain, vomiting, diarrhoea, and blood per rectum.
- There is a wide differential diagnosis including gastroenteritis, parasitic infection, bacterial overgrowth, immunodeficiency, IBD, and vasculitis.
- Diagnosis requires the presence of:
  - Gut symptoms.
  - Eosinophilic infiltrate in on or more areas from the oesophagus to the rectum.
  - Absence of other causes.
- Diagnosis is by biopsy and then clinicopathological correlation.
- It is normal to have some eosinophils present in the lamina propria of the gut mucosa but not the submucosa, muscular, or serosal layers.
- >20 eosinophils per high-power field with infiltration into the submucosa, muscular, or serosal layers is diagnostic in the presence of gut symptoms.
- Peripheral eosinophilia is common in about 50%
- The condition is difficult to treat, and treatment decisions should be based on symptoms rather than histological features alone.
- A proportion of children are food sensitive, most commonly to milk, egg, soya, and wheat. Exclusion of the presumed offending antigen should be on a trial basis with dietetic supervision (4–6 weeks) and careful observation of clinical symptoms. Skin-prick testing and specific IgE T-antibody testing may be helpful in this group food-sensitive group.
- Treatment of the non-food-sensitive group is very difficult, and immunosuppressive including corticosteroids may be required.

Eosinophilic oesophagitis

- Symptoms overlap with GOR with predominance in older atopic males.
- Dysphagia is common secondary to oesophageal dysmotility (this is an unusual symptom in children and should prompt consideration of further investigation).
- Skin-prick testing and IgE RAST antibody testing may be helpful.
- Acid reflux may be present on pH study (usually more prominent during the day than at night).
- Endoscopy is indicated.
- Upper, mid, and lower oesophageal biopsies should be taken.
- Diagnostic criteria on oesophageal biopsy are:
  - Reflux oesophagitis >7 eosinophils per high-power field,
  - Eosinophilic oesophagitis >15–20 per high-power field.
- Treatments include those for GOR, a trial of dietary elimination, corticosteroids, anti-inflammatories, and immunosuppression. Inhaled corticosteroids taken into the mouth then swallowed with nothing to eat or drink for 30 minutes are helpful.
- Dietary elimination should be with milk and soya exclusion in the first instance. Wheat exclusion can be considered (second line). NB Coeliac serology should be performed as a baseline if wheat exclusion is considered.
- The treatment can be difficult and response should be by clinical review and follow-up endoscopy with repeat biopsies in difficult cases.
- The natural history is not well defined, with relapse, remission, and chronicity.

Features suggestive of food allergy as a cause of gastrointestinal disease

- A temporal relationship between characteristic symptoms and ingestion of particular food.
- This is not always clear as non-IgE-mediated food allergies can lead to delayed symptomatology.
- Improvement in symptoms with removal of the implicated food.
- Confirmation of a relationship between ingestion of the specific dietary protein and symptoms by clinical challenge or repeated exposures.
- Evidence of specific IgE antibody/skin-prick test positivity in settings of IgE-mediated disease.
- Associated other atopic features including dermatitis, allergic rhinitis, asthma, and a family history of atopic disease (parents and siblings).

Specific clinical scenarios that may warrant evaluation for food allergy or intolerance

- Immediate GI symptoms (oral, pruritus, vomiting, diarrhoea) after ingestion of particular food(s).
- Mucous/bloody stools in an infant.
- Faltering growth.
- Malabsorption/protein-losing enteropathy.
- Subacute/chronic vomiting, diarrhoea.
- Dysphagia/food bolus obstruction in an older child.
- GI symptoms in a patient with atopy.
- GOR refractory to standard therapies.
- Infantile colic poorly responsive to behavioural interventions.
- Chronic constipation refractory to conventional management.

References and resources

Abdulrahman AA, Storr MA, Shaffer EA. Eosinophilic colitis: epidemiology, clinical features, and current management. Therap Adv Gastroenterol 2011;4:301–9. https://www.ncbi.nlm.nih.gov/pmc/articles/PMC3165205/pdf/10.1177_1756283X10392443.pdf

Furuta GT, Liacouras CA, Collins MN, et al. Eosinophilic esophagitis in children and adults: a systematic review and consensus recommendation for diagnosis and treatment. Gastroenterology 2007;133:1342–63.

Koletzko S, Niggeman B, Aralo A, et al. Diagnostic approach and management of cow's milk allergy in infants and chldren. J Paed Gastro Nutr 2012;55:221–9.

Luyt D, Ball H, Makwana N. BSACI guideline for the diagnosis and management of cow's milk allergy. Clin Exp Allergy 2014;44:642–72.

National Institute for Health and Care Excellence (NICE). Food allergy in children and young people. Clinical Guideline 116. London: NICE; 2011. https://www.nice.org.uk/guidance/CG1160

Papadopoulou A, Koletzko S, Heuschkel R, et al. Management guidelines of eosinophilic oesophagitis in childhood. J Paed Gastro Nutr 2014;58:107–18. http://www.espghan.org/fileadmin/user_upload/guidelines_pdf/Guidelines_2404/Management_Guidelines_of_Eosinophilic_Esophagitis.27.pdf

The pancreas

Background *426*
Pancreatitis *428*
Investigation *430*
Management *432*
Hereditary pancreatitis *434*
Autoimmune pancreatitis *435*
Conclusion *436*
References and resources *436*

Background

The pancreas is a J-shaped, flattened gland located in the upper left abdomen that secretes digestive enzymes into the duodenum and produces several important hormones as part of the endocrine system. Etymologically, the term 'pancreas', derives from the Greek word πάγκρεας (πᾶν ('all', 'whole'), and κρέας ('flesh') meaning all-flesh, due to its fleshy consistency.

Anatomically, the pancreas is divided into the head of pancreas, the neck of pancreas, the body of pancreas, and the tail of pancreas. It has two main ducts, the main pancreatic and the accessory pancreatic duct. These drain enzymes through the ampulla of Vater into the duodenum.

The pancreas is a secretory structure with an endocrine and an exocrine role. As part of its endocrine function the pancreas produces insulin and glucagon, two hormones essential to continuous blood glucose regulation. The digestive enzymes produced as part of its exocrine function in a response to changes in the gut microenvironment and their digestive roles are listed in Table 50.1.

Table 50.1 Pancreatic enzymes and their digestive role

Enzyme	Digestion
Amylase	Starch
Lipase and co-lipase	Triglycerides
Phospholipase	Phospholipids
Trypsin	Peptides
Chymotrypsin	Peptides

Pancreatitis

The incidence of pancreatitis is between 3.6 and 13.2 cases per 100,000 children. It is similar to the incidence in adults but there is a different aetiology, which in adults is mostly associated with lifestyle choices such as smoking and alcohol consumption.

Presenting symptoms of pancreatitis include pain (80–95%) either epigastric or diffuse, nausea and vomiting (40–80%), abdominal guarding, general irritability, abdominal distension, fever, jaundice, ascites, and difficulty in breathing due to pleural effusion.

There are a wide range of medicines associated with pancreatitis with the most commonly reported being azathioprine, 6-mercaptopurine, valproic acid, tetracyclines, aminosalicylic acid, steroids, sulfasalazine, and NSAIDs.

Causes of pancreatitis can be duct obstruction (cholelithiasis), anatomical anomalies (pancreas divisum, long common channel, duodenal diverticulum, biliary obstruction), alcohol, drugs, metabolic conditions (hypertriglyceridaemia, hypercalcaemia, methylmalonic acidaemia), trauma (accidental, child abuse, or iatrogenic (post ERCP)), infection, hereditary causes (PRSS1, SPINK1, CFTR, CPA1), autoimmune, toxins (scorpion venom, pesticides), and idiopathic.

New definitions for pancreatitis were developed during 2011 by the INSSPIRE paediatric working group, which included acute, acute-recurrent, or chronic pancreatitis, and have reclassified the diagnostic criteria.

Acute pancreatitis

Defined as acute-onset abdominal pain mainly in the epigastric region with elevation of serum amylase and/or lipase and evidence of pancreatic tissue inflammation on imaging. The first criteria for acute pancreatitis were agreed in Atlanta, GA, USA, in 1992 and were subsequently revised in 2013. Radiological classification of acute pancreatitis was either acute oedematous interstitial with heterogeneous pancreatic enhancement and peripancreatic fatty changes or acute necrotizing pancreatitis. Peri- and/or pancreatic collections remain controversial in their description. Pancreatic pseudocysts have been clearly differentiated though from acute necrotic collections (<4 weeks from presentation) and walled-off necrosis with pseudocysts appearing after 4 weeks from presentation containing no solid material and having well-formed cyst wall. Some attempts have been made to adopt severity criteria in children including age, white cell count, serum albumin, calcium, urea, lactate dehydrogenase, fluid collections with no general consensus.

Complications of pancreatitis can develop either early (due to a cytokine activation cascade) or late (>1 week after presentation) including pleural effusion, sepsis, coagulopathy, shock, and single or multi-organ failure. Development of local complications includes fat and pancreatic necrosis, abscesses, fluid collections, pseudocysts, and ductal abnormalities. Pancreatic pseudocysts in children usually show spontaneous resolution in 25–50% of cases with up to 50% of cases requiring surgical or endoscopic intervention (usually cyst-gastrostomy depending on their anatomical position). The aetiology is usually pancreatic trauma and they can be complicated by infection, haemorrhage, or spontaneous rupture.

Current therapeutic targets studied have been at both an intracellular and extracellular level. Researchers have been focusing on unfolded protein response (UPR) activators, Ca^{2+} influx inhibitors, mitochondrial depolarization inhibitors, neutrophil migration inhibitors, inflammatory signal inhibitors (protein kinase C+D, nuclear factor kappa B), specific vasoactive agents, neural or vascular response at an extracellular level.

Acute recurrent pancreatitis

Classified when patient has suffered at least two episodes of acute pancreatitis with complete resolution of symptoms and normalization of pancreatic biochemical indices and no evidence of chronic changes on imaging.

Chronic pancreatitis

Diagnosed on the basis of abdominal pain or either endocrine or exocrine insufficiency along with pancreatic imaging suggestive of a chronic inflammatory process. In children, chronic pancreatitis is most commonly associated with genetic, hereditary, or idiopathic conditions.

Investigation

The initial investigations for pancreatitis include serum amylase and lipase, lipid profile and triglycerides, liver function tests and serum calcium. Radiological tests are essential such as ultrasound, MRI pancreas ($\pm$ secretin), MRCP, abdominal CT and if ductal pathology is suspected then ERCP is recommended. Further tests included genetic screening for hereditary causes (PRSS1, SPINK1, and CFTR) and/or a sweat test to exclude cystic fibrosis. Faecal elastase and chymotrypsin are recommended to assess exocrine insufficiency and fat-soluble vitamin (A, D, E, K) levels for malabsorption. Autoimmune profile is advisable (autoantibodies, serum immunoglobulins and IgG subclasses) and pancreatic biopsy either via endoscopic ultrasound or laparoscopy may be considered especially if pancreatic lesions or swelling is confirmed on imaging.

Management

Management of pancreatitis is multidimensional, consisting of pain control, nutrition, dealing with local and systemic complications, and pancreatic rest. For pancreatic rest, treating physicians may consider somatostatin and its analogues although there is conflicting evidence, with no effect on pain but they may work as prophylaxis for further episodes of pancreatitis. Antimicrobials may need to be considered if an infectious cause is suspected. Interventional procedures (such as ERCP if ductal abnormalities) and/or surgery (drainage, pancreatectomy) will need to be discussed with a specialized centre if clinically indicated.

Pain management

Pain control is a key and most troublesome aspect of pancreatitis management more so in chronic cases. The first line of analgesia is currently opioids with dose adjustment as per intensity of symptoms. There is no strong evidence to suggest lipase enzyme replacement for pain management although it supports pancreatic rest. Neuropathic pain agents (such as gabapentin) are a recommended alternative in an attempt to minimize the opioid intake. Other interventions such as transcutaneous electrical nerve stimulation (TENS) are advisable as adjuvant supportive measures. In adults, more invasive techniques such as percutaneous coeliac plexus block (CPB) either via percutaneous or endoscopic ultrasound (EUS)-guided route are an option followed by thoracoscopic splanchnicectomy for more refractory to conservative treatment cases. Endoscopic intervention, extracorporeal shear wave lithotripsy, and surgery have also been utilized for debilitating chronic pain.

Nutrition

Patients with acute severe pancreatitis are considered to be in a hypermetabolic state and nutritional support is essential. Common issues to be addressed in chronic pancreatitis management in children are:

- Faltering growth secondary to increased energy expenditure.
- Malnutrition due to food avoidance, chronic abdominal pain, nausea, and vomiting.
- Patients with biliary involvement may require medium-chain triglyceride fats and additional fat-soluble vitamins.
- Insulin therapy due to pancreatic islet cell destruction to manage diabetes mellitus.
- Gastro-resistant pancreatic enzymes (lipase) may be required. Total daily dose of pancreatic enzyme replacement therapy (PERT) should be tailored to enteral intake but avoid exceeding the maximum daily dose of 10,000IU/kg.

Faecal fat excretion should be measured regularly but the aim should be satisfactory growth and normal fat-soluble vitamin levels.

Initiating small-volume, low-fat oral intake should be attempted within 48–72 hours from presentation and failing that, nasogastric slow-rate continuous low-fat feeds should be the next step. If the child is not tolerating gastric route feeds change to nasojejunal feeding which seems the currently preferred route. If the patient undergoes surgical intervention (Puestow procedure) then enteral feeding may start after 5–7 days from the operation and PN may seem the best option for this interim period. PN can be considered in children once all other routes of enteral feeding have been exhausted. PN fat emulsions are generally well tolerated if there is no current or previous history of hyperlipidaemia.

PN seems to have a higher infection-associated mortality rate and increases gut translocation when compared to enteral feeding. Early nutrition has a protective role in pancreatitis as it reduces the overall rate of infections, surgical interventions, and further complications. Local complications should not be considered as a contraindication for early enteral nutrition and feeding tolerance should be guided by clinical symptoms rather than by elevation of serum amylase and inflammatory markers.

Hereditary pancreatitis

Hereditary pancreatitis has been associated with mutations in the following genes:

- *PRSS1* encoding the cationic trypsinogen, the most abundant isoform of trypsinogen in human pancreatic juice.
- *SPINK1* (serine protease inhibitor) encoding the pancreatic secretory trypsin inhibitor (PSTI), a defensive mechanism against prematurely activated trypsin.
- Chymotrypsin C (*CTRC*) encoding the trypsin-degrading enzyme chymotrypsin C predisposing to pancreatitis by diminishing its protective trypsin-degrading activity.
- *CFTR* encoding an ATP-binding cassette (ABC) transporter that functions as a low conductance chloride-selective channel gated by cycles of ATP binding.
- *CPA1* encoding the A-type carboxypeptidase 1, which hydrolyses the C-terminal bonds in peptide chains with no increase in pancreatic trypsin activation but endoplasmic reticulum misfolding and cellular stress.

The overall management is generic as in other causes of pancreatitis in respect to nutrition, pain control, and indications for interventional procedures. ERCP should be considered if significant ductal changes are identified ± ductal stenting, filling defects and suspected anatomical variations involving the pancreatic ducts.

In cases with persistent pancreatic duct strictures where pancreatic draining is hindered, surgical options can be considered. Longitudinal pancreatojejunostomy (Puestow procedure) should be discussed with surgical colleagues or a Frey procedure considered, where diseased portions of pancreatic head are removed in order to improve drainage and minimize pain. In the current era, total pancreatectomy with islet cell transplantation can be also considered for those patients in whom all other measures to reduce pain and improve quality of life have been unsuccessful. The timing of the respective intervention should be considered carefully. Psychological support has been shown to be effective in patients with chronic pancreatitis and it should be offered early on to them and their families.

Autoimmune pancreatitis

Autoimmune pancreatitis (AIP) is a rare form of chronic pancreatitis in children. It was initially described by Sarles et al. in 1961 as chronic pancreatitis with hypergammaglobulinaemia. Subsequently Toki et al. in 1992 reported further cases and the term AIP was introduced by Yoshida et al. in 1995. Other descriptive names of the condition included chronic pancreatitis with autoimmune features, non-alcoholic duct-destructive chronic pancreatitis, lymphoplasmocytic sclerosing pancreatitis with cholangitis, chronic sclerosing pancreatitis, pseudotumorous pancreatitis, and duct-narrowing chronic pancreatitis. The current accepted definition is histopathological and is classified into type 1 for lymphoplasmacytic sclerosing pancreatitis (LPSP) and type 2 for idiopathic duct centric chronic pancreatitis (IDCP) or AIP with granulocytic epithelial lesion (GEL).

Extrapancreatic lesions have been reported in the form of sclerosing cholangitis, sclerosing sialadenitis, retroperitoneal fibrosis, interstitial nephritis, chronic thyroiditis, interstitial pneumonia, and lymphadenopathy.

Laboratory diagnostic criteria include raised levels of gamma-globulin, IgG or IgG4 subclasses, presence of autoantibodies (smooth muscle, antinuclear, anti-lactoferrin, anti-carbonic anhydrase), raised hepatobiliary and/or pancreatic enzymes, and impaired exocrine and endocrine pancreatic function.

Radiological findings include pancreatic enlargement (mostly of the uncinate process), irregular narrowing of the pancreatic duct, and stenosis of the intrahepatic bile ducts with sclerosing cholangitis-like features.

Pancreatic tissue obtained via EUS or ductal/ampullary sampling via ERCP may be useful to establish the diagnosis. Histological findings include interlobular fibrosis, acinar atrophy, tissue infiltration with IgG4-positive plasma cells, and obliterative phlebitis.

Recommended treatment is oral prednisolone (2mg/kg, max. 60mg once daily) tapered slowly by 5–10mg aiming to keep the patient on a maintenance dose (5–7.5mg/day) for 6 months on average and then review. During the treatment period, patients should be monitored closely for biochemical, clinical, or radiological progress and development of side effects such as hypertension and diabetes.

Conclusion

The pancreas is a vital organ and pancreatic diseases are rare in children but appear to be becoming more prevalent in our current era. Future research on pancreatitis is focused on organ injury at intra- or extracellular level with several severity biomarkers being developed along with interventional procedures and imaging techniques. In adults, where pancreatitis seems to be more severe, timing of organ failure, classification of severity, and duration of disease seem to be important prognostic factors. New genetic causes associated with pancreatitis are identified but there is still a significant proportion where the aetiology remains indeterminate.

References and resources

Afghani E, Pandol SJ, Shimosegawa T, et al. Acute pancreatitis-progress and challenges: a report on an international symposium. Pancreas 2015;44:1195–210.

Troendle DM, Fishman DS, Barth BA, et al. Therapeutic endoscopic retrograde cholangiopancreatography in pediatric patients with acute recurrent and chronic pancreatitis: data from the INSPPIRE (INternational Study group of Pediatric Pancreatitis: In search for a cuRE) Study. Pancreas 2017;46:764–9.

Liver function tests

Aminotransferases *438*
Enzymes of cholestasis *438*
Tests of liver synthetic function *438*

Aminotransferases

- Aspartate aminotransferase (AST)—formerly known as SGOT—is an enzyme that can be found in the mitochondria and the cytosol of many tissues such as the liver, skeletal muscle, cardiac muscle, kidney, brain, and others.
- Alanine aminotransferase (ALT)—formerly known as SGPT—is an enzyme that can be found in the cytosol mostly of the liver.
- Elevated levels of aminotransferases indicate hepatocyte injury, but may also be seen in disorders unrelated to the liver such as myopathies (where the 'biliary' enzymes are normal and creatine kinase is raised).

Enzymes of cholestasis

- Alkaline phosphatase (ALP) is an enzyme for the hydrolysis of organic phosphate esters. It can be found in various tissues, the most important being the liver and the bone. It can be raised in isolation in growing children.
- Gamma-glutamyl transferase (GGT) is a microsomal enzyme found in many tissues not just liver. GGT is raised in a wide variety of liver disorders. It is also induced by many drugs, e.g. phenytoin and phenobarbital. It is not unusual for neonates to have higher levels than children and adults.
- Bilirubin can be unconjugated and conjugated (see Chapter 53).

Tests of liver synthetic function

- Albumin is a serum protein synthesized only in the liver. Low levels of albumin may be due to chronic liver disease, but also to acute infection (albumin is a negative acute phase reactant), nephrotic syndrome, and protein-losing enteropathy amongst others.
- Prothrombin time (PT) assesses the extrinsic pathway of coagulation (involving factors I, II, V, VII, and X). A prolonged PT may be due to disseminated intravascular coagulation, impaired hepatic synthesis, or congenital deficiency of the above-mentioned clotting factors or impaired activation of factors II, VII, IX, and X due to vitamin K deficiency.
- Ammonia is produced mainly in the gut by bacterial urease from dietary amino acids. The majority of it is detoxified by the urea cycle in the liver where it is delivered by the portal vein. High levels of ammonia can be found in acute and chronic advanced liver disease, but also in portosystemic shunts, urea cycle disorders, and Reye syndrome.

Liver biopsy

Introduction *440*
Indications *440*
Contraindications *441*
Practicalities *442*

Introduction

Liver biopsy allows clinicians to view liver tissue on a microscopic scale. It is used as a diagnostic tool in liver disease, but can also be useful for prognosis and monitoring disease progression. It remains a key part of management in specialist liver centres. However, with evolution of diagnostic and laboratory techniques, the role of liver biopsy in children is changing and therefore its indication and benefit in each case needs to be carefully considered.

Indications

Liver biopsy can be performed in a native or transplanted liver. It is commonly used in the diagnosis and monitoring of the following disorders:

- Neonatal cholestasis (e.g. biliary atresia).
- Progressive familial intrahepatic cholestasis.
- Alpha-1 antitrypsin deficiency.
- Alagille syndrome.
- Autoimmune liver disease.
- Lysosomal acid lipase deficiency.
- Cryptogenic hypertransaminasaemia.
- NAFLD.
- Wilson disease.
- Drug-induced liver injury.
- Sclerosing cholangitis.
- Congenital hepatic fibrosis.
- Disorders of glycosylation.
- CMV and EBV viruses.
- Liver tumours.
- Post liver transplantation.

Contraindications

- *Clotting abnormalities*: contraindicated if international normalized ratio (INR) above 1.5, or platelets <60. It should be noted that normal clotting and coagulation does not preclude bleeding, and this can still occur in children with normal platelets and clotting values.
- *Ascites*: biopsy in these patients can cause unpredictable haemodynamic changes and the liver is harder to locate without imaging. In addition, there is an increased risk of bile leak or bleeding which can lead to peritonitis.
- *High-risk groups*: haematological malignancy, hepatic haemangiomas, biliary dilatation, sickle cell disease, haemophagocytic lymphohistocytosis.

Practicalities

Preparation before biopsy

Informed consent should be gained prior to liver biopsy and should be documented in the patient's notes. Information regarding the biopsy should be explained in the parent's native language and an independent interpreter should be used if necessary. The family should be made aware of the indication for biopsy, the procedure, the potential risks, and the benefits. Consent can only be taken by a clinician who has been trained in liver biopsy as per national guidelines.

Blood tests to be done 24 hours prior to procedure:
- Full blood count including platelet count.
- Coagulation screen.
- Fibrinogen.
- Urea and electrolytes.
- Liver function tests.
- Total and direct bilirubin.

Liver biopsy should not be performed if INR is >1.5. In these instances, blood products or vitamin K can be given as supplementation and bloods rechecked prior to procedure. Vitamin K should be given at least 6 hours prior to procedure; FFP can be given immediately before biopsy. FFP volume is calculated at 10–15mL/kg.

Drugs

Any medications interfering with coagulation or platelet function (e.g. aspirin, heparin, warfarin) should be omitted at least 24 hours prior to procedure.

Nil by mouth

Children should remain nil by mouth for at least 4 hours prior to biopsy. This may vary depending on age or medical condition of the child. IV fluid support ($\pm$ glucose) should be provided for small children or those at risk of hypoglycaemia or dehydration.

Ultrasound

It is advised to perform a liver ultrasound scan (USS) prior to biopsy in order to mark an appropriate site for percutaneous biopsy and exclude anatomical variants, e.g. situs inversus.

Antibiotics

Children with high risk of infection should receive at least three doses of prophylactic antibiotics with biopsy.

Sedation

Policies vary between hospitals but it is generally recommended that oral sedation or general anaesthetic should be used for liver biopsy and, if possible, local anaesthetic should be applied to the site of biopsy in order to reduce post-procedural pain.

Procedure

Percutaneous liver biopsy

This method uses percussion of the liver to locate the site of biopsy. The site is usually the area of maximum dullness between the seventh and ninth intercostal spaces in the mid-clavicular line. A USS prior to the biopsy can help to exclude any anatomical variants and provides a marked site for insertion of the needle. After skin preparation and local anaesthetic, the biopsy needle is inserted at this site.

Plugged-track percutaneous biopsy uses the same method as a normal percutaneous biopsy but a 'plugging' agent is inserted into the needle track as the biopsy needle is removed. This is in an attempt to reduce bleeding.

Transjugular liver biopsy

Done in high-risk patients or when percutaneous biopsy is contraindicated. The procedure is performed by interventional radiologists. Its limitations include small or fragmented tissue samples.

Liver biopsy at laparoscopy/laparotomy

Not commonly carried out in children but is still used in certain circumstances. These biopsies are mostly 'wedge biopsies' which obtain peripheral tissue only using a cold knife or electrocautery. With this method the sample site can be more easily selected and a larger sample can be taken. The laparoscopic or open approach also allows for direct vision and easier control of any bleeding from the biopsy site. Alternatively, needle biopsies can be obtained at laparoscopy, offering deeper sampling and a reduced chance of bleeding.

Monitoring

Basic observations including respiratory rate, heart rate, blood pressure, oxygen saturations, and temperature should be taken at least 1 hour prior to liver biopsy.

Complications

The majority of complications post biopsy occur within the first 24 hours of the procedure. These include:

- Pain.
- Infection.
- Bleeding.
- Haemothorax/pneumothorax.
- Organ perforation.
- Haemobilia.
- Bile leak.
- Death.

In studies of liver biopsy in adults, it was found that fatal complications occurred within the first 6 hours after the procedure. For this reason, we monitor children hourly for a minimum of 6 hours after biopsy.

Recommendations post biopsy
- Ensure adequate haemostasis with compression and dressing of the wound site.
- Remain in bed for 1 hour post biopsy.
- Remain nil by mouth for 2 hours after biopsy.
- Blood tests are not necessary immediately after biopsy unless there are signs of haemodynamic instability or concerns about bleeding.
- Avoid contact sports for 1 week after biopsy.

Neonatal jaundice

Epidemiology 446
Unconjugated hyperbilirubinaemia 448
Specific conditions 450
Conjugated hyperbilirubinaemia 452
Idiopathic neonatal hepatitis 458
References and resources 458

Epidemiology

- 30–50% of normal term newborns are jaundiced after birth.
- Physiological and breast milk jaundice account for the majority of cases.
- 1 in 2500 infants has conjugated hyperbilirubinaemia.
- The recommended current practice is to exclude conjugated hyperbilirubinaemia in any infant clinically jaundiced at 14 days if they were born at >37 weeks' gestation or at 21 days if they were born at <37 weeks' gestation.

Unconjugated hyperbilirubinaemia

Bilirubin metabolism

- Unconjugated bilirubin is a product of haem metabolism and is transported by albumin.
- Conjugation is with glucuronic acid by esterification to make it water soluble (enzyme—bilirubin uridine diphosphate glucurony transferase, UGT1A1).
- Secretion occurs against a concentration gradient through the canalicular membrane into the bile.

Causes

(See Table 53.1.)

Most common:
- Physiological jaundice.
- Breast milk jaundice.
- Haemolysis.
- Congenital defects of bile conjugation.

Table 53.1 Causes of neonatal unconjugated hyperbilirubinaemia

Increased production of unconjugated bilirubin from haem	Haemolytic disease (hereditary or acquired):
	• Isoimmune haemolysis (neonatal; acute, or delayed transfusion reaction; autoimmune)
	• Rh incompatibility
	• ABO incompatibility
	• Other blood group incompatibilities
	• Congenital spherocytosis
	• Hereditary elliptocytosis
	• Infantile pyknocytosis
	• Erythrocyte enzyme defects
	• Glucose-6-phosphate dehydrogenase deficiency
	• Pyruvate kinase deficiency
	• Haemoglobinopathy
	• Sickle cell anaemia
	• Thalassaemia
	Others:
	• Sepsis
	• Microangiopathy
	• Haemolytic–uraemic syndrome
	• Haemangioma
	• Ineffective erythropoiesis
	• Drugs
	• Infection
	• Enclosed haematoma
	Polycythemia:
	• Diabetic mother
	• Fetal transfusion (recipient)
	• Delayed cord clamping

Table 53.1 (*Contd.*)

Decreased delivery of unconjugated bilirubin (in plasma) to hepatocyte	Right-sided congestive heart failure Portacaval shunt
Decreased bilirubin uptake across hepatocyte membrane	Presumed enzyme transporter deficiency Competitive inhibition: ● Breast milk jaundice ● Lucy–Driscoll syndrome ● Drug inhibition (radiocontrast material) Miscellaneous: ● Hypothyroidism ● Hypoxia ● Acidosis
Decreased biotransformation (conjugation)	Physiological jaundice Inhibition (drugs) Hereditary (Crigler–Najjar): ● Type I (complete enzyme deficiency) ● Type II (partial deficiency) Gilbert disease Hepatocellular dysfunction
Enterohepatic recirculation	Intestinal obstruction: ● Ileal atresia ● Hirschsprung disease ● Cystic fibrosis ● Pyloric stenosis Antibiotic administration
Breast milk jaundice	

Kernicterus may result from high levels of unconjugated bilirubin.

Management strategy is with phototherapy (if serum bilirubin >250μmol/L in term babies; standard charts available for the preterm), adequate hydration, identifying and treating the underlying causes.

Specific conditions

Physiological jaundice

- 50% of term and 80% of preterm babies are jaundiced in the first week.
- Jaundice within the first 24 hours of life is always pathological and cannot be attributed to physiological jaundice.
- Aetiology of physiological jaundice is not precisely known but probably reflects immaturity of bilirubin uridine diphosphate glucuronyl transferase (UGT) activity.
- Jaundice peaks on day 3 of life.

Breast milk jaundice

- Occurs in 0.5–2% of newborn babies.
- Develops after day 4 (early pattern) or day 7 (late pattern).
- Jaundice peaks around the end of second week.
- May overlap with physiological jaundice or be protracted for 1–2 months.
- Diagnosis is supported by a drop in serum bilirubin (≥50% in 1–3 days) if breastfeeding is interrupted for 48 hours.

Haemolysis

- Commonly due to isoimmune haemolysis (Rh, ABO incompatibility), red cell membrane defects (congenital spherocytosis, hereditary elliptocytosis), enzyme defects (glucose-6-phosphate dehydrogenase or pyruvate kinase deficiency), or haemoglobinopathies (sickle cell anaemia, thalassaemia).
- Finding of jaundice in the presence of anaemia and a raised reticulocyte count necessitate further investigation for cause of haemolysis.

Inherited disorders of unconjugated hyperbilirubinaemia

- This spectrum of disease depends on the degree of bilirubin UGT deficiency.
- Liver function tests and histology are normal.
- Autosomal recessive inheritance. Gilbert syndrome and Crigler–Najjar type II can also have autosomal dominant transmission.

Gilbert syndrome

- Mild, 7% of population.
- Polymorphism with TA repeats in the promoter region (TATA box) in white patients compared to exon mutations in Asian patients on chromosome 2q37.
- Higher incidence of neonatal jaundice and breast milk jaundice.
- Usually presents after puberty with an incidental finding of elevated bilirubin on blood tests or jaundice after a period of fasting or intercurrent illness.
- More common in males.
- No treatment required, compatible with normal life span.

Crigler–Najjar type I
- Severe deficiency of UGT.
- High risk of kernicterus.
- Require life-long phototherapy or even liver transplantation.

Crigler–Najjar type II
- Moderate deficiency.
- May require phototherapy and phenobarbital.

Conjugated hyperbilirubinaemia

Definition
- Conjugated (direct) bilirubin >15% of total serum bilirubin level or
- Conjugated bilirubin > 25μmol/litre (NICE guidelines 2010).
- Conjugated jaundice is always pathological and needs prompt diagnosis and therapy.

Pathophysiology

The defect lies at the hepatocyte level or in the biliary drainage system. Disorders affecting the major bile ducts are usually amenable to surgical correction while the management of the defects at the hepatocyte or bile canalicular level is mainly medical. Liver transplantation may be necessary for those who progress to end-stage liver disease.

Causes of conjugated jaundice
(See Table 53.2.)
Common causes:
- 'Idiopathic' neonatal hepatitis (40%).
- Biliary atresia (25–30%).
- Intrahepatic cholestasis syndromes (20%), e.g. Alagille syndrome, progressive familial intrahepatic cholestasis (PFIC).
- Alpha-1 antitrypsin deficiency (7–10%).

If biliary atresia is suspected, the child should be referred to a liver unit for further investigation.

Clinical features
- Jaundice.
- Dark urine.
- Pale stools (not always).
- Hepatomegaly or hepatosplenomegaly.
- Variable degree of liver failure—hypoglycaemia, ascites, acid–base imbalance, electrolyte imbalance, coagulopathy.

Table 53.2 Causes of neonatal conjugated hyperbilirubinaemia

Biliary tree disorders	Biliary atresia
	Biliary hypoplasia (non-syndromic)
	Mucous plug
	Bile duct stenosis/stricture
	Spontaneous perforation of common bile duct
	Neonatal sclerosing cholangitis
	Caroli disease
	Compression of bile duct by a mass
	Inflammatory pseudotumour at porta hepatis

Table 53.2 (*Contd.*)

Infections	Bacterial:
	• Urinary tract infection
	• Septicaemia*
	• Syphilis
	• Listeriosis
	• Tuberculosis
	Parasitic:
	• Toxoplasmosis
	• Malaria
	Viral:
	• Cytomegalovirus
	• Herpes simplex*
	• Human herpes virus type 6*
	• Herpes zoster
	• Adenovirus
	• Parvovirus*
	• Enterovirus
	• Reovirus type 3
	• Human immunodeficiency virus
	• Hepatitis B*
	• ?Hepatitis A
	• ?Rotavirus
Metabolic disorders	Carbohydrate metabolism:
	• Galactosaemia*
	• Fructosaemia*
	• Glycogen storage disease type 4
	• Carbohydrate deficient glycoprotein*
	Protein metabolism (amino acid):
	• Tyrosinaemia*
	• Hypermethioninaemia
	Urea cycle defects (arginase deficiency)
	Lipid metabolism
	Niemann–Pick disease (type C)
	Cholesterol ester storage disease (Wolman disease)*
	Gaucher disease
	Bile acid metabolism disorders (primary/secondary)
	Zellweger syndrome
	Bile acid transport disorder
	Rotor syndrome
	Dubin–Johnson syndrome
	Fatty acid oxidation defects*
	Disorders of oxidative phosphorylation*
	Other mitochondrial disorders*
Endocrine disorders	Hypothyroidism
	Hypopituitarism (with or without septo-optic dysplasia)

(*Continued*)

Table 53.2 (*Contd.*)

Chromosomal disorders	Trisomy 21 (Down syndrome)
	Trisomy 18 (Edward syndrome)
	Trisomy 13 (Patau syndrome)
	Cat-eye syndrome
	Leprechaunism
Other genetic metabolic defects	Alpha-1 antitrypsin deficiency
	Cystic fibrosis
Familial cholestasis syndromes	Alagille syndrome
	Byler's syndrome (PFIC1)
	Bile salt export protein defect (BSEP defect, PFIC2)
	Multidrug resistant 3 deficiency (MDR3, PFIC3)
	Hereditary cholestasis with lymphoedema (Aagenaes syndrome)
Metals and toxins	Neonatal haemochromatosis*
	Copper related cholestasis*
	Parenteral nutrition
	Fetal alcohol syndrome
	Drugs
Haematological disorders	Haemophagocytic lymphohistiocytosis*
	Langerhans' cell histiocytosis
	Inspissated bile syndrome
Immunological disorders	Neonatal lupus erythematosus
	Giant cell hepatitis with Coombs positive haemolytic anaemia*
	Graft-versus-host disease
	Adenosine deaminase deficiency
Vascular anomalies	Haemangioendothelioma
	Budd–Chiari syndrome
	Congenital portocaval anomalies
Idiopathic	Familial
	Non-familial (good prognosis)
Miscellaneous	Hypoperfusion of liver*
	ARC syndrome (arthrogryposis, renal tubular dysfunction and cholestasis)

* Conditions that can present as acute liver failure.

Investigation
(See Box 53.1.)
- Confirm conjugated hyperbilirubinaemia.
- Look for evidence of sepsis or liver failure.
- Look for cause of conjugated jaundice.

Perform an extended metabolic screen if there is evidence of:
- Hypoglycaemia.
- Increased lactate or pyruvate.
- Steatosis on liver biopsy.

Box 53.1 Investigations for hyperbilirubinaemia

Urgent investigations at first contact
- Liver function tests.
- PT.
- Blood sugar.
- Serum electrolytes, urea and creatinine.
- Full blood count, reticulocyte count, peripheral blood smear, and direct Coomb's test if evidence of haemolysis.
- Blood and other body fluid cultures if indicated (unwell baby).
- Urine culture.
- Urine for reducing substances.

Subsequent investigations to consider
- Alpha-1 antitrypsin phenotype.*
- Galactose-1-phosphate uridyl transferase.*
- Urine succinyl acetone.
- Serum TSH and T_4.
- Serum cortisol (short Synacthen® test if cortisol low).
- Immunoreactive trypsin (<4 weeks of age).
- Serum and urine amino acid.
- Urine organic acids.
- Urine bile acids (child must be off ursodeoxycholic acid for 2–3 weeks).
- Serum triglyceride.
- Serum fibrinogen.
- Serum ferritin.
- TORCH screen, VDRL.
- Serology for HIV, human herpesvirus 6, and parvovirus B19.
- Hepatitis B antigen, hepatitis C antibody.
- Ultrasound of liver and biliary tree.
- Radiograph long bones and spine.
- Ophthalmic examination (anterior chamber, lens and retina).
- Liver biopsy.
- Endoscopic/percutaneous/MRCP, hepatobiliary scintigraphy (depending on local expertise) to demonstrate biliary tree patency.
- Bone marrow examination (to exclude storage disorders particularly Niemann–Pick type C, haemophagocytic lymphohistiocytosis or other haematological conditions).
- Exploratory laparotomy and operative cholangiography.

* Test should be carried out on parents if baby received blood products in last 6 weeks.

Management

- Identify treatable cause urgently and institute treatment.
- Manage vitamin K deficiency.
- Manage acute liver failure.
- Optimize nutrition.

Coagulopathy

PT can be prolonged due to:

- Vitamin K deficiency leads to deficient gamma-carboxylation of factors II, VII, IX, and X, resulting in the failure to trigger the clotting cascade. Administer 1mg/year of age (max. 5mg) of IV vitamin K and recheck PT 4–6 hours later. PT should normalize.
- Acute liver failure results in decreased synthesis of factors II, V, VII, IX, and X. Deficiency of factor VII and V is the most prominent as they have the shortest half-lives. Administration of vitamin K does not correct this coagulopathy.

Special dietary requirements

- Exclude galactose from diet until galactosaemia is excluded.
- If baby not thriving while awaiting investigations, start feed based on medium-chain triglycerides.
- Give fat-soluble vitamins (A, D, E, and K), twice recommended daily allowance. Can be a combination of Ketovite® liquid 5mL and three tablets with 1mg of Konakion MM® once daily, or Abidec® 1.2mL and vitamin E 100mg/kg daily with 1mg Konakion MM®.

Idiopathic neonatal hepatitis

- Diagnosis of exclusion (see Table 53.3).
- Associated with low birth weight or prematurity.
- Histology:
  - Hepatocellular swelling (ballooning), focal hepatic necrosis, and multinucleated giant cells.
  - Bile duct proliferation and bile duct plugging are usually absent.
- Factors predicting poor prognosis:
  - Severe jaundice beyond 6 months.
  - Acholic stools.
  - Familial occurrence.
  - Persistent hepatosplenomegaly.
- 90% do well with no long-term liver disease.

Table 53.3 Clinical clues to the diagnoses

Signs	Conditions
Cleft lip/palate, micropenis, optic nerve hypoplasia	Septo-optic dysplasia
Peripheral pulmonary stenosis, triangular facies, posterior embryotoxon	Alagille syndrome
Cataract	Galactosaemia
Cutaneous haemangioma	Haemangioendothelioma
White hair	Haemophagocytic lymphohistiocytosis (HLH)
Rickets	Tyrosinaemia
Coagulopathy	Tyrosinaemia, galactosaemia, HLH
Inverted nipples, lipoatrophy	Congenital disorders of glycosylation

References and resources

Moyer V, Freese DK, Whitington PF, et al. Guideline for the evaluation of cholestatic jaundice in infants: recommendations of the North American Society for Pediatric Gastroenterology, Hepatology and Nutrition. J Paed Gastro Nutr 2004;39:115–28.
National Institute for Health and Care Excellence (NICE). Jaundice in babies under 28 days old. Clinical Guideline CG98. London: NICE; 2016. https://www.nice.org.uk/guidance/cg98

Chapter 54

459

Biliary atresia

Definition *460*
Incidence *460*
Types *460*
Pathogenesis *460*
Clinical presentation *461*
Diagnosis *461*
Treatment *461*
Complications *462*
Prognosis *462*
References and resources *462*

Definition

Biliary atresia (BA) is a progressive cholangiopathy of unknown aetiology affecting the extra- and intrahepatic biliary system presenting within the first several weeks of life.

Incidence

The condition is sporadic with an estimated worldwide incidence of around 1/10,000–17,000 live births. It has been described in isolation in twin and triplet pregnancies, with no seasonal pattern. Children are typically born at term, with no gender predominance.

Types

There are three macroscopic types of BA:
- Type I—affecting the distal part of the common duct.
- Type II—affecting the common hepatic duct, common bile duct, and gallbladder.
- Type III—affecting right and left hepatic ducts and the gallbladder.

Some 10–15% of patients with BA have other congenital anomalies, including splenic abnormalities (asplenia, polysplenia, lobulated spleen), partial or complete situs inversus, mediopositioned liver, intestinal malrotation, atretic inferior vena cava, preduodenal portal vein and congenital heart defects. These 'syndromic' children may represent a separate aetiological subgroup, which has been termed biliary atresia splenic malformation (BASM) syndrome due to the universal presence of the splenic pathology.

Pathogenesis

The cause of BA is unknown. Several viruses have been suspected of triggering inflammatory response in this condition, including reovirus, rotavirus type C, CMV, human papilloma virus (HPV), and human herpes virus type 6 (HHV-6). It is conceivable that BA may represent a final phenotypic pathway of neonatal liver injury caused by diverse aetiologies, including developmental, infectious, or vascular factors, which could be operational antenatally or within the first several weeks of life. It is also tempting to speculate that aberrant host immune reactivity, related to physiologically reduced immune competence at this age, may play a role in this condition, unique to early infancy.

Clinical presentation

Most of children with BA have clinical features, indistinguishable from other causes of conjugated hyperbilirubinaemia in infancy. These include jaundice, mild hepatosplenomegaly, dark urine, and acholic stools, which could initially contain some pigment. Blood tests indicate non-specific elevation of conjugated (direct) bilirubin, transaminases, GGT, and alkaline phosphatase. Ascites or cutaneous signs of chronic liver disease are rarely detected. Coagulopathy, if present, readily responds to IV vitamin K. Early referral to specialist centres is essential. The initial good general condition and appropriate weight gain of the infant with BA can be misleading, resulting in late referral to specialist centres.

Diagnosis

Expert ultrasonography can point to BA by demonstrating an irregularly shaped or absent gallbladder. A skilfully performed and interpreted percutaneous liver biopsy under local anaesthesia using the Menghini technique is diagnostic in up to 90% of cases. Histological features of BA include expansion of portal tracts, cholestasis, and bile duct damage and reduplication with various degree of fibrosis. In ambiguous cases, ERCP or intraoperative cholangiography may be required. Radionuclide dynamic studies such as a HIDA (hepatobiliary iminodiacetic acid) scan are not specific enough to distinguish biliary atresia from other causes of prolonged neonatal cholestasis.

Treatment

If untreated, BA leads to complete biliary obstruction, cirrhosis, and death in infancy. The treatment of biliary atresia is surgical. The complete excision of the atretic biliary tree is followed by re-anastomosis, using approximately 40cm of the patient's bowel to form a Roux-en-Y loop, connecting viable bile ducts at the resected surface of the liver with proximal jejunum (portoenterostomy or Kasai procedure). Because of the progressive nature of BA, the earlier operation has better chances of establishing the effective bile flow. Approximately 50–60% of the patients will have a successful operation, completely clear the jaundice, and avoid liver transplantation in the short term. What proportion of them will require liver transplantation during adulthood has not been yet established.

The operated patients receive initial antibiotic prophylaxis (1 month) to minimize the likelihood of ascending infection from the gut and long-term fat-soluble vitamin supplementation. Development of portal hypertension and blood supply to the liver is monitored by regular ultrasound Doppler studies.

Liver transplantation in patients with BA should be complementary to Kasai portoenterostomy. Primary transplantation should be reserved only for infants in whom decompensated cirrhosis has developed because of delayed diagnosis.

Complications

The main complications of BA are:
- Ascending cholangitis.
- Portal hypertension.
- Synthetic hepatic failure.
- Chronic encephalopathy.
- Hepatopulmonary syndrome.

The successful management of these complications by standard means such as IV antibiotics or banding and sclerotherapy of oesophageal varices, when necessary, contributes to the improved long term outcome.

Prognosis

Around 20–30% of operated children will require liver transplantation during the first 2 years of life. Another 20–30% have established compensated chronic liver disease and may need liver transplantation later in childhood. It is unknown for certain, but a small proportion of long-term survivors may need consideration for liver transplant in adulthood. Overall, combined surgico-medical management with sequential Kasai portoenterostomy and liver transplantation provides long-term survival with a good quality of life for 95% of the patients referred early and treated in specialist centres.

References and resources

Patient. Biliary atresia. 2014. https://patient.info/doctor/biliary-atresia

Alpha-1 antitrypsin deficiency

Definition *464*
Genetics and epidemiology *464*
Clinical disorders *464*
Pathogenesis of liver disease *464*
Clinical features of homozygous PiZ A1AT deficiency *465*
Management *465*
Liver disease in other forms of A1AT deficiency *466*
References and resources *466*

Definition

Alpha-1 antitrypsin (A1AT) is a 55 kD glycoprotein, produced predominantly in the hepatocytes, but also by alveolar macrophages and intestinal endothelial cells. It acts as a protease inhibitor during acute phase response.

A1AT variants

A1AT protein can be electrophoretically differentiated into four main (PiM—normal; PiZ; PiS; and Pi null—abnormal), and >80 other rare, clinically irrelevant, variants.

Genetics and epidemiology

- A1AT deficiency affects predominantly Caucasians. Phylogenetically, the PiZ allele originates from Northern Europe, and PiS allele from Iberian peninsula.
- The inheritance is autosomal codominant. The estimated prevalence of PiMZ (carrier) state is 1/30 among white Europeans.

Clinical disorders

- A1AT deficiency is the commonest genetic indication for the liver transplantation in children.
- Aberrant polymerization leads to retention of the abnormal PiZ protein in the liver and, in ~10–15%, to chronic liver disease of varying severity. PiZ, PiS, and Pi null variants can induce chronic obstructive pulmonary disease in the third or fourth decade of life, particularly in smokers. PiS and Pi null variants do not cause liver disease.
- Other conditions described in association with A1AT deficiency are vasculitis, glomerulonephritis and panniculitis.

Pathogenesis of liver disease

The polymers of abnormally folded PiZ A1AT are retained in the endoplasmic reticulum of the hepatocytes since early infancy. By several yet incompletely understood pathogenetic processes they inflict a progressive liver injury. The liver damage ranges from a mild non-specific hepatitis to advanced fibrosis and cirrhosis. In the most severe cases the cirrhosis may decompensate during first 2 years of life, necessitating liver transplantation. The pathogenesis of chronic obstructive pulmonary disease is completely different and related to low levels of the protein in homozygous PiZ and PiS and Pi null variants.

Clinical features of homozygous PiZ A1AT deficiency

- The typical presentation of liver disease secondary to PiZ A1AT deficiency is of prolonged neonatal jaundice, pale stools, dark urine, elevated liver enzymes, and, sometimes, vitamin K-responsive coagulopathy. These features are clinically indistinguishable from other hepatic disorders presenting early in infancy such as biliary atresia, progressive familial cholestasis, neonatal hepatitis, and others. The remaining 15% of the symptomatic homozygous PiZ children present later during childhood with the signs of established liver disease, such as impaired liver synthetic function, hepatosplenomegaly, and portal hypertension.

- The liver histology usually demonstrates non-specific hepatitis with variable cholestasis, mild biliary features, and slender fibrosis. These appearances can sometimes mimic BA. The presence of periportal microvesicular fat, indicative of intrahepatic trafficking problem, could be an important diagnostic clue. Periodic acid–Schiff stain-positive, diastase-resistant granules and globules in the periportal hepatocytes of older children are highly suggestive of A1ATD, but they are usually not evident before 3–6 months of age. Conventional electrophoretic serum phenotyping or molecular genotyping are diagnostic golden standards.

- Of the symptomatic PiZ children, approximately one-quarter will progress to end-stage chronic liver disease and require the liver replacement during childhood. The presence of fibrosis in the liver biopsies and jaundice after 6 months of age are associated with a higher risk of developing end-stage liver disease. Chronic liver disease can lead to hepatocellular carcinoma, which is often serum alpha-fetoprotein negative.

Management

- There is no effective medical treatment for A1AT deficiency, short of liver replacement. Standard therapy for complications of the chronic liver disease such as banding ligation or sclerotherapy for bleeding varices, diuretics, and albumin, and vitamin supplementation may temporarily control the disease.

- Overall liver transplant results are not different from other indications for elective liver replacement, approaching >90% for 5-year patient survival. Transplant recipients may be at risk of hypertension in the immediate postoperative period and calcineurin inhibitor-related nephrotoxicity in the long term due to subclinical A1AT deficiency-related renal involvement.

Liver disease in other forms of A1AT deficiency

Homozygous PiS A1AT deficiency can be identified incidentally in children with various liver disorders, related to the estimated high PiS allele prevalence of 4–10 % in Europe. Abnormal polymerization of A1AT in PiSS individuals can be demonstrated *in vitro*, but does not lead to its retention in the hepatocytes and consequent liver damage during childhood.

Homozygous and heterozygous forms of PiZ A1AT deficiency are increasingly recognized in adults with cryptogenic liver disease or associated with other co-morbid conditions such as alcoholism, iron overload, auto-immunity, or chronic viral hepatitis. It is possible that possession of one PiZ allele may represent an initial risk factor in the 'multiple hit' pathogenesis of the liver injury. Therefore, family screening is important in order to suggest lifestyle modifications, such as avoiding active and passive smoking and heavy drinking.

References and resources

Children's Liver Disease Foundation. Alpha-1 antitrypsin deficiency. https://childliverdisease.org/liver-information/childhood-liver-conditions/alpha-1-antitrypsin-deficiency/

Silverman EK, Sandhaus RA. Clinical practice. Alpha1-antitrypsin deficiency. N Engl J Med 2009;360:2749–57.

Alagille syndrome

Definition 468
Incidence 469
Pathogenesis 469
Clinical presentation 469
Diagnosis 469
Complications 470
Treatment 471
Prognosis 472
References and resources 472

Definition

Alagille syndrome (ALGS) is a genetic multisystemic condition whereby most recognized patients have liver disease associated with characteristic features. Their features and frequency are summarized in Table 56.1.

Genetic abnormalities are defined in the Online Mendelian Inheritance in Man (OMIM) database: ALGS1: 118450; ALGS2: 610205.

DNA/chromosome segments JAG1 (Jagged 1 gene; locus 20p12.2; disease ALGS1); NOTCH2 (Notch 2 gene; locus 1p12–p11; disease ALGS2).

The Jagged 1–Notch 2 system is an evolutionary ancient mechanism for embryogenesis, with effects on development of brain, eye, heart, kidney, GI tract, vascular structures, cartilage, bone marrow cell lines, and liver where it is required for morphogenesis rather than for biliary cell specification. Notch 2 appears to influence development of tubules from hepatic ductal plate structures and promote subsequent involution of non-tubular structures. After liver injury, predominant activation of either Notch or Wnt/β-catenin signalling leads to myofibroblasts and macrophages promoting the divergent specification of bipotent hepatic progenitor cells towards biliary or hepatocellular lineage of recovering cells respectively, and so promote or subdue subsequent hepatic fibrosis.

The inheritance has been described as autosomal dominant with variable penetrance and poor genotype–phenotype correlation even within families with phenotype discordance described between monozygotic twins. 15% are estimated to be new mutations.

Table 56.1 Features of Alagille syndrome

Criteria	Description
Cholestasis 89–100%	Typically presenting as jaundice in the neonatal period, often with pale stools
Facies 70–98%	Broad forehead, deep-set eyes, straight nose with a bulbous tip, pointed chin giving the face a characteristic triangular appearance and prominent or 'bat' ears
Heart disease including murmur 85–98%	Most often peripheral pulmonary artery stenosis and in 30% structural defects such as atrial septal defect, ventricular septal defect, Fallot's tetralogy or pulmonary atresia
Vertebral anomalies, 33–87%	Characteristically butterfly vertebrae, a radiological appearance due to incomplete fusion of the anterior arches of the vertebrae, with other reported anomalies being hemi-vertebrae, fusion of the adjacent vertebrae, and spina bifida occulta
Posterior embryotoxon 56–88%	A prominent Schwalbe's ring at the junction of the cornea and the iris, also seen in 8–15% of normal subjects
Renal anomalies—not included as major diagnostic criteria by all authorities 19–73%	Renal tubular acidosis, renal cysts, dysplasia, horseshoe kidney

Incidence

The incidence of ALGS is estimated to be 1 in 70,000 live births. However, as not all patients with ALGS present with neonatal cholestasis, the phenotype is variable and the condition underdiagnosed; the incidence of ALGS could be 1 in 30,000–50,000 live births.

Pathogenesis

The characteristic liver biopsy finding is of paucity of interlobular bile ducts with cholestasis, but it is unclear if the primary defect is duct hypoplasia or a disappearing bile duct syndrome. Up to 30% of early liver biopsies may show ductular proliferation or non-specific features. There is typically less biliary fibrosis than duration and severity of cholestasis would lead one to expect.

Clinical presentation

Most patients present with neonatal cholestasis with or without pale stools. Faltering growth and a cardiac murmur may already be evident. Facial features may initially be overlooked. Patients may also present with cholestasis associated with congenital heart disease or cholestatic chronic liver disease often with faltering growth, or later onset of pruritus.

Diagnosis

The diagnosis depends on three of the major features (characteristic facies, cardiac lesions, posterior embryotoxon, butterfly vertebrae) with cholestasis. Two features plus an affected first-degree relative or one feature with a compatible genetic abnormality have also been proposed.

Complications

The main complications of ALGS are:

- Faltering growth and short stature. Patients are constitutionally short, compounded by the severity of liver disease, and rickets if present. Delayed puberty is characteristic of the condition so that final height is generally within the normal range.
- Pruritus tends to be severe and may be intractable. It is necessarily subjective, but patients and families suffer severely impaired quality of life from it. A Clinician Scratch Scale (visible damage to the skin on a 5-point scale) and a visual analogue score of 0 (no pruritus) to 10 (the worst pruritus imaginable) can be helpful for objective assessment of treatment.
- Xanthomas/xanthelasmas are associated with hypercholesterolaemia, tending to form in areas of skin trauma. Apart from cosmetic considerations they can be exquisitely tender and may prevent wearing normal shoes. Cholesterol-lowering drugs have not been used because of concerns about hepatotoxicity. They respond to external biliary diversion if successful and liver transplantation.
- Metabolic bone disease results from fat-soluble vitamin deficiency, severity of liver disease, and renal tubulopathy. Treatment requires prolonged normalization of vitamin D, calcium, phosphate, bicarbonate, and parathyroid hormone. Pathological fractures may be an indication that the liver disease warrants liver transplantation.
- The congenital cardiac lesions in ALGS are most often right sided, particularly with peripheral pulmonary artery stenosis also present. Non-correctable lesions such as pulmonary atresia have a poor prognosis in their own right and preclude liver transplantation worsening the prognosis overall.
- Renal complications. Renal dysplasia is seen in 39% but renal tubular acidosis is often overlooked and probably more common especially with vitamin D deficiency. Patients require careful correction of plasma bicarbonate. Nephropathy often worsens as a result of immunosuppression after transplantation.
- Complications of portal hypertension. Most children with ALGS appear protected from fibrosis and cirrhosis in comparison with their peers with biliary diseases such as BA. Therefore variceal bleeding in childhood is uncommon.
- Hepatocellular carcinoma has been reported in children with ALGS with and without cirrhosis.
- Spontaneous or post-surgical bleeding in various organs is reported in 22%, while bleeding associated with moyamoya syndrome suggests a vasculopathy.
- An increased frequency of infections is described particularly of the respiratory tract. An abnormality of complement–T-cell interactions through Jagged–Notch–CD46 function may be the mechanism.

Treatments

- Nutrition—cholestasis is often profound with fat malabsorption and fat-soluble vitamin deficiencies. Essential fatty acids may be deficient but are difficult to monitor. Feeds of up to 150% of RDA calories for weight, with up to 30% medium-chain triglycerides and carbohydrate as short-chain polymers may necessitate tube feeding. Essential fatty acid-rich oils and specific vitamin supplements based on plasma levels require close nutritional supervision.
- Growth depends on optimizing nutrition. Thereafter, patients tend to remain short during childhood and do not respond well to growth hormone treatment.
- Pruritus—no treatment is universally efficacious. Ursodeoxycholic acid 15–20mg/kg/day in two doses tends to be first-line treatment followed by rifampicin 4–7mg/kg/day in two doses. Third line is naltrexone 0.2–1mg/kg/day. Sertraline may be beneficial. Sedative antihistamines may buy brief respite but itch becomes refractory. Biliary diversion, external and internal, is considered later in this list. Liver transplantation is the ultimate treatment for very poor quality of life with itch.
- Renal disease tends to be under-recognized. Apart from structural defects and dysplasia, patients are particularly at risk of renal tubular acidosis requiring close monitoring and supplementation with oral bicarbonate, calcium, and phosphate to maintain normal plasma levels.
- Biliary diversion. Partial external diversion via a short ileal loop from the gallbladder has been shown to improve itch and xanthomas in a selected cohort. Patients without significant fibrosis and with residual bile flow to divert seem to benefit most. Complications include infection and lithiasis of the externalized system, infection worsening cholestasis and problems of stoma care.
- Liver transplantation can transform the impaired health and quality of life of children with ALGS, even those who do not have cirrhosis. Apart from resolution of itch and xanthomas, energy levels, appetite, growth and development, and metabolic bone disease respond well to transplantation.
- The right-sided cardiac pressures are a major determinant of the risk of transplantation. Interventional cardiological procedures to ensure that the right ventricular pressure is less than half of aortic and that the patient is able to increase cardiac output by at least 50% in response to 20mg/kg/min infusion of dobutamine have ensured that significant perioperative events are now rare in ALGS.

Prognosis

- Prognosis for the liver is as highly variable as the phenotype.
- Recognized indicators of prognosis include:
    - Severity of congenital heart disease predicts medium-term survival, including suitability for liver transplantation in severe liver disease.
    - Severity and persistence of jaundice in the first year of life predicts severity of liver disease and need for transplantation.
    - Speculation on spontaneous remission of liver disease at puberty has little objective evidence.

References and resources

Mouzaki M, Bass LM, Sokol RJ, et al. Early life predictive markers of liver disease outcome in an International, Multicentre Cohort of children with Alagille syndrome. Liver Int 2016;36:755–60.
Subramaniam P, Knisely A, Portmann B, et al. Diagnosis of Alagille syndrome – 25 years of experience at King's College Hospital. J Pediatr Gastroenterol Nutr 2011;52:84–9.

Familial and inherited intrahepatic cholestatic syndromes

Definition 474
Nomenclature and current changes 475
Epidemiology 476
Pathophysiology 478
Clinical features 480
Management 482
References and resources 486

Definition

The presence of persistent cholestasis or remitting cholestasis that has relapsed on at least one occasion with:

- Direct or indirect evidence of an inherited aetiology (or a single remitting episode with direct evidence of heredity).
- Supportive histological features.

Onset may be at any time from the neonatal period into adolescence. Early-onset cases typically present as neonatal cholestasis; later-onset cases may present as unexplained or drug-related cholestasis.

Nomenclature and current changes

Early recognized conditions falling within this spectrum had names derived from their description, with characteristic syndromic features. Among these are Aagenaes syndrome and North American Indian cholestasis. Others have names derived from their pathophysiological mechanisms such as bile salt export pump (BSEP) deficiency or from their gene markers, PFIC1 disease. Table 57.1 (p. 477) shows a classification of familial intrahepatic cholestasis variants that combines clinical features with available genetic knowledge.

As definitive tests even for the variants of PFIC with accepted markers are becoming generally clinically available, allocation of patients to a genetic classification is becoming clearer, and while diagnostic and therapeutic uncertainty persists particularly among heterozygotes, if in doubt we ultimately continue to fall back to the phenotypic features for a management strategy.

New cholestasis gene panels derived from the application of next-generation sequencing have been developed by many of the international paediatric liver centres and are offered in the best circumstances with the additional benefit of clinical interpretation. Our own consists of 27 genes associated with disorders having features that overlap with intrahepatic cholestatic diseases such as neonatal hepatitis/cholestasis, acute and chronic cholestasis, cryptogenic liver disease with cholestatic overtones, etc. The tests are not individually expensive in the context of a firm diagnosis being made in one from a variety of possible rare diseases. However, there is not currently capacity or resource to apply them at an early stage in clinical contexts such as neonatal hepatitis syndrome when most results will be negative and a proportion unhelpfully ambiguous. There is also a reporting delay of 4–6 weeks which is occasionally clinically important. Thus we have yet to clarify the exact application of these panels in the existing phased investigation of cholestatic syndromes or if they will lead to a paradigm change in the initial investigation of newly presenting liver disease.

Epidemiology

Recent attention to cholestatic syndromes facilitated by understanding of their genetics and pathophysiology has revealed that they are more common than previously recognized, and has shed light on the pathophysiological mechanisms of cholestasis. Inheritance and gene markers are in favour of autosomal recessive aetiology in most types (see Table 57.1). Clearer understanding of the breadth of possible phenotypes has shown that cases of neonatal hyperbilirubinaemia, particularly those that recur or have a poor prognosis for chronic liver disease, or some patients with cryptogenic chronic liver disease, fall within this spectrum. Obstetric cholestasis, although genetically and pathophysiologically related to some variants, is not considered in this paediatric text.

Table 57.1 Classification of PFIC types

Phenotype	Current condition name	Previous names	Gene marker/defect
Infantile cholestasis			
Low GGT—may have diarrhoea, short stature, and short digits	PFIC1 disease	Byler disease	FIC1–ATP8B1
Low GGT	BSEP deficiency	PFIC2	ABCB11
Low GGT, hypercholanaemia, neurological and respiratory problems	TJP2 defects		TJP2–ZO2 deficiency
High GGT ± cholangiopathy	MDR3 deficiency	High GGT neonatal intrahepatic cholestasis	ABCB4
High GGT ± cholangiopathy, tubulopathies/renal cysts, hearing defects, dyslexia	Ciliopathies DCDC2 defects	–	–
Neonatal sclerosing cholangitis	NSC	–	DCDC2 defects for some
Neonatal sclerosing cholangitis with ichthyosis	NISCH syndrome	–	CLDN1
Infantile cholestasis	EPHX1 deficiency	Hypercholanaemia	EPHX1
(Benign) recurrent cholestasis			
Low GGT ± pancreatitis	BRIC1	Summerskill–Walshe–Tygstrup syndrome	ATP8B1
Low GGT	BRIC2	Summerskill–Walshe–Tygstrup syndrome	BSEP mutations of ABCB11 E186G, V444A
High GGT	–	–	ABCB4
Severe cholesterol gallstone formation	MDR3 deficiency	–	ABCB4
Pregnancy/oral contraceptive-induced cholestasis	Cholestasis of pregnancy	–	ABCB4, ATP8B1D2S1374

Pathophysiology

Primary pathophysiological mechanisms of cholestasis may occur at hepato-cellular, basolateral membrane, or canalicular levels. A key, common mechanism in the progress of liver disease appears to be local concentration of free bile acids with detergent effects on hepatocyte and/or biliary canalicular cell and intracellular membranes, with normal 1000-fold concentration gradients disrupting unprotected intra or extracellular areas. Remitting or benign recurrent variants have inducible or suppressible critical enzymes or steps within the bile acid transport pathway.

Most patients with liver disease progress towards end-stage either progressively or with variable episodes of remission. Even cases initially identified as benign fibrosis tend to accumulate insidiously over time. Patients proceed towards either biliary cirrhosis or a reticulate porto-portal fibrosis. Copper-associated protein is frequently seen in periportal areas as evidence of chronic cholestasis.

Aetiologies and subtypes

Low serum values of GGT in the setting of cholestasis usually allude to the diagnosis of progressive familial intrahepatic cholestasis. The aetiology of the cholestasis must lie upstream of the canalicular membrane since GGT was not being released and circulated in the blood. It has also been shown that the low GGT subgroup has a worse prognosis, with 50% dying or coming to liver transplantation within 5 years.

Some subtypes are associated with syndromic features that may be helpful in making the diagnosis and indicating the prognosis. Among these are PFIC1 associated with short stature, diarrhoea, short fingers with lichenification of skin, and renal tubular acidosis. Aagenaes syndrome is associated with lymphoedema that may develop over months or years. North American Indian cholestasis is associated with pancreatitis and 'paper-money skin'. Nephropathies are associated with the fibrosis and cholangiopathy of DCDC2 defects while TJP2 defects result in a whole body permeability of tight junctions that may have respiratory and neurological features.

Disease pathophysiology

Deficiency of the bile salt export pump (BSEP) results in rapid onset of cholestasis, typically with aggressive liver disease. Remitting or recurrent types are described but the condition presents as progressive intrahepatic cholestasis complicating neonatal hepatitis/cholestasis. The condition PFIC1 results from deficiency of an ATP-dependent membrane transporter, accounting for later-onset cholestasis requiring the accumulation of synthesized bile salts within hepatocytes. The various extrahepatic manifestations and the persistence of features, particularly diarrhoea, renal tubular acidosis, and fatty liver after liver transplantation, are accounted for by transporter defects expressed in other organs. BSEP deficiency results in failure of bile salt transport across the canalicular membrane. A third defect, MDR3 deficiency, is explained by the relative absence of phospholipid to protect the canalicular membrane from detergent effects of biliary bile acids. Canalicular membrane and bile duct damage with cholestasis and possible cholangiopathy result. TJP and claudin defects of tight junctions probably contribute a small proportion of the total cases. Undoubtedly other important mechanisms for low and high serum GGT cholestasis remained to be discovered with perhaps 20% of low-GGT variants still lacking a gene marker.

Clinical features

Presentations

- *Progressive intrahepatic cholestasis* as a complication of neonatal cholestasis or neonatal hepatitis syndrome. High- and low-serum GGT types can present in this way. At presentation, stools may have a variable degree of pallor, occasionally mimicking BA. Histology of low GGT subtypes such as BSEP deficiency is more likely to be giant cell hepatitis whereas that of high GGT types such as MDR3 deficiency or neonatal sclerosing cholangitis may have giant cell hepatitis but is more likely to have portal tract expansion with bile ductular reduplication. Other known causes of progressive cholestasis complicating neonatal cholestasis not falling within this definition must be excluded.
- *Cholestasis of later onset in infancy.* Patients may present for the first time with jaundice at 3–6 months of age or later. Histology may be of bland cholestasis with little inflammation or giant cell transformation. 'Byler bile' may be present on electron microscopy, suggestive of PFIC1 disease.
- Patients may present with a *first or second episode of acute cholestasis* with jaundice, pale stools, and dark urine and ultimately itch at any age in childhood or adolescence. Precipitating factors such as drugs, particularly penicillin antibiotics, and oestrogens, may be recorded up to 2 months before the onset of jaundice. Puberty may be a contributing factor. Previous episodes may have been misinterpreted as viral hepatitis including hepatitis A. Low-serum GGT types predominate. Drugs associated with cholestasis are shown in Table 57.2.
- *Cholestasis in pregnancy* can present at any time from late in the first trimester onwards, although it is commoner in the second and third trimesters. Itch is the predominant symptom and jaundice follows (if present) by ~2 weeks. Serum transaminases are usually minimally elevated or in the normal range. Glucose intolerance may be associated. Histological features typically show bland cholestasis with occasionally bile plugs but little inflammation. There is an increased risk of premature delivery and fetal death. The reader should look to an adult text for further information on this topic.

Benign recurrent cholestasis

- Patients with full clinical, biochemical and histological remission after two or more cholestatic episodes may be said to have *benign recurrent cholestasis* (BRIC). Serum GGT is usually low. Drug cholestasis may be suspected initially and drugs may be a trigger as previously mentioned. This diagnosis requires extreme caution as many cases prove not to be benign with progression insidious, or precipitate after long periods without apparent progression.
- Syndromic features related to the whole body nature of the defects such as tight junction or ciliary dysfunction may provide diagnostic clues unless they are evident significantly later than presenting cholestasis.

Table 57.2 Drugs associated with cholestasis

Group	Examples
Antibiotics	Amoxicillin, flucloxacillin, macrolides, rifampicin
Steroids	Glucocorticoids, oestrogens, androgens
Psychotropic/neurology	Chlorpromazine, phenothiazines, methyldopa
Cardiology	Verapamil, nifedipine, amiodarone
Antimetabolites	Methotrexate
Immunosuppressants	Ciclosporin

Natural history

Occasional cases of both high and low GGT intrahepatic cholestasis complicating neonatal cholestasis follow an unremitting course with nutritional impairment, fat-soluble vitamin deficiency, portal hypertension and its complications, and finally decompensation of liver synthetic function sometimes at an age as early as 8 months to 2 years comparable with deterioration following missed BA.

Later-onset infantile cases, those presenting as drug-related cholestasis but with a poor prognosis, and apparent benign recurrent cholestasis cases who have subsequently declared themselves as having progressive disease, all tend to have a remitting and relapsing course. Pruritus, faltering growth, and fat-soluble vitamin deficiencies require close monitoring and vigorous treatment. Loose stools or diarrhoea often complicate classical PFIC1 disease and short stature is particularly problematic.

Management

Extrahepatic consequences of cholestasis, particularly nutritional, including growth faltering and essential fat-soluble vitamin deficiencies, are frequent. Vitamin D and E deficiencies are common, but vitamin A deficiency is less so. Supplementation is mandatory even among patients without jaundice. Medications for treatment and prophylaxis of deficiency are shown in Table 57.3. Essential fatty acid deficiency may be detected following prolonged cholestasis. Its significance for neurodevelopment is unclear.

Our institutional regimen for the management of pruritus is shown in Table 57.4. Non-cirrhotic patients with residual bile flow may respond to external or internal biliary diversion. Both of these methods involve interrupting the intrahepatic recirculation of bile salts at a point between the extrahepatic biliary system and the point of a bile salt re-uptake in the terminal ileum. External diversion may be by the insertion of a loop of ileum

Table 57.3 Nutritional supplements—vitamins and minerals

Nutritional element	Daily requirement	Means of administration	Comments/ monitoring
Vitamin A	<10kg 50,00IU >10kg 10,000IU IM–50,000IU	Oral	IM supplement only in severe refractory deficiency Serum retinol/ RBP ≤0.8
Vitamin D	10,000–40,000 units per day IM–30,000IU 1–3-monthly	Oral/IM	Supplementation with oral products containing calciferol may suffice. Refractory cases may require 25-OHD or IM preps 25-OHD serum levels >20ng/mL
Vitamin E	TPGS* 25IU/kg IM 10mg/kg (max. 200mg) every 3 weeks	Oral	Vitamin E/total lipids ≤0.6mg/g Vitamin E <30g/mL Look for reflexes!
Vitamin K	2mg/day Weekly 5mg: 5–10kg 10mg: >10kg IM—5–10mg every 2 weeks	Oral IM	Prothrombin time PIVKA II <3ng/mL
Water-soluble vitamins	Twice RDA	Oral	Supplement as needed
Minerals Calcium Selenium Zinc Phosphate	25–100mg/kg 1–2µg/kg 1mg/kg 25–50mg/kg	Oral	Supplement as needed

IM, intramuscular; PIVKA-II, protein induced in vitamin K absence assay.

Table 57.4 The sequence of medical management of pruritus of cholestasis

Number	Medicine	Dose range
1	Colestyramine	4g sachets (1–4/day)
2	Ursodeoxycholic acid	15–30mg/kg/day in 2 doses
3	Rifampicin	7–10mg/kg/day in 2 doses
4	Naltrexone	0.3–0.6mg/kg/day in 1 dose
5	Ondansetron	2–8mg/day in 2 doses as for antiemetic treatment
6	UVA light treatment or acupuncture may be offered with benefit for some patients.	

between the gallbladder brought out as a stoma usually in the right iliac fossa. Alternatively, the preterminal ileum may be brought out as a double-barrel stoma. Internal diversion involves the formation of distal ileum to colon fistula with the terminal ileum in a blind loop. This latter diversion avoids a stoma but may cause bile-salt-related diarrhoea and has a theoretical increased risk of colonic carcinoma in the long term. The second and third methods will require regular provision of vitamin B_{12} since its terminal ileal uptake will be interrupted. Excellent results for improvements of pruritus, jaundice, and liver histology have been described. Our institutional experiences have been less good, probably because of selection of patients who were cirrhotic and with very poor bile flow.

Liver transplantation

Indications for liver transplantation include:
* Management of poor quality of life.
* Faltering growth.
* Intractable pruritus.
* Dysplastic hepatic nodules with raised alpha-fetoprotein.
* Risk of hepatic cellular carcinoma.
* Established hepatocellular carcinoma <5cm.
* Failure of synthetic function.

Patients with PFC1 disease may have very severe intra- and extrahepatic complications after transplantation. Their longitudinal growth improves initially after transplantation but very short stature may persist. Diarrhoea may worsen considerably and tacrolimus or ciclosporin treatment may unmask severe renal tubular acidosis and risk of dehydration with electrolyte disturbance. A prolonged and intractable hepatic steatosis is frequently seen in the early months to years after successful transplantation.

Monitoring for hepatocellular carcinoma

Intrahepatic cholestasis due to BSEP deficiency has a risk of hepatocellular carcinoma in excess of other causes of PFIC or biliary cirrhosis. Many patients continue to have raised alpha-fetoprotein levels suggesting hepatocyte dysplasia. Patients require regular monitoring of alpha-fetoprotein and liver ultrasound 6 monthly for early recognition.

Benign recurrent cholestasis

Cases with more than one episode of cholestasis where symptoms recede fully and liver function tests, ultrasonography, and liver biopsies return entirely to normal between episodes may be considered benign. Episodes of cholestasis may last up to several months and treatments for pruritus and fat-soluble vitamin deficiency should be given as described previously. There is no evidence that earlier treatment with choleretics cuts short the duration of the episodes. However, temporary biliary diversion by nasal biliary intubation and drainage has been shown to cut short episodes very rapidly. Patients should be labelled benign with extreme caution as they may have low-grade chronic liver disease that can take years to declare itself. Recognized precipitants such as antibiotics or oestrogens should be avoided in such patients.

References and resources

Grammatikopoulos T, Sambrotta M, Strautnieks S, et al. Mutations in DCDC2 (doublecortin domain containing protein 2) in neonatal sclerosing cholangitis. J Hepatol 2016;65:1179–87.

Sambrotta M, Strautnieks S, Papouli E, et al. Mutations in TJP2 cause progressive cholestatic liver disease. Nat Genet 2014;46:326–8.

Srivastava A. Progressive familial intrahepatic cholestasis. J Clin Exp Hepatol 2014;4:25–36.

Drug-induced liver injury

Introduction *488*
Epidemiology *488*
Pathophysiology *489*
Clinical features *490*
Investigation *494*
Management *496*
Prevention/prognosis *498*
References and resources *498*

Introduction

Drug-induced liver injury (DILI) in children is a rare, adverse, drug reaction that can result in a wide spectrum of clinical manifestations. Making a diagnosis can be difficult due to its range of presentations and lack of objective diagnostic tests. The diagnosis is, therefore, based on clinical history and exclusion of other causes. Due to the liver's central role in drug metabolism, most drugs have the potential to cause liver injury.

Epidemiology

- DILI in children is relatively rare due to the fact that most children take few medications but also due to under-recognition and under-reporting.
- DILI as a cause of acute liver failure (ALF) accounts for 19% (14% due to paracetamol; 5% due to other drugs) of all cases of ALF in children.
- Among the most commonly implicated agents are paracetamol, antibiotics, antiepileptics, and antineoplastic agents.
- DILI caused by herbal and dietary supplements is increasing.

Pathophysiology

The liver plays a pivotal role in the metabolism of drugs through complex metabolic pathways. There are two principal enzymatic pathways:

- Phase 1 reactions (cytochrome p450 system) of oxidation, reduction, hydrolysis, dehalogenation, etc.
- Phase 2 reactions of sulfation, transferation (as in glucuronosyltransferase for bilirubin conjugation), etc.

Disruption of the balance between phase 1 and phase 2 pathways due to the offending drug, concurrent infection, co-administered drugs, nutrition, and genetic differences is integral in causing hepatotoxicity.

Patterns of DILI can be divided into:

- Direct *cytotoxic* picture whether the damage be in the hepatocytes, endothelial cells, or bile duct epithelial cells. This leads to impaired cellular function and ultimately cell death.
- *Immune-mediated* hepatotoxicity where there are systemic symptoms of fever and extrahepatic organ inflammation. This can lead to DRESS syndrome (drug reaction with eosinophilia and systemic symptoms) and ALF.

Clinical features

The diagnosis of DILI is clinical and should be considered if no other underlying cause of abnormal liver function can be found. Diagnostic tools have been developed in adults (e.g. RUCAM) but lack proven accuracy. A thorough history and examination is, therefore, essential. It is important to remember that DILI can occur in a *predictable, intrinsic, dose-related* manner as well as in an *unpredictable, idiosyncratic, dose-unrelated* fashion.

History and physical examination

- Gender, age, and ethnicity.
- Exposure time of drug and temporal relationship between drug intake and onset of clinical picture up to 6 months or even 1 year prior to the onset of symptoms.
- Enquire about herbal and dietary supplements (Table 58.1).
- Co-morbidities and other liver disorders (e.g. NAFLD).
- History of other drug reactions (e.g. cross-reactivities with antiepileptics).
- Symptoms: lethargy, weakness, nausea, abdominal pain, jaundice, dark urine, pruritus, and rash.
- Signs: fever, rash, hepatomegaly, hepatic tenderness, and signs of chronic liver disease.

Table 58.1 Examples of herbal and dietary supplements and DILI

Herbal or dietary supplement	Hepatic effect
Aloe vera	Very rare, idiosyncratic hepatocellular injury
Catechin (green tea)	Very rare, hepatocellular injury
Comfrey	Hepatic veno-occlusive disease
Chinese herbal medicine	Multiple agents have been implicated in hepatocellular injury
Creatine	Hepatotoxic when used long term
Echinacea	CNS stimulation, anaphylaxis
Fenugreek	Not implicated in liver injury
Ginseng	Not implicated in liver injury
Lavender	Not implicated in liver injury
Melatonin	Not implicated in liver injury
Pennyroyal oil	Acute hepatic necrosis and liver failure
Peppermint oil	Hepatotoxic in high doses
St John's wort	Not implicated in liver injury
Valerian	Very rarely hepatotoxicity

It is useful to consider the clinical features of DILI in the following forms.

Hepatocellular
- This is the most common form where the damage is primarily in the hepatocytes leading to elevation in aminotransferases. The patient may simply be asymptomatic, experience some malaise or develop frank ALF.
- ALT and AST elevation greater than three times the ULN.
- Bilirubin and ALP can be normal or elevated.

Cholestatic
- The damage is primarily in the bile ducts leading to an obstructive picture with jaundice and pruritus.
- Elevation in bilirubin, ALP, and GGT
- Takes longer to resolve but has good prognosis

Mixed hepatocellular-cholestatic
- Multiple cell types are affected in this setting causing findings of both hepatocellular and cholestatic forms.

Table 58.2 lists the common drugs implicated in paediatrics.

Table 58.2 Patterns of drug-induced liver injury by commonly used drugs in children

Drug	Pattern of injury
Co-amoxiclav	Cholestatic or mixed hepatocellular-cholestatic, idiosyncratic
Antineoplastic drugs	Hepatocellular, cholestatic or mixed and vaso-occlusive disease
Aspirin	Hepatocellular, dose related
Azathioprine	Hepatocellular or mixed hepatocellular-cholestatic
Carbamazepine	Hepatocellular or cholestatic
Ceftriaxone	Cholestatic or mixed hepatocellular-cholestatic, dose related
Ciclosporin	Cholestatic, dose related
Erythromycin	Mixed hepatocellular-cholestatic
Fluconazole	Hepatocellular or mixed hepatocellular-cholestatic, idiosyncratic
Infliximab	Cholestatic or mixed hepatocellular-cholestatic
Isoniazid	Hepatocellular, idiosyncratic
Methotrexate	Hepatocellular and liver fibrosis, idiosyncratic
Non-steroidal anti-inflammatory drugs	Hepatocellular or mixed hepatocellular-cholestatic, idiosyncratic
Oral contraceptive pill (oestrogen)	Cholestatic, dose related
Paracetamol	Hepatocellular, dose related
Phenobarbital	Hepatocellular or mixed hepatocellular-cholestatic, can be idiosyncratic
Phenytoin	Hepatocellular or mixed hepatocellular-cholestatic and DRESS syndrome
Retinoids	Hepatocellular or cholestatic, dose related
Sulfasalazine	Hepatocellular or mixed hepatocellular-cholestatic
Valproic acid	Hepatocellular or mixed hepatocellular-cholestatic, idiosyncratic

Investigation

- AST, ALT, GGT, and ALP.
- Conjugated and unconjugated bilirubin.
- Coagulation profile.
- Full blood count, eosinophils, and blood film.
- Drug levels where appropriate.
- Hepatitis A, B, C, and E serology/antigen tests.
- EBV, CMV, HSV, adenovirus and enterovirus viral serology/antigen tests, and PCR.
- Autoantibodies and immunoglobulins including IgE.
- Alpha-1 antitrypsin phenotype.
- Caeruloplasmin, serum copper, and penicillamine challenge.
- Liver USS.
- MRI ± MRCP should be considered if the USS is abnormal.
- Liver biopsy should also be considered. It is indicated when there is uncertainty in the diagnosis and other disorders need to be excluded or when the extent of liver damage needs to be assessed.

.

Management

- The most important treatment is to suspect and withdraw the offending drug. Patients should be treated supportively according to their presentation. In clinically well patients with abnormal LFTs, the withdrawal of the offending drug should be sufficient. Patients who present with ALF should be treated according to specialist guidelines and should be referred to a liver unit.
- Re-challenging with the offending drug is not advocated in children.
- It is important to remember that DILI may unmask other underlying pathology such as autoimmune hepatitis and mitochondrial cytopathies.

Management of paracetamol overdose

- If a paracetamol overdose is suspected or known, the child must be treated immediately with acetylcysteine at the local hospital whatever the time between the alleged overdose and visit to the hospital.
- The 'high-risk treatment line' is used in all cases once a level is known (see Fig. 58.1).
- Acetylcysteine should be continued until the INR is normal (<1.3) bearing in mind that 'transaminitis' may take longer to resolve.
- IV fluid should be used to provide adequate hydration and avoid hypoglycaemia. Higher than 10% concentrations of dextrose may be needed.

Investigations

- Liver function tests, urea and electrolytes, and INR.
- Blood gas, lactate and blood sugar level.
- INR, blood sugar, renal function and blood gases must be repeated at least twice a day and, if abnormal, three times a day. Immediately start broad-spectrum antibiotics if INR abnormal (piperacillin/tazobactam) and in the presence of abnormal renal function, fluconazole, or liposomal amphotericin IV.

Prognosis

- The most important prognostic parameter is acidosis on day 2. If despite acetylcysteine and good hydration, the child becomes acidotic, the prognosis is poor. Acidosis is the best prognostic factor independent from all other factors. Even in the presence of a very prolonged INR, a patient who is not acidotic will have an 80% chance of surviving. If the pH is <7.25, there is a 95% mortality, therefore, the child should be emergency listed for transplantation.
- Other factors predicting a poor outcome are the development of grade III hepatic encephalopathy with oliguric renal failure (which usually occurs 3 or 4 days after ingestion), and/or a PT of >100 seconds and a raised plasma lactate.

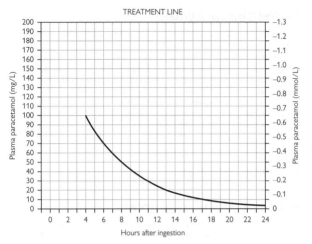

Fig. 58.1 High-risk treatment line for paracetamol overdose.

Prevention/prognosis

- Liver function tests should be routinely performed on a regular basis in drugs known to cause DILI.
- Patients should be informed about the side effects of the drugs they are taking and patients should be made aware of the clinical signs of DILI.
- Suspected DILI cases should be reported to a central database.
- Recognition and identification of DILI and the removal of the offending drug is paramount in preventing further liver injury.
- Re-challenging the patient with the offending drug or drugs from the same family is not advocated in children.
- The prognosis of DILI depends on the severity and the pattern of the insult but is usually completely reversible when the offending drug is removed.
- Presentation as ALF predicts poor outcome.

References and resources

Chalasani NP, Hayashi PH, Bonkovsky HL, Navarro VJ, Lee WM, Fontana RJ. ACG clinical guideline: the diagnosis and management of idiosyncratic drug-induced liver injury Am J Gastroenterol 2014;109:950–66.

Murray K, Hadzic N, Wirth S, Bassett M, Kelly D. Drug-related hepatotoxicity and acute liver failure. J Pediatr Gastroenterol Nutr 2008;47:395–405.

National Institute of Diabetes and Digestive and Kidney Disease (NIDDK) and the National Library of Medicine: LiverTox (http://www.livertox.nih.gov) for a free, online DILI resource.

Squires RH Jr, Shneider BL, Bucuvalas J, et al. Acute liver failure in children: the first 348 patients in the pediatric acute liver failure study group. J Pediatr 2006;148:652–8.

Chapter 59

Autoimmune liver disease

Introduction *500*
Autoimmune hepatitis *502*
Autoimmune hepatitis/sclerosing cholangitis overlap syndrome *504*

Introduction

In paediatrics, two forms of autoimmune liver disease are recognized:
- Autoimmune hepatitis (AIH).
- AIH/sclerosing cholangitis overlap syndrome (autoimmune sclerosing cholangitis, ASC).

Autoimmune hepatitis

- AIH is a progressive inflammatory liver disorder, preferentially affecting females, characterized serologically by high levels of transaminases and IgG and presence of autoantibodies, and histologically by interface hepatitis in the absence of a known aetiology.
- AIH is divided into two types according to the autoantibody profile:
  - Type 1 is positive for antinuclear (ANA) and/or anti-smooth muscle (SMA) antibody.
  - Type 2 is positive for anti-liver kidney microsomal antibody type 1 (anti-LKM-1) and/or anti-liver cytosol type 1 (anti-LC1).
- AIH-1 represents two-thirds of the cases. Severity of disease is similar in the two types. AIH-2 patients are younger and have a higher tendency to present with ALF, but the duration of symptoms before diagnosis and the frequency of hepatosplenomegaly are similar in the two groups. Both have a high frequency of associated autoimmune disorders (~20%) and a family history of autoimmune disease (40%).
- The presentation of AIH is variable. Up to 40–50% of patients present with symptoms of acute hepatitis, some 40% with an insidious onset, characterized by progressive fatigue, relapsing jaundice, headache, amenorrhea, anorexia, and weight loss, and some 10% with complications of portal hypertension, such as splenomegaly, haematemesis from oesophageal varices, bleeding diathesis, chronic diarrhoea, and weight loss. The disease should therefore be suspected and excluded in all children with symptoms and signs of prolonged or severe liver disease. The course of disease can be fluctuating, with flares and spontaneous remissions, a pattern that may result in delayed referral and diagnosis.
- On physical examination, clinical signs of an underlying chronic liver disease, i.e. cutaneous stigmata (spider naevi, palmar erythema, leukonychia, striae), firm liver, and splenomegaly are common.
- On ultrasound scanning, the liver parenchyma is often nodular and heterogeneous.
- Children with AIH-2 have higher levels of bilirubin and transaminases at presentation than those with AIH-1 and present more frequently with fulminant hepatic failure. Most patients have increased levels of IgG, but ~20% do not, particularly those presenting with a severe acute hepatitis picture, indicating that normal IgG values do not exclude the diagnosis of AIH. Partial IgA deficiency is significantly more common in LKM1-positive than in ANA/SMA-positive patients.
- Histologically, the severity of interface hepatitis at diagnosis is similar in both types, but cirrhosis on initial biopsy is more frequent AIH-1 than in AIH-2, suggesting a more chronic course of disease in the former. Progression to cirrhosis during treatment is also more frequent in AIH-1.
- AIH is exquisitely responsive to immunosuppression except from the children presenting with ALF with encephalopathy, in which case liver transplantation is usually the only option.

Standard treatment at King's College Hospital, London, UK

- *Prednisolone* is started at a dose of 2mg/kg per day (max. 60mg daily), which is gradually decreased over the next 4–8 weeks to a minimum dose of 2.5–5mg depending on the age. It is important to monitor the blood tests (liver function tests, full blood count, and clotting profile) weekly and aim to an 80% transaminase decrease in 6 weeks to avoid steroid side effects.
- *Azathioprine* can be introduced as a steroid-sparing agent, but should not be used as first-line treatment because of its potential hepatotoxicity, particularly in jaundiced and/or cirrhotic patients. Because of its myelosuppressive effect, a starting dose of 0.5mg/kg is used, to be increased to maximum 2mg/kg per day. Blood tests are done weekly to start with, then monthly, and then at least 3-monthly for the first year of treatment. Daily treatment is advisable for effective control of disease, and does not impair growth.

Alternative management

- Mycophenolate mofetil has been used both in children and adults who were intolerant to azathioprine, with good response.
- Ciclosporin has been used to induce remission with no added benefit over standard treatment (see earlier) and both ciclosporin and tacrolimus have been used in patients who did not respond to standard treatment.

Treatment should be continued for 3–4 years. Cessation of treatment can be discussed when liver function tests and serum IgG have been within normal limits for at least 1 year with negative or low-titre auto antibodies. A liver biopsy should be performed to assess the degree of inflammation. If there is no inflammation present, first the dose of azathioprine and subsequently the dose of prednisolone should be discontinued gradually under frequent monitoring of the blood tests. Treatment withdrawal is not advisable just before or during puberty, when the risk of relapse is higher.

In our experience, children with AIH-2 usually relapse and have to be restarted on treatment, and only 20% with AIH-1 can stay off immunosuppression. Despite the efficacy of standard immunosuppressive treatment, severe hepatic decompensation may develop even after many years of apparently good biochemical control, leading to transplantation 10–15 years after diagnosis in 10% of the patients. In our analysis, bilirubin levels and INR at diagnosis were found to be independent risk factors of death and/or transplantation.

Autoimmune hepatitis/sclerosing cholangitis overlap syndrome

- A prospective study at our centre was conducted over a period of 16 years, in which all children with serological (i.e. autoantibodies, high IgG levels) and histological (i.e. interface hepatitis) features of autoimmune liver disease underwent a cholangiogram at the time of presentation. Approximately 50% of these patients had alterations of the bile ducts characteristic of sclerosing cholangitis, though generally less advanced than those observed in adult primary sclerosing cholangitis. A quarter of the children with ASC, despite abnormal cholangiograms, had no histological features suggesting bile duct involvement and the diagnosis of sclerosing cholangitis was only possible because of the cholangiographic studies.
- Virtually all patients (55% of whom were female) were seropositive for ANA and/or SMA. The mode of presentation was similar to that of typical AIH-1.
- IBD was present in about 45% of children with ASC compared to about 20% of those with typical AIH. IBD can be asymptomatic and should be sought and treated in all children/adolescents with autoimmune liver disease, as its presence is associated with progression of hepatic damage.
- Increased serum IgG levels were found in 90% of children with ASC. At the time of presentation, standard liver function tests did not help in discriminating between AIH and ASC, though the alkaline phosphatase/aspartate amino transferase ratio was significantly higher in ASC. Atypical pANCA were present in 74% of patients with ASC compared to 45% of patients with AIH-1 and 11% of those with AIH-2.
- Children with ASC respond to the same immunosuppressive schedule used in AIH, liver test abnormalities resolving within a few months after starting treatment in most patients. Steroids and azathioprine, although beneficial in abating the parenchymal inflammatory lesion, appear to be less effective in controlling the bile duct disease. Ursodeoxycholic acid is usually added at a dose of 15–20mg/kg per day, although its usefulness in arresting the progression of ASC has not been proved.
- The medium-term prognosis is good, with a reported 7-year survival of 100%, though 15% of the patients required liver transplant during this period of follow-up. Recurrence of ASC after transplant is frequent (30–60%), particularly in the presence of active IBD. Evolution from AIH to ASC has been documented but whether the juvenile autoimmune form of sclerosing cholangitis and AIH are two distinct entities, or different aspects of the same condition, remains to be elucidated.

Metabolic liver disease

Background *506*
Clinical features *507*
Clinical presentations of metabolic disorders *508*
Investigation *514*
General management *516*
References and resources *518*

Background

The diagnostic approach to a child with metabolic liver disease requires a high degree of suspicion, detailed history and physical examination, and extensive blood and urine tests; liver, skin, and muscle biopsies are usually necessary to establish the diagnosis.

Important features in the history
- Family history of a metabolic condition or genetic disorder.
- Unexplained early neonatal deaths, stillbirths, and recurrent miscarriages.
- Consanguinity.
- Developmental delay or neurological regression.
- Recurrent episodes of vomiting of unknown aetiology.
- Episodes of encephalopathy.

There are six major modes of clinical presentation in a patient with liver disease of metabolic origin:
- Acute liver failure (ALF).
- Infantile cholestasis.
- Neonatal ascites.
- Abnormal liver enzymes or fatty liver reported on USS performed incidentally.
- Hyperammonaemia.
- Acidosis.

Clinical features

There is a wide variety of clinical signs and symptoms strongly associated with specific metabolic disorders affecting the liver including:

- *Coarse facies:* mucopolysaccharidosis (MPS), GM1 gangliosidosis.
- *Corneal clouding:* MPS.
- *Macroglossia:* GM1 gangliosidosis.
- *Diarrhoea:* Wolman disease, cystic fibrosis, mitochondrial disorders, congenital disorder of glycosylation (CDG).
- *Lymphadenopathy:* Wolman disease, Gaucher disease.
- *Cherry-red spot:* Niemann–Pick C, GM1 gangliosidosis.
- *Ichthyoids or collodion skin:* Gaucher disease.
- *Hypotonia and seizures:* urea cycle defect (UCD), long chain acyl-co A dehydrogenase deficiency (LCHAD), CDG, mitochondrial disorders.
- *Hypertrophic cardiomyopathy:* glycogen storage disorders (GSDs), fatty acid oxidation disorders (FAODs).
- *Abnormal fat distribution:* CDG.
- *Sweaty feet:* glutaric acidaemia, isovaleric acidaemia.
- *Rancid, fishy, or cabbage-like smell:* tyrosinaemia.

Clinical presentations of metabolic disorders

The following is an approach to metabolic liver disease according to the presenting clinical picture.

Acute liver failure

- *Galactosaemia (galactose-1-phosphate uridyltransferase deficiency)*: autosomal recessive (AR) inherited disorder; patients can present with faltering growth, vomiting, diarrhoea, renal tubular aminoaciduria, coagulopathy, and bleeding. There is exacerbation of jaundice in the neonate after lactose ingestion. Cirrhosis may be evident at birth, with cerebral oedema and cataracts; patients demonstrate predisposition to Gram-negative sepsis. The management is lactose exclusion from the diet, usually a soya-based formula with appropriate calcium supplementation is given.
- *Neonatal haemochromatosis*: syndrome defined by the coexistence of liver disease of antenatal onset with excess iron deposition at the extrahepatic sites but with the reticuloendothelial components remaining iron free. Liver disease is usually apparent at birth or shortly after. Lip mucosa biopsy can be supportive of the diagnosis. Liver transplantation is the treatment of choice. Pregnant mothers with a previous affected child are offered weekly IV immunoglobulin infusions with reassuring results.
- *Mitochondrial hepatopathies*: nuclear and mitochondrial genes encode for mitochondrial proteins and enzymes. Mutations in these genes can lead to mitochondrial DNA to be quantitatively decreased and result in mitochondrial liver disease including ALF. The infant may exhibit lactic acidosis and multisystem disease involvement: brain, muscle, heart, and kidneys. Panel screening for mutations in *DGUOK, POLG1, MPV17,* and *TRMU* are usually carried out early when suspected.
- *Fatty acid oxidation disorders*: beta oxidation of fatty acids takes place in the mitochondrial matrix and is essential for energy production. Defects in the metabolism of fatty acids can result in hypoketotic hypoglycaemia, dicarboxylic aciduria, encephalopathy, and liver dysfunction. The diagnosis is made by acylcarnitine profile and confirmed by genotyping. Management is primarily the avoidance of decompensation by the use of glucose polymer drinks.
- *Haemophagocytic lymphohistiocytosis*: there is a sporadic and a familial form (AR) presenting at various ages. Associated with EBV infection. Can present with fever, hepatosplenomegaly, jaundice, lymphadenopathy, encephalopathy, seizures, and a maculopapular rash. There is evident hypertriglyceridaemia, hypofibrinogenaemia and the diagnosis is established with histiocyte erythrophagocytosis evident in bone marrow aspirate. Treatment includes immunoglobulins, dexamethasone, and chemotherapy; prognosis is generally poor.

- *Congenital disorder of glycosylation*: this is a rare and heterogeneous group of disorders where the defect lies in glycosylation—a form of post-translational modification. Usually the disease is multisystemic and symptoms appear at birth. The prototype CDG is phosphomannomutase deficiency or CDG1a. Diagnosis is detected by isoelectric focusing of serum transferrin and confirmed by mutational analysis.
- Wilson disease (see Chapter 62).

Infantile cholestasis

- *Alpha-1 antitrypsin deficiency* (see Chapter 55).
- *Cystic fibrosis* (see Chapter 25).
- *Congenital hypothyroidism*: thyroxine can affect bile flow and cause prolonged unconjugated hyperbilirubinaemia. Patients will have a suboptimal response to thyroid-releasing hormone test and symptoms usually resolve within a few weeks of supplementation with levothyroxine.
- *Congenital hypopituitarism*: presenting usually within the first few weeks of life and is associated with dysmorphic facial features (frontal bossing, depressed nasal bridge, and hypotelorism) and nystagmus indicating septo-optic dysplasia. Patients can present with hypoglycaemia, hypothermia, hypotension, and conjugated hyperbilirubinaemia. Biochemical findings include low early morning cortisol level and abnormal short tetracosactide test. Patients can also have a suboptimal thyroid-releasing hormone response. Treatment is with hydrocortisone and levothyroxine where appropriate. Patients may require growth hormone supplementation after the first year. Cholestasis usually resolves within 6 months of treatment.
- *Tyrosinaemia type 1*: AR inherited disorder caused by deficiency of fumarylacetoacetate hydrolase, the last enzyme of tyrosine degradation. It can also present as ALF with hypoglycaemia, coagulopathy, and a raised serum alpha fetoprotein. Can also present with porphyric crises, renal tubular acidosis, faltering growth, and rarely with hypertrophic cardiomyopathy. It is diagnosed by hypertyrosinaemia, hypermethioninaemia, and raised urinary succinylacetone and gamma aminolaevulinic acid. Raised incidence of hepatocarcinoma. Restriction of dietary protein intake (1g/kg/day) to maintain tyrosine and phenylalanine level within range. Ensure adequate intake of other essential amino acids (special metabolic protein mix). Administration of 2-(2-nitro-4-trifluomethylbenzoyl)-1,3-cyclohexanedione (NTBC) has revolutionized the outcome of tyrosinaemia.
- *Fructosaemia (fructose-1, 6-diphosphatase deficiency)*: presentation is usually before 6 months of age with enlarged and fatty liver, muscle hypotonia, severe ketotic hypoglycaemia, and hyperventilation with severe metabolic acidosis All infant formulas (except Glactomin 19® and Isomil®) can be used and all feeds (except Pediasure®). The main aim is to eliminate all sources of fructose from their diet but an intake of 1–2g per day is acceptable. Supplementation is required for vitamin C, folic acid, and fibre due to dietary restrictions.

- *Peroxisomal disorders*: diagnosis is made by skin fibroblast studies, plasma assays of very long-chain fatty acids, plasmalogens, phytanic acid, L-pipecolate, and bile acid intermediates by gas chromatography/mass spectrometry.
  - *Zellweger syndrome*: this is the most severe form among the peroxisomal disorders comprising of neonatal adrenoleucodystrophy and infantile Refsum disease. The infant may present with neonatal non-immune hydrops or later in infancy with hepatosplenomegaly. There is multisystem involvement with severe neurological impairment. Treatment is primarily supportive.
  - *Neonatal adrenoleucodystrophy*: a X-linked inherited disorder associated with dysmorphic features, deafness, developmental delay, hypotonia, seizures and characteristic hepatomegaly. Survival is greater than in Zellweger syndrome.
  - *Infantile Refsum disease*: an AR disorder with a milder clinical picture than in Zellweger syndrome with sensorineural deafness and pigmentary retinopathy (Leber's congenital amaurosis). Hepatomegaly and cholelithiasis have been reported.
  - *Primary hyperoxaluria type I*: secondary to the deficiency of the enzyme alanine-glyoxylate aminotransferase; characterized by continuous high urinary oxalate excretion and progressive bilateral oxalate urolithiasis and nephrocalcinosis. No characteristic craniofacial features. Liver transplantation is the treatment of choice with renal transplantation at a later stage in patients with end-stage renal disease.
- *Glycogen storage disease type IV (1,4 glucan-6-glycosyl transferase deficiency)*: AR inherited disorder presenting with hydrops fetalis, hepatomegaly, faltering growth, liver cirrhosis with associated complications, cardiac failure, skeletal muscle weakness, hypoglycaemia, metabolic acidosis, and raised cholesterol and triglycerides. Diagnosis confirmed by branching enzyme deficiency in leucocytes and cultured fibroblasts. Liver transplantation has been performed but neurological prognosis remains guarded.
- *Glycogen storage disease type VI (liver phosphorylase deficiency)*: patients present with hepatomegaly, faltering growth, and mild hypoglycaemia. Progression to cirrhosis is uncommon.
- *Bile acid synthesis defect*: this is a very rare group of disorders of sterol (cholesterol) metabolism that present with cholestasis and malabsorption. It forms part of your differential diagnosis when presented with a case of low GGT cholestasis with lack of pruritus. Diagnosis is based on spectrometry of bile acids—fast atom bombardment ionization mass spectrometry (FAB-MS) and liquid-gas chromatography. On liver biopsy there is giant cell transformation with bile duct proliferation and canalicular plugging progressing to cirrhosis. Prognosis is excellent with bile acid therapy.

Neonatal ascites

- *Niemann–Pick type C*: This is characterized by an abnormality in cholesterol transport causing accumulation of sphingomyelin and cholesterol in the lysosomes and a secondary reduction in sphingomyelinase activity. Patients can present with massive hepatosplenomegaly in severe cases, a cherry-red spot on retinal examination and vertical supranuclear gaze palsy. Diagnosis can be established from storage cells in bone marrow aspirate and rectal ganglion cells.
- *Wolman disease*: AR lysosomal storage disease caused by deficiency of the acid lipase and accumulation of cholesterol esters and triglycerides in histiocytic cells of most visceral organs. Other salient features are diarrhoea, fat malabsorption, and adrenal calcification.
- *Zellweger syndrome*: see p. 508.
- *Gaucher type II (acute neuronopathic disease)*: AR disease caused by β-glucosidase deficiency, which results in the accumulation of glucosylceramide-laden macrophages. It can present with hypersplenism, gross hepatosplenomegaly, bone marrow infiltration, and skeletal disease.
- *GM1 gangliosidosis*: AR lysosomal storage disorder characterized by the generalized accumulation of GM1 ganglioside, oligosaccharides, and the mucopolysaccharide keratin sulfate (and their derivatives). There are three clinical subtypes classified according to the age of presentation: the infantile, juvenile, and adult types.

Incidental finding of abnormal liver enzymes

Incidental findings of abnormal liver transaminases should be further investigated to exclude metabolic liver disorders. It is important to measure creatine kinase to exclude muscle as a source of transaminase elevation. However, elevation of GGT and conjugated bilirubin are specific to liver pathology. Metabolic conditions that are commonly picked up in this manner are Wilson disease, paediatric fatty liver disease, and FAODs. Age-appropriate and disease specific investigations are recommended.

Hyperammonaemia

Urea cycle defects usually present in the first days of life with irritability, poor feeding, vomiting, lethargy, hypotonia, and respiratory distress. If left untreated it can lead to seizures, coma, and death. There are five enzyme defects affecting the liver which are all AR inheritance apart from ornithine transcarbamylase deficiency (OTC) which is X-linked. The other four affected enzymes are carbamoyl phosphate synthetase, arginosuccinic acid synthetase, arginosuccinic lyase, and arginase. The treatment in suspected cases is haemodialysis within a few hours after birth and a limited protein intake diet. Liver transplantation could be beneficial but is associated with high mortality and morbidity. Poor neurological outcome once patients suffer hyperammonaemic coma.

Acidosis and ketosis

Organic acidaemias

- *Methylmalonic acidaemia:*
  - Episodic metabolic ketoacidosis with the most severe defect presenting in the first week of life; hyperammonaemia in up to 80% of patients and hypoglycaemia in 40% of patients. These episodes can be associated with neutropenia and thrombocytopenia. Some patients can develop a severe extrapyramidal disorder.
  - Elevated plasma glycine levels and raised plasma and urine methylmalonate levels. There is a low free carnitine level accompanied by a larger percentage of short-chain acylcarnitine levels.
- *Propionic acidaemia:*
  - Patients present with episodic metabolic ketoacidosis. In the newborn period the ammonia levels may stimulate urea cycle defects; episodes possibly associated with neutropenia and thrombocytopenia.
  - Investigations: elevated plasma glycine, propionic acid, and methylcitrate levels. Low free carnitine levels accompanied by a larger percentage of acylcarnitine; fatty liver
- *Isovaleric acidaemia:*
  - Recurrent episodes of metabolic ketoacidosis progressing to coma, with 50% of patients presenting at 3–14 days of age. Characteristic odour of sweaty feet during these episodes from sweat, urine, blood, and saliva. Refusal to eat; possible alopecia; some patients may develop pancreatitis during acute episodes.
  - Investigations: during an acute episode there could be hyperglycaemia or hypoglycaemia, neutropenia, thrombocytopenia, or pancytopenia with elevated urinary isovalerylglycine; part of the Expanded Newborn Screening programme in the UK.

Investigation

First-line investigations

Blood
- Full blood count, urea and electrolytes, liver function tests, and INR.
- Blood gas.
- Glucose, ammonia, and uric acid.
- Lactate and pyruvate (L:P ratio).
- Ketones.
- Amino acids.
- Acylcarnitines.
- Alpha-1 antitrypsin level and phenotype.

Urine
- Organic acids.
- Electrolytes, calcium, and phosphate for tubular dysfunction.

Blood film
- Vacuolated white blood cells on blood film:
  - Wolman disease.
  - GM1 gangliosidosis.
  - Niemann–Pick C.
  - Mucopolysaccharidosis.
  - Glycogen storage disease.

Second-line investigations
- Galactose-1-phosphate uridyltransferase levels if suspecting galactosaemia.
- Serum copper, caeruloplasmin, and penicillamine challenge if suspecting Wilson disease.
- Chitotriosidase as a screening biomarker for storage disorders.
- White cell enzymes if suspecting a storage disorder.
- Transferrin isoforms for congenital disorder of glycosylation.
- Lysosomal acid lipase levels on dried blood spot card.
- MRI brain, echocardiography, renal USS, and electromyography if multiorgan involvement is suspected.
- Skin biopsy for fibroblast culture: can be used to carry out specific enzyme assays as well as providing a source of DNA.
- Muscle biopsy for electron transport chain enzymology for the assessment of mitochondrial hepatopathies.
- Bone marrow aspirate: for identification of storage cells, e.g. Niemann–Pick C.

Liver biopsy
- Periodic acid–Schiff ± diastase resistant granules: alpha-1 antitrypsin deficiency, GSD type IV, and afibrinoginaemia.
- Iron deposition: neonatal haemochromatosis, Zellweger syndrome.
- Microvesicular steatosis: non-specific finding in metabolic disorders but particularly those related to mitochondrial disorders and FAODs.

- Glycogen and plant-like cells: GSD.
- Copper: Wilson disease, Indian childhood cirrhosis, and other copper toxicity states.

Ophthalmology

- Kaiser Fleisher rings—Wilson disease.
- Corneal clouding—MPS.
- Cataracts—galactosaemia, peroxisomal and mitochondrial disorders.
- Pigmentary retinopathy—mitochondrial disorders and FAODs.
- Cherry-red spot—sphingolipidoses.

Radiology

- MRI brain if suspecting a multisystemic disorder.
- Stippled epiphyses, periosteal cloaking of long bones and ribs: GM1 gangliosidosis.
- Dysostosis multiplex: MPS and advanced GSD.
- Calcified adrenal glands: Wolman disease.

Genetics

- Next-generation sequencing is a high throughput sequencing technology that can rapidly generate masses of DNA sequence data.
- Targeted sequencing can be carried out to specifically examine genes of interest.
- At King's College Hospital, London, UK, we carry out in-house, genetic panel testing comprising of 26 disorders of cholestasis. This panel is constantly being expanded.

General management

Avoidance of catabolic states

- Avoid fasting—can be fatal.
- Strict feeding regimen (timing, prescribing diet).
- Every patient should have an individual feeding plan.

Early detection of catabolic states

- Vomiting is an alarming symptom; fluid losses may need to be replaced or administer emergency regimen.

Detecting loss of metabolic control

This could be associated with any of the following conditions:
- Abnormal behaviour.
- Hypo- or hyperglycaemia.
- Metabolic acidosis/lactic acidosis.
- Hepatic encephalopathy.
- Cerebral oedema.
- Abnormal coagulation studies and subsequent bleeding.
- Seizures.
- Hyperammonaemia.
- Dehydration and severe electrolyte imbalances.
- Cardiac arrhythmias.
- Loss of temperature control.
- Respiratory depression.
- Renal impairment.
- Pancytopenia.
- Myocardial insult.

Managing acute illnesses and regaining metabolic control

- Close monitoring of target-to-background ratio, blood pressure, and oxygen saturation.
- Check blood sugars regularly.
- Some patients may require neuro-observations.

Emergency regimen

- This consists of a high-energy, protein-free, and fat-free drink which should be offered frequently and in small amounts either orally or via a NGT.
- High concentration in carbohydrates for energy (e.g. Maxijul®) but more tolerable substitutes can also be used (e.g. Lucozade®).
- If the oral regimen is not tolerated or the child has persistent ketoacidosis, an IV infusion of 10% or higher concentration of glucose will be required.
- Electrolytes should be monitored regularly and managed by fluid resuscitation (hypovolaemic hypernatraemia) and/or electrolyte supplementation (hypokalaemia due to vomiting).
- Patients with protein metabolism disorders should not stay off protein for a prolonged time as this may cause an endogenous release of protein.
- Working closely with an experience dietitian in the field is advisable.

Acute hypoglycaemic event

- Prompt treatment is essential in order to avoid subsequent neurological damage.
- Initially in a conscious child, who is feeding, glucose 10–20g is given by mouth in a liquid form (GlucoGel®, milk etc.). This may need to be repeated after 10–15 minutes.
- Alternatively, 2mL/kg of IV 10% glucose (200mg/kg of glucose) may be given IV into a large vein, following a saline flush as the preparation is a potential irritant and may cause an extravasation injury or even lead to venous thrombosis.
- Hypoglycaemia that is not responding to the above measures or hypoglycaemia that causes loss of consciousness or fitting requires intramuscular or IV administration of glucagon.
- No response to glucagon should raise the suspicion of a GSD or a FAOD.

Management of hyperammonaemia

- Sodium benzoate and sodium phenylbutyrate conjugate glycine and glutamine respectively. In doing so, they become water soluble to be excreted by the kidneys, reducing the nitrogen load on the kidneys.
- Dialysis is required if hyperammonaemia is not controlled.

Management of other systems

- Invasive monitoring of the acutely unwell patient is recommended.
- Patients may develop an oxygen requirement and some may also need to be intubated and ventilated.
- Peritoneal dialysis, haemofiltration, or exchange transfusion may be required in order to remove harmful metabolites and restore haemostasis

References and resources

British Inherited Metabolic Disease Group (BIMDG): http://www.bimdg.org.uk/site/index.asp
Hoffmann G, Zschocke J, Nyhan W. Inherited metabolic diseases. Berlin: Springer; 2010.

Non-alcoholic fatty liver disease

Definition *520*
Epidemiology *520*
Risk factors *520*
Pathophysiology *521*
Clinical presentation and diagnosis *522*
Natural history *526*
Management *527*
Current areas of research *528*
References and resources *528*

Definition

Non-alcoholic fatty liver disease (NAFLD) is a condition characterized by the presence of liver steatosis with or without inflammation (steatohepatitis) and fibrosis. It is a diagnosis of exclusion and made in the absence of other possible metabolic or toxic causes of fat accumulation. It was first described in children in 1983 shortly after it was recognized in adults. Histologically, it is similar to alcoholic liver disease; however, it occurs in the absence of significant alcohol consumption. It is almost always seen in the presence of overweight/obesity or the metabolic syndrome, the absence of which may suggest an alternate diagnosis. The umbrella term NAFLD encompasses both bland steatosis and non-alcoholic steatohepatitis (NASH) which can involve both inflammation and fibrosis.

Epidemiology

NAFLD is the most prevalent chronic liver disease in children and young people, the rise in which is closely linked to the obesity epidemic. NAFLD is thought to be present in 9% of children and young people with NASH in 3% based on a study using a histological diagnosis. In overweight/obese children, the prevalence of NAFLD may be as high as 50–80%.

Risk factors

In general, boys are more at risk and prevalence increases with age. Those of Hispanic ethnicity are most susceptible, followed by Asian ethnicity, then Caucasian and finally black, non-Hispanic children. Familial clustering of NAFLD is also commonly seen. Other genetic susceptibility factors have been identified by genome-wide association studies including single nucleotide polymorphisms of which the gene for adiponutrin (*PNPLA3*) is the best characterized as associated with the presence of the disease.

The strongest risk factor is the presence of visceral adiposity and other features of the metabolic syndrome; obesity, hyperlipidaemia, and hypertension or a family history of such.

Nutrition and physical activity are important environmental factors determining risk with specific dietary factors playing either a protective (polyunsaturated fatty acids, vitamin D, fibre, vitamin C and vitamin E) or harmful role (fructose consumption, saturated fats) in the development and progression of NAFLD.

More recent hypotheses regarding susceptibility to NAFLD include the influence of intrauterine priming in the form of maternal obesity with deposition of excess fatty acids in the fetal liver. Infant feeding may also have a role, with breastfeeding a protective factor and infant overfeeding a risk factor.

Pathophysiology

NAFLD is the hepatic manifestation of the metabolic syndrome. Insulin resistance is found in up to 80% of children with NAFLD, similarly to adults with the condition. The pathogenesis of NAFLD is still incompletely understood. The 'two-hit hypothesis' proposed in 1998 suggests that the imbalance of fatty acid supply and demand in the liver cell initiates steatosis, making the cell vulnerable to injury. A second hit in the form of oxidative stress, inflammation, or small bowel bacterial overgrowth is then required for progression to steatohepatitis and fibrosis. A more recent hypothesis suggests that fat accumulation in the liver is a protective mechanism but when the capacity of the cell to accumulate triglycerides is overwhelmed, steatohepatitis follows.

Hyperinsulinism

Hyperinsulinism results in increased delivery of lipids to the hepatocyte, increased *de novo* lipogenesis, and decreased export via very low-density lipoprotein and decreased oxidation, all resulting in the production and release of toxic free fatty acids into the circulation.

Oxidative stress

Oxidative stress is also implicated in the pathophysiology of NAFLD. The mitochondria are overwhelmed by free fatty acids requiring oxidation and may not function as effectively. There is an increase in reactive oxygen species which results in damage to the hepatocytes.

Inflammation

NAFLD is closely associated with central or visceral obesity characterized by an increased waist circumference. This is well known to be a chronic inflammatory state predisposing to ischaemic heart disease and cancer. Adipocytokines produced by adipocytes and infiltrating macrophages are mediators of this inflammation. Increased production of adipokines such as leptin, visfatin, and decreased production of adiponectin have been found in patients with NAFLD.

Apoptosis

The principal mechanism of cell death in NAFLD is apoptosis which may be intrinsically or extrinsically mediated and in the liver may give way to an inflammatory response.

Fibrosis

The final common pathway of inflammation, oxidative stress, and apoptosis is fibrosis; the accumulation of excessive extracellular matrix in the liver parenchyma with distortion of the architecture. Classic complications of chronic liver disease such as impaired synthetic function, portal hypertension, and hepatocellular carcinoma may follow as a consequence. Therefore, more information about pathophysiology of liver injury in NAFLD may lead to better understanding of chronic liver injury, irrespective of the cause.

Clinical presentation and diagnosis

Children and young people with NAFLD are often asymptomatic or present with vague non-specific symptoms or incidental findings such as abdominal pain or fatigue. Most children and young people will come to medical attention due to an incidental blood test showing elevated AST/ALT or GGT or an abdominal USS showing a bright liver. The majority of children have visceral adiposity and a true diagnosis of NAFLD in a child of normal weight should only be made after careful consideration of alternative causes (Table 61.1).

Table 61.1 Differential diagnosis of steatosis

Clinical condition	Diagnostic clues
Wilson disease	Low caeruloplasmin, high urinary or tissue copper, mutational analysis
Alpha-1 antitrypsin deficiency	Phenotype or genotype
Drugs: steroids, amiodarone, alcohol, methotrexate, ecstasy, L-asparaginase, vitamin E, valproate, tamoxifen, antiretrovirals	History
Cystic fibrosis-associated liver disease	History/sweat test or mutational analysis
Malnutrition	History
Coeliac disease	Tissue transglutaminase, jejunal biopsy
Hepatitis C	Hepatitis C virus antibody status
Parenteral nutrition-associated liver disease	History
Mitochondrial disease/fatty acid oxidase deficiency	Lactate, acylcarnitines, respiratory chain enzymes, mutational analysis
Metabolic disease: lysosomal acid lipase deficiency (cholesterol ester storage disease)	White cell enzymes, mutational analysis
Galactosaemia	Gal-1-PUT
Fructosaemia	Enzymology
Glycogen storage disease	White cell enzymes, mutational analysis
Peroxisomal disorders	Very long-chain fatty acids, mutational analysis
Mauriac syndrome	History of type 1 diabetes
Hypobetalipoproteinaemia/ abetalipoproteinaemia	Low lipid levels, reduced/absent Apo1B, mutational analysis
Lipodystrophies	Mutational analysis
Shwachman syndrome	Pancreatic insufficiency/mutational analysis

Even in the presence of overweight, NAFLD is less common in children <10 years and is extremely rare in children <3 years and an alternative metabolic diagnosis should be strongly considered in these cases. Mild hepatomegaly and splenomegaly may be present on examination in addition to acanthosis nigricans (black pigmentation of axilla, skinfolds, and neck) often seen in children with insulin resistance.

The majority of children with NAFLD have insulin resistance with 10–25% in some series having glucose intolerance. There is often a positive family history of the metabolic syndrome. NICE guidelines suggest that children with type 2 diabetes should be screened for the condition. Some centres also screen children who are overweight or obese. Even in the presence of other features of the metabolic syndrome, NAFLD is a diagnosis of exclusion and many other conditions leading to steatosis must be considered at presentation. As 25% of the paediatric population is now classified as overweight or obese, the consideration of other treatable liver diseases such as Wilson disease in an otherwise 'simply' overweight child is essential.

Liver biopsy is the criterion standard for diagnosis of NAFLD and also for differentiation of steatosis without inflammation from steatohepatitis and fibrosis. Liver biopsy is not always practical or acceptable as a screening tool however, and at present there is no consensus on which children should undergo the procedure. Biopsy is most useful for excluding other diseases (particularly Wilson disease, for example) in those who may have other parameters pointing towards an alternative diagnosis, children under the age of 10 and children with normal or near normal BMI for age. Biopsy is also useful in children in whom significant or severe disease is suspected, e.g. children with persistently abnormal biochemistry (>1.5 times the ULN of ALT/AST/GGT), persistent splenomegaly, or evidence of portal hypertension. Children with a very abnormal oral glucose tolerance test or those with a family history of severe NAFLD are also candidates for liver biopsy. Of note though elevated transaminases are used as a screening tool for NAFLD, ALT may be normal in 40% of cases of significant fibrosis secondary to the disease. Diagnosis of is based on a pattern of histopathological findings including macrovesicular steatosis, mixed or polymorphonuclear portal inflammation, ballooning degeneration of hepatocytes, and fibrosis. In adults, the pattern of inflammation is largely lobular and fibrosis perivenular (type 1 NASH), whereas in children, periportal disease is common (type 2 NASH). The reason for this difference in histological pattern is not clear. Type 2 NASH in both children and in adults when present, is associated with more severe disease.

In view of the fact that biopsy is not universally used for diagnosis and is impractical for use as a longitudinal measure of disease, non-invasive biomarkers of disease are of much interest. Algorithms of simple biomarkers have been developed and validated in mostly adult cohorts. The paediatric NAFLD fibrosis index (PNFI) was developed and validated using a paediatric cohort. Markers of apoptotic cell death such as CK18 M30 have demonstrated some use in assessment of disease activity in both adults and children. Though NICE recommend ELF (enhanced liver fibrosis) as a screening and monitoring tool in both children and adults with

NAFLD, it has not been adequately validated in a paediatric population. Imaging techniques such as transient elastography and acoustic radiation force imaging, both of which use shear waves to determine liver stiffness, have been shown to have a useful sensitivity and specificity for more significant fibrosis in both adult and paediatric patients. Newer techniques such as using magnetic resonance technology are also promising; however, cost may be prohibitive.

See Table 61.2 for examination and investigation findings.

Table 61.2 What to look for in the child with NAFLD

Examination	Investigation
Height and weight	Liver function tests
Waist circumference	Full lipid profile
Hepatosplenomegaly may be present	Oral glucose tolerance test including fasting insulin
Acanthosis nigricans	
Blood pressure	Ultrasound scan
	Liver biopsy if indicated
	Screening tests for other diagnoses (see Table 61.1)

Natural history

NAFLD is well recognized to progress to end-stage liver disease and/or hepatocellular carcinoma. End-stage liver disease due to NAFLD is likely to become the most frequent indication for liver transplantation by the year 2020. Adult data have shown that progression of disease varies greatly and the challenge is in identifying those individuals who are likely to progress from those who are not. Meta analyses in adult patients with NAFLD have shown that those with simple steatosis only rarely go on to develop significant liver disease or die a liver-related death, although the mortality from cardiovascular disease is higher than that of controls. The natural history of paediatric NAFLD is not yet well defined. Paediatric longitudinal studies are rare, however in one 20-year follow-up, fibrosis progression was shown in four of five patients who underwent a second liver biopsy and a liver transplant was required in two teenagers with cirrhosis secondary to NAFLD. Several other case series have reported severe fibrosis or cirrhotic change in young teenagers with a risk of progression to end-stage liver disease and hepatocellular carcinoma during young adulthood though this is extremely rare.

Management

The mainstay of management of NAFLD in both children and adults is adoption of a healthy lifestyle. Several case series and uncontrolled trials have demonstrated the effect of weight loss on improvement of NAFLD. Children and young people who underwent a 5–10% decrease in BMI demonstrated significant improvements in liver echogenicity on ultrasound steatosis with smaller studies demonstrating an improvement in liver histology. Particular factors in the diet may be important, with an emphasis on reducing sugar (especially fructose which has been implicated in pathogenesis) and saturated fat. No one specific dietary intervention has proven superior, however. Other methods of weight loss such as bariatric surgery have been found to have inconclusive effects on NAFLD.

There is uncertainty about the optimal pharmacological treatment of paediatric NAFLD. Insulin sensitizers such as metformin are used to improve insulin sensitivity. Recent randomized controlled trials in both adults and children, however, have failed to demonstrate any difference to placebo. Thiazolidinediones have been used in adults but not extensively evaluated in children in view of reported early safety concerns. The PIVENS trial in adults did not find that pioglitazone was superior to placebo for non-diabetic patients with NAFLD.

Antioxidants such as vitamin E have also been evaluated. In both the paediatric TONIC trial and the PIVENS adult trial, vitamin E at large doses (800IU/day in adults and 400IU/day in children) was found to improve histological severity when compared to placebo. Ursodeoxycholic acid has also been investigated but a recent Cochrane meta-analysis concluded that it did not have any significant therapeutic advantage.

Polyunsaturated fatty acids (PUFAs) have become a particular focus of interest with a number of small trials demonstrating promising effects in patients with NAFLD. PUFAs such as docosahexaenoic acid may increase beta oxidation and decrease lipogenesis, improving both steatosis and progression to steatohepatitis. Probiotics are also a promising therapy in light of the evidence that the gut/liver axis and bacterial overgrowth have a role in the development of NAFLD. Several small studies including two in children have suggested their therapeutic effect.

Though there is little evidence for any one approach to date, it is likely that a personalized, family-based approach to lifestyle intervention will most benefit patients with NAFLD. Specialist advice tailoring their diet and activity to their beliefs and their circumstances seems optimal. In addition, given the high prevalence of anxiety and depression in these young people, a psychologically minded approach to their management is essential. The ideal approach is multidisciplinary with dietician, psychologist, and physical therapist working with medical and nursing staff to engage and encourage lifestyle change.

Long-term monitoring is important as prognostic factors for development of end-stage liver disease and/or hepatocellular carcinoma in early adult hood are unknown. Surveillance with ultrasound and biochemistry (liver function tests, alpha-fetoprotein) is recommended. Though the average interval required to progress one fibrosis stage is estimated to be 7 years in adults, the rate of progression in children and young people is unknown. Therefore it is prudent to monitor with on an annual or biannual basis.

Current areas of research

NAFLD is the most common chronic liver disease in the Western world and with the current trend in overweight and obesity is likely to remain as such. A better understanding of the condition and improvement in management are urgently needed in order to avoid a potential epidemic of end-stage liver disease in early adulthood. It is also a marker of future risks for endocrine, cardiovascular, and skeletal pathology. The pathophysiology of the condition and key differences from the adult disease need to be explored. Prevention is an important focus but needs to be a multifaceted approach at a societal level. Though lifestyle change remains the cornerstone of management, many new compounds and molecules are under investigation for their potential therapeutic benefit. Focus on microbiota, bile acids as metabolic regulators, and several transcription factors are current areas of research focus. Methods of non-invasively making a positive diagnosis and monitoring response to treatment are also under development.

References and resources

National Institute for Health and Care Excellence (NICE). Non-alcoholic fatty liver disease (NAFLD): assessment and management. NICE Guideline NG49. London: NICE; 2016. https://www.nice.org.uk/guidance/ng49

Vajro P, Lenta S, Socha P, et al. Diagnosis of nonalcoholic fatty liver disease in children and adolescents: position paper of the ESPGHAN Hepatology Committee. J Pediatr Gastroenterol Nutr 2012;54:700–13.

Wilson disease

Introduction *530*
Clinical features *530*
Diagnosis *531*
Management *532*
Indications for liver transplantation *534*
References and resources *534*

Introduction

- Wilson disease (WD) is an autosomal disorder of copper metabolism. The gene *ATP7B* codes for a copper carrier which both exports copper from hepatocyte to bile, and enables caeruloplasmin synthesis.
- WD occurs worldwide with reported incidences of 5–30 per million population. WD may present with almost any variety of liver disease in the age group 3–12 years, with psychiatric and/or neurological disease in adolescence or young adults, with combined hepatic and neurological problems, or less commonly with haemolysis or arthritis.
- Low plasma caeruloplasmin, a positive penicillamine challenge test, and raised hepatic copper concentration suggest the diagnosis. There are numerous diagnostic pitfalls.
- If diagnosed early, it is readily treatable with zinc or chelators, and has a good long-term prognosis.
- Fulminant hepatic disease has a poor outcome without transplantation. Molecular methods now aid diagnosis, but pose new management dilemmas.

Clinical features

WD has protean clinical presentations. Approximately 40% present with liver disease, usually between the ages of 3 and 12 years. Approximately 50% have a psychiatric or neurological presentation, usually in adolescence or early adult life. Approximately half of this group will have clinically detectable liver disease. The remainder present with skeletal, renal, or haemolytic disease, and these features may also be present in the other clinical categories. Younger siblings should be detected by screening.

Liver disease in Wilson disease

The first indication of liver disease in WD may be ALF, acute hepatitis, chronic hepatitis, asymptomatic enlargement of the liver, the serendipitous finding of abnormal liver function tests, variceal haemorrhage from unsuspected portal hypertension, or signs of decompensated chronic liver disease. Therefore, since WD may present with almost any clinical variety of hepatic abnormality, the important message is to suspect WD in any child with undiagnosed liver disease. Other patients are discovered to have liver disease having presented with neurological, ophthalmic, haemolytic, skeletal, or, rarely, renal problems. Clinical awareness of WD is therefore all-important.

In all of these hepatic presentations, the absence of Kayser–Fleischer rings means that the diagnosis of WD will rest upon laboratory tests.

Diagnosis

The first essential in making the diagnosis of WD is to think of it. The WD diagnostic score takes into account:

- Presence or absence of Kayser–Fleischer rings.
- Neuropsychiatric symptoms (or typical brain MRI changes).
- Coombs-negative haemolytic anaemia (with a high serum copper).
- Raised urinary copper, particularly if >25μmol/24 hours following penicillamine—the penicillamine challenge.
- Raised hepatic copper, >250mg/g dry weight.
- Rhodanine-positive hepatocytes on biopsy.
- Low plasma caeruloplasmin, <0.2g/L.
- Presence of disease causing mutations on one or both chromosomes.

The presence of mutations without other abnormalities—clinical or biochemical—may not constitute WD.

Penicillamine challenge

Basal urine copper is an unreliable parameter, showing both poor sensitivity and poor specificity, though values >5μmol/24 hours are highly suggestive. A penicillamine challenge test gives greater discrimination. Following penicillamine 0.5g 12-hourly × 2, urine copper >25μmol/24 hours is found in 88% of patients with WD and 2% of those with other liver disorders.

Management

Diet

There is no clinical evidence that copper content of the diet influences the age of onset or the severity of WD, but there is some circumstantial evidence that it affects the severity of liver disease in animal models of WD. It is therefore appropriate to avoid excessive use of high-copper foods such as chocolate, shellfish, and liver.

Drugs

Three drugs are available to treat WD: penicillamine, trientine, and zinc. Both penicillamine and trientine may cause initial deterioration of neurological function on commencement of treatment. A fourth agent, ammonium tetrathiomolybdate, remains under clinical investigation.

Penicillamine

Penicillamine 'detoxifies' the copper possibly by inducing metallothionein by augmenting the bile pool or by a direct anti-inflammatory action. Toxic effects include skin rash, usually urticarial occurring soon after commencing treatment, and responding to cessation of treatment; proteinuria, in most cases mild and not requiring cessation of treatment but in a small number of patients proceeding to immune complex nephrotic syndrome; and bone marrow depression. Pyridoxine deficiency is a theoretical risk in childhood. A more serious and fortunately rare side effect is systemic lupus erythematosus.

Trientine

Trientine was initially introduced as a second-line drug for patients intolerant of penicillamine. The most commonly reported side effect is sideroblastic anaemia.

Zinc

Zinc, by inducing metallothionein in intestinal cells, reduces absorption and, by inducing metallothionein in hepatocytes, binds copper. It is of low toxicity and cheap, but its principal disadvantage is poor palatability.

The initial management of WD must be tailored to the clinical presentation. Patients with fulminant hepatic failure (patients with encephalopathy) have a poor prognosis, and must be transferred to a centre where they can be offered liver transplantation. A prognostic score can help to predict the need for urgent liver transplantation in patients who present with decompensated liver disease (see Table 62.1).

For the treatment of young children identified on screening, there is no consensus on the best drug or the age when treatment should be instituted. Our practice is to treat children with zinc acetate only after the age of 2 years.

Table 62.1 Revised King's Wilson Disease Index for predicting mortality

Score	Bilirubin (μmol/L)	INR	AST (IU/L)	WCC (10⁹/L)	Albumin (g/L)
0	0–100	0–1.29	0–100	0–6.7	>45
1	101–150	1.3–1.6	101–150	6.8–8.3	34–44
2	151–200	1.7–1.9	151–300	8.4–10.3	25–33
3	201–300	2.0–2.4	301–400	10.4–15.3	21–24
4	>301	>2.5	>401	>15.4	<20

Score of 11 or more indicates high mortality and need for liver transplantation. WCC, white cell count.

Reprinted from Dhawan A. et al (2005) Wilson's disease in children: 37-Year experience and revised King's score for liver transplantation Liver Transplantation 11(4):441–448 with permission from the American Association for the Study of Liver Diseases and Wiley.

Indications for liver transplantation

Liver transplantation is indicated for patients with fulminant liver failure with an adverse prognostic score (Table 62.1) and for those patients who do not respond to therapy, or who have advanced liver failure and/or intractable portal hypertension.

References and resources

Ferenci P, Caca K, Loudianos G, et al. Diagnosis and phenotypic classification of Wilson disease. Liver Int 2003;23:139–42.

Dhawan A, Taylor RM, Cheeseman P, De Silva P, Katsiyiannakis L, Mieli-Vergani G. Wilson's disease in children: 37-year experience and revised King's score for liver transplantation. Liver Transpl 2005;11:441–8.

Hepatitis B

Epidemiology 536
Transmission 537
Clinical features 537
Interpretation of HBV serology 538
Complications 540
Prevention 541
Management of chronic HBV infection 542
References and resources 544

Epidemiology

- About 2 billion people (one-third of the world population) show evidence of exposure to hepatitis B virus (HBV) infection, with 300–400 million showing evidence of chronic HBV infection.
- There are seven genotypes, A–G (A and G predominates in Europe and the US, B and C in Asia, E in Africa).
- HBV carrier rate varies from 1% to 20% of the normal population worldwide (Table 63.1).

Table 63.1 Geographical distribution and the mode of transmission of HBV infection

	Rate, %	Areas	Mode of transmission
Low	0.1–2	Canada, Western Europe, Australia, New Zealand	Sexual and parenteral
Intermediate	3–5	Eastern Europe, Mediterranean basin, Middle East, South America, Central Asia	Sexual and parenteral
High	10–20	South-east Asia, China, sub-Saharan Africa	Perinatal

Transmission

HBV infection is commonly transmitted by percutaneous (i.e. puncture through the skin) or mucosal (i.e. direct contact with mucous membranes) exposure to infectious blood or to body fluids containing blood. Serum, semen, and saliva have been demonstrated to be infectious.

Perinatal transmission is the most common route of transmission in children, followed by horizontal transmission from infected household contacts. Adolescents are at risk of HBV infection primarily through unprotected high-risk sexual activity and IV drug use.

The risk for chronic HBV infection in a newborn infant born to an HBsAg and HBeAg positive mother with a high HBV viral load is 90% in the absence of postexposure immunoprophylaxis. The risk decreases to <10% in the absence of postexposure immunoprophylaxis if the mother is HBsAg positive but HBeAg negative. Rarely HBV infection can present as acute liver failure in perinatally infected infants born to a mother who is HBsAg positive but HBeAg negative.

Clinical features

- Incubation period 50–150 days.
- *Acute hepatitis B:* mostly asymptomatic. If symptomatic, mainly constitutional symptoms such as anorexia, nausea, vomiting, low-grade fever, myalgia, fatiguability, right upper quadrant pain, and/or jaundice. Although acute liver failure has been reported in 2% of cases, viral clearance occurs in >95% of infected adolescents and adults.
- *Chronic hepatitis B:* defined by presence of HBsAg in serum for >6 months. Usually patients are healthy carriers without any evidence of active disease. Sometimes they can present with constitutional symptoms as described for acute hepatitis B. The risk of chronicity depends on the age of acquiring infection (90% in infants, 25–50% in children, 5% in adults).

Interpretation of HBV serology

- HBV core antigen (HBcAg):
  - Not detected in serum.
- HBc antibody (anti-HBc):
  - Presence of anti-HBc IgM indicates acute infection/reinfection.
  - Anti-HBc IgG suggests previous exposure to HBV and is detected in children who are immune or have chronic HBV infection.
- HBV early antigen (HBeAg):
  - 'Early' appearance during acute HBV infection.
  - Marker of a high degree of HBV infectivity.
  - Correlates with a high level of HBV replication.
- HBe antibody (anti-HBe):
  - Associated with decreasing levels of HBV DNA and liver enzymes in the blood marking the end of the replicative phase of the disease.
  - High HBV DNA with positive HBeAb suggests precore mutants.
- HBV surface antigen (HBsAg):
  - Presence in serum for at least 6 months indicates chronic infection.
- HBs antibody (anti-HBs):
  - Indicates an effective immune response to HBV infection or vaccination, or the presence of passively acquired antibody (hepatitis B immunoglobulin—HBIG).
- HBV DNA (viral load):
  - Best indicator of active viral replication.
- The pattern of HBV infection and HBV serology is shown in Table 63.2.

Table 63.2 Pattern of HBV infection and HBV serology

	Acute infection	Chronic HBV infection				Vaccinated	Resolved infection
		Immunotolerant	Immunoactive	Precore mutant	Low infectivity carrier		
HBsAg	+	+	+	+	+	–	–
HBeAg	+/–	+	+	–	–	–	–
Anti HBc IgM	+	–	–	–	–	–	–
Anti HBc IgG	+/–	+	+	+	+	–	+
Anti-HBs	–	–	–	–	–	+	+
Anti-HBe	+/–	–	–	+	+	–	–/+
HBV DNA	+/–	+++	++/+++	++/+++	+/–	–	–
Serum ALT	↑↑↑	N	↑/↑↑	↑/↑↑	N	N	N

Complications

- Cirrhosis: high risk in patients who continue to be HBeAg +ve; usually takes several years before decompensation.
- Hepatocellular carcinoma.
- Membranous glomerulonephritis.
- Polyarteritis nodosum.
- Panniculitis.

Prevention

Hepatitis B immunoprophylaxis
- Universal immunization against HBV is recommended.

Postexposure prophylaxis
- Term babies born to mother with hepatitis B infection: see Table 63.3.
- Babies with a birthweight of 1500g or less, born to mother infected with hepatitis B, should receive HBIG in addition to the vaccine regardless of the e-antigen status of the mother.
- Recommended vaccine schedule is the accelerated immunization schedule with vaccine at birth, 1 and 2 months, and 1 year of age.
- Children should be tested for HBsAg at 1 year of age at the time of the fourth dose to check if the vaccination has been successful or not.
- Response to vaccine (done 1–4 months after completing the schedule):
  - Anti-HBs concentration >100mIU/mL—responder, no further dose required.
  - Anti-HBs concentration >10 but <100mIU/mL—responder but requires an additional dose at that time.
  - Anti-HBs concentration <10mIU/mL—non-responder, repeat course of vaccine followed by another test to check the response.
- Accidental exposure/contamination from blood from a known HBsAg +ve person:
  - Previously immunized and responder: booster dose.
  - Previously immunized but non-responder: HBIG and a booster dose with second dose of HBIG after 1 month.
  - Previously unimmunized: accelerated course of HBV vaccine with HBIG one dose.
- Individuals at continuing risk of infection should be offered a single booster dose of vaccine, once only, ~5 years after primary immunization.
- Patients with chronic renal failure on haemodialysis should have antibody levels checked annually and if anti-HBs concentration <10mIU/mL, they should receive a booster dose.

Table 63.3 Prevention in term babies born to mother with hepatitis B infection

Hepatitis B status of mother	Hepatitis vaccine	HBIG
Mother is HBsAg +ve, HBeAg +ve (usually have high HBV DNA)	Yes	Yes
Mother is HBsAg +ve, HBeAg –ve but high HBV DNA	Yes	Yes
Mother is HBsAg +ve but e-markers unknown and/or HBV DNA unknown	Yes	Yes
Mother had acute hepatitis B infection in pregnancy	Yes	Yes
Mother is HBsAg +ve, HBeAg –ve and anti-HBe +ve and low HBV DNA	Yes	No

Management of chronic HBV infection

- Therapy currently recommended only for patients with chronic active disease (HBsAg +, HBeAg +, high HBV DNA and abnormal AST/ALT).
- Patients with HBeAg seroconversion and low/undetectable HBV DNA have improved outcome with prolonged survival without complications, reduced rate of hepatocellular carcinoma, and clinical and biochemical improvement.

Antiviral therapy

Immunomodulators

Interferon alfa

- Antiviral and immunomodulatory protein.
- About 30–40% of adults achieve HBeAg seroconversion.
- High pre-treatment AST/ALT levels, low pre-treatment HBV DNA, late acquisition of HBV infection and hepatocellular inflammation are the factors predicting good response.
- Side effects—flu-like symptoms, depression, bone marrow suppression, autoantibody induction, anorexia and weight loss, hair loss.
- If a severe reaction occurs, dose should be halved or discontinued.

Pegylated interferon alfa 2a

- Structurally modified interferon to ensure a long half-life.
- Dose—100mcg/m^2 subcutaneously once a week.
- Not yet licensed in children as yet for chronic HBV infection.
- Currently in a phase III trial as monotherapy in children with chronic HBV infection with abnormal liver function tests.
- Side effects—similar to interferon *alfa*.

Oral antiviral agents

Lamivudine

- Nucleoside analogue which inhibits DNA synthesis.
- Rapidly reduces HBV DNA levels to undetectable, however comes back to pre-treatment levels after cessation of the medications.
- Dose – 3mg/kg once daily (max. 100 mg once daily)
- Side effects—GI symptoms (nausea, vomiting, abdominal pain, diarrhoea), malaise, fatigue, pancreatitis, cough, headache, dizziness, neutropenia, elevation of transaminases, myalgia, urticarial rash.
- Development of YMDD (tyrosine–methionine–aspartate–aspartate) mutants increases with duration of the therapy (17% after 1 year to 63% after 5 years).
- Not recommended as a monotherapy treatment option.

Adefovir

- Nucleotide analogue of adenosine.
- Inhibitor of HBV reversed transcriptase and DNA polymerase.
- Effective in YMDD mutations.
- Side effects: nephrotoxicity, development of resistance mutations.
- Approved for treatment of children (>12 years) with immune-active chronic HBV though not highly recommended as a monotherapy.
- Dose—10mg once daily.

Entecavir
- Oral guanosine (nucleoside) analogue.
- Selective inhibitor of HBV DNA polymerase.
- Approved for monotherapy treatment of children (>3 years) with immune-active chronic HBV.
- Dose:
  - 0.015mg/kg once daily (max. 0.5mg) in nucleoside-naïve patients.
  - 0.025mg/kg once daily (max. 1mg) in nucleoside-experienced patients.
- Advantages:
  - Very potent antiviral activity.
  - Low drug resistance rate in nucleos(t)ide treatment-naïve patients.
  - Role is debatable in patient with lamivudine resistance.
  - Side effects are minimal.

Tenofovir
- Nucleotide analogue (adenosine monophosphate).
- A potent reverse transcriptase and viral polymerase inhibitor.
- Effective in YMDD mutations.
- Dose—300 mg once daily.
- Advantages:
  - Very potent antiviral activity.
  - Low drug resistance rate in nucleos(t)ide treatment-naïve patients.
- Side effects: nephrotoxicity, changes in bone mineral density.

Future potential therapies
- Pegylated interferon + nucleos(t)ide analogue.
- Gene therapy: antisense oligonucleotide, ribozyme, interfering proteins.
- Immunomodulatory therapy: thymosin, DNA vaccine.
- Concept of 'HBV cure'—using a combination of different direct antiviral agents ± immunomodulators.

References and resources

Defresne F, Sokal E. Chronic hepatitis B in children: therapeutic challenges and perspectives. J Gastroenterol Hepatol 2017;32:368–71.

Jonas MM, Lok AS, McMahon BJ, et al. Antiviral therapy in management of chronic hepatitis B viral infection in children: a systematic review and meta-analysis. Hepatology 2016;63:307–18.

Man Cho S, Choe BH. Treatment strategies according to genotype for chronic hepatitis B in children. Ann Transl Med 2016;4:336.

Nannini P, Sokal EM. Hepatitis B: changing epidemiology and interventions. Arch Dis Child 2017;102:676–80.

Hepatitis C

Epidemiology *546*
Risk of transmission *546*
Clinical features *547*
Specific viral tests *547*
Diagnosis of HCV infection in infants born to
    HCV +ve mother *547*
Management *548*
References and resources *550*

Epidemiology

- Hepatitis C virus (HCV) is an RNA virus of the Flaviviridae family.
- More than 150 million people are infected with HCV worldwide.
- UK prevalence of chronic HCV is 0.4%.
- There are seven different genotypes (1–7) with subtypes (see Table 64.1).
- In England and Wales, genotypes 1 and 3 are most prevalent.

Table 64.1 Subtypes of HCV

HCV genotypes	Sub types	Geographical distribution
1	1a, 1b	Europe, North America
2	2a, 2b	Western Africa
3	3a–f	South East Asia
4	4a–j	Central Africa
5	5a	South Africa, Asia
6	6a	South East Asia
7	–	Congo (Central Africa)

Risk of transmission

- Vertical transmission is the most common.
- Transmission from mother to child is ~5% but it increases if the mother is co-infected with HIV.
- Risk is negligible if mother is HCV antibody positive but HCV RNA negative.
- Mode of delivery does not affect the risk of transmission unless the mother is co-infected with HIV, when Caesarean section may have a protective role.
- Though HCV RNA can be detected in breast milk and colostrum, breastfeeding does not appear to increase the rate of HCV transmission.
- Other routes of transmission include parenteral, sexual, or blood-product transfusion.

Clinical features

- Incubation period: average 6 weeks, range 2–26 weeks.
- Symptoms: usually asymptomatic, non-specific illness such as fatigue, headache present in 30–40%, 20–30% may develop jaundice.
- Extrahepatic manifestations: membranous glomerulonephritis, autoimmune hepatitis, thyroiditis, polyarteritis nodosa, polymyositis, cryoglobulinaemia.
- Chronic HCV infection is defined by persistence of HCV RNA in serum for >6 months.
- Patients with chronic HCV have intermittent abnormalities of liver enzymes.
- 75% of adults with HCV develop chronic infection with increased lifetime risk of cirrhosis (10–20% after 20 years) and hepatocellular carcinoma (1%).
- Children with transfusion-acquired chronic HCV infection have a higher chance of spontaneous resolution (27–48%) as compared to the vertical transmission (5.6–10%).
- Severe fibrosis leading to cirrhosis is very rare in the paediatric population.

Specific viral tests

- Anti-HCV antibody: positive enzyme-linked immunosorbent assay (ELISA) test confirms exposure to HCV but not persistence of infection; in infancy it can represent transplacental passage of maternal anti-HCV antibodies.
- HCV RNA positivity confirms ongoing infection.
- HCV genotype influences the outcome and duration of the interferon-based treatment regimen, however it will probably not influence the treatment duration or the outcome of the newer direct antiviral agents.

Diagnosis of HCV infection in infants born to HCV +ve mother

Check HCV RNA at 2–3 months of age:
- If HCV RNA −ve, infection is unlikely; confirm by repeating at 6–12 months of age.
- If HCV RNA +ve, most likely the child is infected; confirm by repeating test in 6–12 months.

Management

All children >3 years with chronic HCV infection should be offered treatment. Current approved treatment is interferon-based treatment, however multiple trials of different combinations of directly acting antiviral agents (DAAs) are being carried out in children with chronic HCV infection. In near future, the mainstay of treatment will be DAAs. Children not responding to interferon-based treatment can be offered treatment with DAAs.

Directly acting antiviral agents

- In adults, current recommended treatment regimen is combination of different DAAs.
- Harvoni® (sofosbuvir 400 mg + ledipasvir 90mg): approved by US Food and Drug Administration for children (age 12–17 years) with chronic HCV infection with genotype 1, 4, 5, or 6:
  - Duration: 12 weeks.
  - Side effects: similar to placebo group.
- Sofosbuvir 400mg + ribavirin (15mg/kg in two divided doses, max. total dose 1400mg): approved for treatment of children (age 12–17 years) with chronic HCV infection with genotype 2 and 3.
- Duration:
  - Genotype 2: 12 weeks.
  - Genotype 3: 24 weeks.
  - Side effects: similar to placebo group.
- The newer DAAs are shown in Table 64.2.

Table 64.2 Newer DAAs

NS3/4A protease inhibitors (Drugs ends with … previr)	Grazoprevir
	Paritaprevir
	Simeprevir
	Voxilaprevir
NS5A inhibitors (Drugs ends with … asvir)	Daclatasvir
	Elbasvir
	Ledipasvir
	Ombitasvir
	Velpatasvir
	Pibrentasvir
NS5B RNA-dependent RNA polymerase inhibitors (Drugs ends with … buvir)	
Nucleot(s)ide polymerase inhibitor (NPI)	Sofosbuvir
Non-nucleot(s)ide polymerase inhibitor (NNPI)	Dasabuvir

Interferon-based treatment

- For children <12 years old with chronic HCV infection, combination of pegylated interferon + ribavirin is the recommended treatment with sustained viral clearance in about 50–60% in genotype 1 and 80–100% in genotypes 2 and 3.
- Dose:
  - Pegylated interferon ($100mcg/m^2$) subcutaneously once a week
  - Ribavirin: 15mg/kg in two divided doses (max. 1400mg).
- Duration of treatment:
  - Genotypes 1, 4, 5, 6: 48 weeks (check HCV RNA at 24 weeks, if negative, continue for another 24 weeks).
  - Genotypes 2 and 3, duration is 24 weeks.
- Side effects:
  - Pegylated interferon: neutropenia, thrombocytopenia, hypothyroidism, autoimmune disorder, mood swings, depression, etc.
  - Ribavirin: haemolytic anaemia.
- Good prognostic factors for antiviral treatment are absence of cirrhosis, young age at acquisition, and absence of co-morbidity (HBV and/or HIV).

References and resources

Abdel-Hady M, Bansal S, Davison SM, et al. Treatment of chronic viral hepatitis C in children and adolescents: UK experience. Arch Dis Child 2014;99:505–10.

Sokal E, Nannini P. Hepatitis C virus in children: the global picture. Arch Dis Child 2017;102:672–5.

Bacterial, fungal, and parasitic infections of the liver

Introduction *552*
Bacterial sepsis *554*
Spirochaetal infections *558*
Rickettsial infections *559*
Fungal infections *559*
Parasitic infections *560*
Granulomatous hepatitis *564*

Introduction

Infectious agents can affect the liver either via direct invasion or by release of toxins. The liver's dual blood supply renders it uniquely susceptible to infection, receiving blood from the intestinal tract via the hepatic portal system, and from the systemic circulation via the hepatic artery. Due to this unique perfusion, the liver is frequently exposed to systemic or intestinal infections or the mediators of toxaemia. The biliary tree provides a further conduit for gut bacteria or parasites to access the liver parenchyma.

Infections of the liver with a wide range of organisms present variously from asymptomatic biochemical abnormalities to symptomatic hepatitis, or space-occupying lesions (e.g. abscesses), or granulomata producing biochemical cholestasis but rarely significant jaundice. Some of these infections have a high mortality if not treated promptly.

Bacterial sepsis

There are two main bacterial sepsis-associated clinical manifestations: hypoxic hepatitis and jaundice. The latter is well recognized particularly in neonates and infants in the context of sepsis.

Aetiology and pathological changes

- Liver dysfunction is mainly due to systemic or microcirculatory disturbances, spillovers of bacteria and endotoxin (lipopolysaccharide, LPS), and subsequent activation of inflammatory cytokines as well as mediators.
- A diverse group of organisms are responsible for hepatic dysfunction following bacteraemia:
  - Gram-negative organisms: *Escherichia coli*, *Klebsiella pneumoniae*, *Pseudomonas aeruginosa*, *Proteus* spp., *Paracolon bacteria*, *Bacteroides*, *Salmonella typhi*.
  - *Haemophilus influenzae*.
  - Aerobic and anaerobic streptococci.
  - *Staphylococcus aureus*.
  - *Streptococcus pneumoniae*.

The exact pathogenesis of hepatic insult is not known, but may be multifactorial;

- Direct invasion of liver parenchyma by blood-borne pathogens.
- Non-specific injury secondary to hypoxia, fever, and malnutrition.
- Certain drugs or organisms can cause haemolysis (e.g. *Clostridium perfringens*, or in malaria). It can be precipitated in the presence of underlying cell abnormalities such as glucose-6-phosphate dehydrogenase deficiency.
- Ascending cholangitis is an important cause of jaundice to exclude in the septic patient.
- Endotoxin-induced cholestasis (see Fig. 65.1)

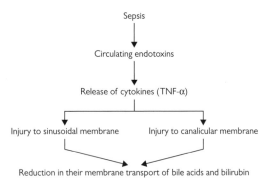

Fig. 65.1 Sepsis-induced cholestasis. TNF-α, tumour necrosis factor alpha.

Laboratory diagnosis and treatment

Clinical evaluation and microbiological investigation may identify the source of sepsis and antimicrobial therapy usually results in complete resolution. Cytology and biopsies should be performed where indicated.

Liver abscess

Pyogenic liver abscess (PLA) in infancy and childhood is rare, with up to 40–50% occurring in immunocompromised children.

- Predisposing factors include immunosuppression, quantitative or qualitative granulocyte abnormalities such as chronic granulomatous disease, trauma, umbilical vein catheterization, omphalitis, sickle cell disease, biliary tract surgery, hepatic artery thrombosis (post-liver transplantation), liver biopsy, percutaneous or endoscopic biliary drainage, diabetes, worm infestation, and protein–energy malnutrition especially in developing countries.
- Pyogenic bacteria can reach the liver through various routes:
  - Portal: secondary to gut pathologies such as appendicitis, IBD.
  - Biliary: caused by extrahepatic biliary tract disease such as stricture, calculus, or malignancy.
  - Blood borne, from an infected focus anywhere in the body.
  - Contiguous extension from gallbladder or perinephric abscess.
  - Following penetrating wounds of liver.
  - Cryptogenic.

PLA may present as a single large lesion or multiple abscesses, the latter often secondary to biliary tract infection.

- Gram-negative aerobes, anaerobes, and microaerophilic streptococci are common cause but *Staphylococcus aureus* is the most common isolate in children with chronic granulomatous disease. Less frequent causes include *Pseudomonas* spp., *Clostridium* spp., *Salmonella typhi*, *Yersinia enterocolitica*, and *Pasteurella*.

Clinical presentation

- The classic presentation is pyrexia, chills, right upper quadrant abdominal pain, hepatomegaly, and leucocytosis, but may be non-specific.
- Unusual presentations include an abdominal mass or acute abdomen secondary to rupture into the peritoneal cavity or portal hypertension secondary to portal pyaemia and portal vein thrombosis.

Diagnosis

- Liver function tests may be unhelpful, with non-specific changes.
- USS, CT, and MRI are all sensitive but cannot always differentiate abscesses from other lesions such as cysts, tumours, or haemorrhage.
- USS- or CT-guided drainage of as much pus as possible (from as many abscesses as possible) confirms diagnosis, and is central to management.
- Contraindications to drainage include ascites and inaccessible lesions.
- Complications of aspiration include haemorrhage, hepatic laceration, fistula formation, peritonitis, and additional abscess formation.
- Indications for open drainage procedure are biliary obstruction, loculated or highly viscous abscesses, persistence of fever for >2 weeks despite percutaneous catheter drainage and appropriate antimicrobial therapy.

Treatment and prognosis
- Aspiration under USS guidance is helpful.
- Initial treatment is conservative with broad-spectrum antibiotics (e.g. cephalosporins plus metronidazole or clindamycin) and should be adjusted when culture results are available. Duration of treatment is usually 3–6 weeks.
- Patients with multiple abscesses have to be on conservative treatment after a diagnostic tap, and up to 3–4 months of antibiotic therapy has been recommended to prevent relapses.
- Prognosis is worse in multiple abscesses.
- Most reports emphasize the good outcome after percutaneous drainage, which should be USS or CT guided.

Cholangitis

The normal biliary tract is sterile and, in children, acute cholangitis rarely occurs in the absence of congenital abnormalities or interventions in the biliary tract.

Aetiology and pathogenesis
The children at highest risk include:
- Those with porto-enterostomy or choledochal cyst, and those who have non-operative biliary manipulations such as transhepatic cholangiography or endoscopic retrograde cholangiography with stent placement.
- Risk of cholangitis in children after Kasai operation is 40–50%.

Diagnosis and treatment
- Clinical diagnosis is based on fever, abdominal pain, jaundice, pale stools, or hepatic tenderness.
- Leucocytosis is common, but changes in liver function tests are non-specific; the serum bilirubin may be normal.
- In recurrent cholangitis liver biopsy may be indicated for confirmation and microbiological examination.
- Treatment requires supportive care and an urgent USS or CT to help establish whether obstruction requires drainage. Broad-spectrum antibiotics should be administered, such as an acylureidopenicillin (piperacillin, mezlocillin, or piperacillin-tazobactam) or late-generation cephalosporin (e.g. ceftazidime), plus an aminoglycoside. Duration of treatment is generally 3 weeks, but prolonged therapy for recurrent cholangitis.

Tuberculosis (TB)

Liver involvement alone by *Mycobacteria* is common in endemic areas. TB of the liver is almost invariably a complication of miliary disease, and occurs in 50% and 75% of patients with pulmonary or extrapulmonary TB respectively. The site of primary focus usually dictates presentation. Rarely the liver appears to be the sole site of infection such as in congenital TB acquired via the placenta.

Brucellosis

Granulomatous hepatitis may occur in acute or chronic disease and manifests as non-specific changes in liver function tests.

Listeriosis

Listeria monocytogenes may cause liver disease as part of systemic intra-uterine infection of the fetus (granulomatosis infantiseptica) at birth or later in the neonatal period and in older immunocompromised children after ingestion of contaminated food or water. The major hepatic manifestation is granuloma; jaundice is rare.

Tularaemia

Francisella tularensis: in some cases a hepatitis-like picture follows with raised aminotransferases. Hepatomegaly is rare and biopsy may show necrosis. Diagnosis is usually serological as the bacterium is difficult to recover in culture. Treatment with streptomycin or gentamicin is effective.

Spirochaetal infections

The spirochaetal infection which affect the liver are:
- Leptospirosis.
- Borreliosis.
- Congenital syphilis.

Leptospirosis

Epidemiology and clinical manifestations
- Human infection follows exposure to leptospires excreted in the urine of chronically infected animals including rats, cattle, and dogs, or water contaminated with urine.
- The incubation period is 5–15 days and in 90% of patients there is a self-limiting anicteric disease but 5–10% develop jaundice (Weil disease).
- Weil disease is characterized by hepatic, renal, and vascular dysfunction with persistent fever, profound jaundice, abdominal pain, renal failure, confusion, epistaxis, haematuria, GI bleeding, and other haemorrhagic phenomena.
- Death may follow cardiovascular collapse, renal failure, and GI or pulmonary haemorrhage, though with supportive therapy mortality should be <10%.

Diagnosis and treatment
- Liver histology and culture; leptospires may be recovered from blood, urine, or cerebrospinal fluid (CSF) during the first week of illness, and from urine thereafter.
- Diagnosis is usually serological, however, PCR can detect leptospiral DNA in blood, serum, CSF, urine, or aqueous humour.
- Penicillin or doxycycline are recommended and most beneficial if started early in the disease.

Borreliosis
- Also known as Lyme disease; caused by *Borrelia burgdorferi*, a tick-borne spirochaete.
- The hepatic involvement is part of systemic disease, abnormal liver function tests are seen in up to 19% of patients, particularly serum transaminases are raised. Rarely there is hepatomegaly and right upper quadrant tenderness.
- Diagnosis is based on clinical suspicion, positive serology, and histopathology.
- In the early stages of disease, amoxicillin for children <9 years and tetracycline for children >9 years of age are the treatments of choice. In late stages of the disease, IV cefotaxime or ceftriaxone are recommended.

Congenital syphilis
- Hepatomegaly is seen in 50–90% of symptomatic infants. Neonatal death is caused by liver failure, severe pneumonia, or pulmonary haemorrhage.
- The diagnosis is made by detecting IgM-specific antibodies and detection of antigen.
- Penicillin is the drug of choice and is risk free in the neonate; alternatively, ceftriaxone can be used.

Rickettsial infections

Q fever

- The causative organism is *Coxiella burnetii*.
- Infection results from inhalation of dust from infected animals, consumption of raw milk, or via transplacental transmission or blood transfusion.

Clinical manifestations

- The incubation period is 1–2 weeks, usual course is self-limiting. There are three major presentations:
  - Atypical pneumonia.
  - Flu-like syndrome.
  - Hepatitis.
- Hepatitis occurs in 3–4% of cases, jaundice in one-third of cases, and fever and hepatomegaly in >70% of cases. The abnormal liver function tests are noted in up to 70–80% of patients. Commonest abnormality of liver function test is an elevation of the alkaline phosphatase.

Diagnosis

- History of contact with an animal host is a vital clue.
- Diagnosis is made by detection of phase I and phase II antibodies of *Coxiella burnetii*.
- Seroconversion usually detected 7–15 days after onset of clinical symptoms; 90% of patients have detectable antibodies by third week.

Treatment

- Doxycycline has been the agent most frequently investigated and currently the treatment of choice.
- Fluoroquinolones can be used as alternative antibiotic agents. Ofloxacin and pefloxacin have been used with success in patients then ciprofloxacin.
- Macrolides, especially azithromycin and clarithromycin, can also be used as alternative agents, but some strains of *Coxiella burnetii* show resistance.
- Trimethoprim-sulfamethoxazole (TMP-SMZ) has also been used
- Macrolides or TMP-SMZ may be options in children <8 years.
- Adjuvant corticosteroid treatment has been used in antimicrobial-nonresponsive hepatitis.

Fungal infections

- Fungal infections of the liver are usually seen in the immunocompromised, including those with acute liver failure.
- Although *Candida albicans* predominates, other *Candida* spp. and *Aspergillus* spp. infections are increasingly reported.
- Other rare fungal infections of the liver include cryptococcosis, mucormycosis, histoplasmosis, blastomycosis, coccidioidomycosis, and paracoccidioidomycosis.

Parasitic infections

Hepatic amoebiasis

- *Entamoeba histolytica* is most commonly encountered in the tropics and subtropics.
- Hepatic abscess is a major complication of invasive amoebiasis and seen in 3–9% of adult cases but is less common in children.
- Amoebic trophozoites reach the liver via the portal vein and induce hepatocyte apoptosis and a leucocyte response, resulting in abscesses containing viscous brown pus.

Clinical manifestations and diagnosis

- The hepatic lesion can manifest as multiple or single.
- Multiple abscesses may be associated with more severe disease.
- The abscess is commonly seen in the right lobe of liver.
- A typical presentation is with pyrexia (75%) and right upper quadrant pain radiating to the right shoulder.
- Tenderness in the hypochondrium (85%), tender hepatomegaly (80%), and localized swelling over the liver (10%) may be elicited.
- Less specific symptoms include nausea, vomiting, concurrent diarrhoea or dysentery (10%), and loss of weight.
- Jaundice is present in up to 8% of cases. The white blood cell count is usually elevated.
- Hepatic abscesses can be demonstrated by USS or CT scanning.
- Demonstrating cysts in stool may contribute to diagnosis, but serum antibodies are present in >95% of patients.
- Aspiration under USS guidance may yield 'anchovy sauce' pus; rarely amoebae are seen in necrotic abscess wall or adjacent parenchyma.

Complications

- Abscesses may rupture in to the peritoneal cavity, pleural cavity or lungs, pericardium, portal vein, or biliary tract, intraperitoneal rupture being more common than intrathoracic.

Treatment

- Extra-intestinal amoebiasis should be treated with metronidazole or dehydroemetine for at least 2 weeks.
- To prevent continued intraluminal infection, a luminal amoebicide, such as paromomycin or diloxanide furoate, should be given.
- Percutaneous needle aspiration along with medical treatment is recommended if the abscess is large (>6cm), or does not respond to medical treatment within 72 hours, if there is imminent risk of abscess rupture.
- Surgical intervention is required in cases complicated with abscess rupture.

Schistosomiasis

Patients present with pyrexia, urticaria, eosinophilia, hepatosplenomegaly, or upper GI tract bleeding from oesophageal varices.

- The diagnosis is made by demonstrating ova in stool and urine and may be identified in liver or rectal mucosal biopsy. Serological tests cannot distinguish past from active infection but a negative ELISA excludes the diagnosis.
- Praziquantel is the drug of choice; oxamniquine an alternative for *Schistosoma mansoni*.

Hydatid disease

- The liver is the most common site for cyst formation and in 60–85% of cases the cyst is located in the right lobe.
- The signs and symptoms of hepatic echinococcosis may include hepatic enlargement, with or without a palpable mass, epigastric pain, nausea, and vomiting.
- Rare presentations secondary to pressure effects or rupture of the cyst include portal hypertension, inferior vena cava compression or thrombosis, secondary biliary cirrhosis, biliary peritonitis, or pyogenic abscess.
- USS of the liver reveals round, solitary or multiple, cysts of variable size with multiple internal daughter cysts; calcification may be noted.
- Diagnosis requires demonstration of specific antibody.
- The primary treatment is surgical removal of the cysts. Both mebendazole and albendazole can cross the cyst wall and have the potential to treat small uncomplicated cysts.

Ascariasis

- Rarely ascariasis can invade the biliary tree and cause biliary obstruction.
- Ultrasonography may show worms in the common duct, or abscess formation may be noticed. ERCP shows the adult worms as a filling defect or a worm protruding through the papilla.
- Treatment is with anthelmintic drugs, but endoscopic removal of the worm may be necessary in patients with persisting biliary symptoms.

Toxocariasis

- Hepatosplenomegaly, lymphadenopathy, or pruritic skin lesions may be present.
- Serodiagnosis is available by the ELISA technique.
- The treatment is tiabendazole 50mg/kg per day in two divided doses for 5 days.

Liver flukes (*Fasciola hepatica*)

- Hepatic invasion is by penetration of the hepatic capsule by metacercariae which migrate through liver parenchyma and enter bile ducts causing cholangitis and hepatomegaly.
- The diagnosis is made by demonstrating ova in stool and on the basis of positive serology.
- ERCP shows filling defects due to the inflammatory response; worms can also be aspirated.

Clonorchis sinensis infection

- *Clonorchis sinensis* is a flat worm which inhabits the biliary tree.
- Cysts from infected fish are ingested and migrate from the duodenum into the bile ducts. Ova are excreted from the stools.
- The intermediate host is a snail, which completes the life cycle by infecting fish.
- Humans are infected by eating raw fish.
- The biliary epithelium becomes inflamed from constant irritation, leading to cholangitis, ductal fibrosis, stricturing, and stone formation.

Clinical manifestations and diagnosis

- The classic symptoms are recurrent pyogenic cholangitis.
- There are recurrent attacks of right upper quadrant pain, jaundice, and pyrexia.
- Examination may reveal tender hepatomegaly and splenomegaly if portal hypertension exists.
- Imaging of the biliary tree by MRI or ERCP is essential to delineate the distribution of stones and strictures. Ova are demonstrated in faeces or duodenal aspirate.

Treatment

- The drug of choice is praziquantel. Surgery is indicated if stones or strictures are present.

Toxoplasmosis

Congenital toxoplasmosis

- Severely infected neonates present with cholestasis, purpura, and hepatosplenomegaly.
- Other associated symptoms and signs can be hydrocephalus, retinochoroiditis, intracranial calcification, and hydrops fetalis.
- The diagnosis of acute infection in the newborn is made on the basis of presence of IgA and IgM antibodies from peripheral blood of newborn. *Toxoplasma gondii*-specific DNA is detected in body fluids (blood, urine, and CSF) by using PCR. Histologically, liver biopsy shows giant cell hepatitis and extramedullary haematopoiesis.
- Pyrimethamine plus sulfadiazine twice daily plus folinic acid supplement for 3 weeks, alternating with spiramycin daily in two divided doses for 3 weeks. Continue the alternating therapy for 1 year.

Granulomatous hepatitis

Common infectious causes of granuloma in liver
- Bacterial causes:
  - Tuberculosis.
  - Brucellosis.
  - Listeriosis.
  - Yersiniosis.
  - *Mycobacterium avium intracellulare.*
  - BCG infection.
  - Tularaemia.
  - Rickettsia.
  - Q fever.
  - Chlamydia.
  - Psittacosis.
  - Cat scratch disease due to *Bartonella.*
- Fungal infections:
  - Histoplasmosis.
  - Nocardiosis.
  - Blastomycosis.
  - Coccidioidomycosis.
  - Candidiasis.
- Parasitic infections:
  - Schistosomiasis.
  - Visceral larva migrans.
  - Visceral leishmaniasis.
  - Toxoplasmosis.

Liver tumours

Introduction 566
Infantile haemangiomata 566
Mesenchymal hamartoma 567
Focal nodular hyperplasia 567
Nodular regenerative hyperplasia 567
Hepatoblastoma 568
Hepatocellular carcinoma 568
References and resources 568

Introduction

Liver tumours in children are rare, accounting for 0.5–2% of all neoplasms in the paediatric age group.

Infantile haemangiomata

- Benign vascular tumour.
- Occurs almost exclusively in the first year of life.
- Relatively common in the skin and mucous membranes but can affect any organ system.
- In the liver, two histological types of lesions have been described:
  - Capillary haemangioma (or haemangioendothelioma).
  - Cavernous haemangioma.
- Presenting features are hepatomegaly and abdominal distension.
- Involvement can be as a single tumour or multifocal.
- Complications include high-output cardiac failure, often life-threatening, due to the presence of significant shunting; Kasabach–Merrit syndrome (anaemia, consumptive coagulopathy, cholestasis); vascular malformation involving other organs, and rarely intraperitoneal haemorrhage secondary to rupture. Hypothyroidism can occur associated with increased activity of type 3 iodothyronine deiodinase within the tumour.
- Diagnosis is made on imaging including USS with Doppler, CT, and MRI. Needle liver biopsy is contraindicated because of the high risk of bleeding. Liver tissue can be obtained at laparotomy in selected cases, when malignancy cannot be excluded on imaging.

Management

- Asymptomatic: does not warrant treatment because of the spontaneous resolution of the lesion over time.
- Symptomatic: depends on its severity.
- Medical treatment consists of symptomatic treatment of high-output cardiac failure with digoxin or angiotensin-converting enzyme inhibitors and diuretics.
- Treatment with beta blockers (propranolol) has been shown to promote the involution of the lesions and is well tolerated. Other treatments such as corticosteroids, interferon, and chemotherapy with vincristine have also been used.
- Surgical management includes resection of the lesion by hepatic lobectomy or hepatic artery ligation, depending on the size and localization of the lesion.
- Liver transplantation should be reserved for cases that do not respond to any of the above-listed treatment options.

Mesenchymal hamartoma

- Rare benign tumour.
- Multicystic appearance.
- Typically affects children during the first 2 years of life.
- Presentation can be with symptoms of abdominal distension but is often an incidental finding on clinical examination or imaging and is rarely symptomatic.
- Biochemically, AFP can be mildly raised, liver function tests usually normal.
- Imaging with USS, CT, and MRI.
- Final diagnosis is made on the basis of histology, usually obtained at the time of resection. Spontaneous regression has been described.

Focal nodular hyperplasia

- Benign epithelial tumour is considered to be a hyperplastic response to increased blood flow in normal liver.
- The lesion, typically well circumscribed and lobulated, can vary in size and be single or multiple. On imaging, a central scar can be seen.
- The presence of an underlying porto-systemic shunt (Abernethy malformation) needs to be excluded.
- Seen in all age groups, more common in females, has been reported in older patients with glycogen storage disease type 1.
- Associations with other vascular abnormalities including cardiac have been reported.
- Presentation with abdominal pain is common.
- Imaging with USS including contrast US, CT, and MRI are usually diagnostic.
- Management strategies:
  - Closure of the porto-systemic shunt needs to be considered either by interventional radiology or surgery.
  - In isolated focal nodular hyperplasia, conservative management with regular clinical and radiological follow-up or surgical excision of the mass should be considered.
- Beta-catenin mutations in the tumour have been associated with malignant transformation in which case liver transplantation might be considered.

Nodular regenerative hyperplasia

- Rare in paediatric age group.
- Usually asymptomatic; hepatosplenomegaly is detected fortuitously.
- CT and MRI usually suggest the diagnosis.
- Can involve the whole liver and lead to portal hypertension and its complications.
- Treatment is management of the complications.

Hepatoblastoma

- Embryonic tumour derived from the epithelial cells of the fetal liver and characterized by a rapid growth.
- Most frequent malignant liver tumour in children, most commonly diagnosed in the first 3 years of life.
- Male preponderance.
- Association with genetic cancer syndromes, prematurity and very low-birth-weight children
- Spreads by vascular invasion, typically in the lungs.
- Presentation usually with abdominal distension, abdominal pain, and faltering growth.
- Anaemia and thrombocytosis are common; very high AFP levels are characteristic and are a marker of response to therapy.
- CT or MRI is necessary for an accurate differentiation between tumour and normal liver tissue. PRETEXT classification is used.
- Liver histology can contribute to the diagnosis.
- Treatment consists of chemotherapy and complete tumour resection by partial hepatectomy or, if the tumour is unresectable, by liver transplantation.
- Adverse prognostic factors are low serum AFP (<100ng/mL), lack of response to chemotherapy, and presence of metastases at diagnosis.

Hepatocellular carcinoma

- Rare in paediatric age group, but when present, is typically seen in older children/teenagers.
- Most commonly, hepatocellular carcinoma develops in the presence of an underlying liver disease such as chronic viral hepatitis (e.g. hepatitis B) or a metabolic disorder (e.g. tyrosinaemia or progressive familial intrahepatic cholestasis syndromes).
- Typical presentation is with abdominal pain and an abdominal mass.
- AFP is often elevated, though not as much as in hepatoblastoma.
- CT and MRI can help to determine whether tumour resection is an option.
- Liver biopsy under USS guidance is indicated if no underlying liver pathology is present.
- Treatment consists of resection or liver transplantation, ± chemotherapy, but the prognosis is poor, particularly for those with metastatic disease and the fibrolamellar variant.

References and resources

Aronson DC, Meyers RL. Malignant tumors of the liver in children. Semin Pediatr Surg 2016;25:265–75.

Avagyan S, Klein M, Kerkar N, et al. Propranolol as a first-line treatment for diffuse infantile hepatic hemangioendothelioma. J Pediatr Gastroenterol Nutr 2013;56:e17–20.

Hadzic N, Finegold MJ. Liver neoplasia in children. Clin Liver Dis 2011;15:443–62.

Sorkin T, Strautnieks S, Foskett P, et al. Multiple β-catenin mutations in hepatocellular lesions arising in Abernethy malformation. Hum Pathol 2016;53:153–8.

Complications of chronic liver disease

Cirrhosis 570
Growth failure and malnutrition 571
Hepatic encephalopathy 572
Coagulopathy 574
Portal hypertension and variceal bleeding 574
Ascites 575
Spontaneous bacterial peritonitis 576
Hepatorenal syndrome 577
Pulmonary complications 578
Cirrhotic cardiomyopathy 580
Pruritus 580
Hepatic osteodystrophy 581
Endocrine dysfunction 582
Hepatocellular carcinoma 582

Cirrhosis

Definition

Cirrhosis is a histopathological term used to describe microscopic and/or macroscopic changes in liver characterized by aberrant nodule formation, vascular changes, and totally disturbed architecture associated with fibrosis. It is an end result of progressive fibrosis irrespective of the insult to the parenchyma or biliary tree.

The complications of chronic liver disease and cirrhosis are a consequence of the impaired metabolic and synthetic function and structural alteration of the parenchyma leading to elevated portal pressure (see Box 67.1).

Box 67.1 Complications of cirrhosis in children

- Growth faltering and malnutrition.
- Hepatic encephalopathy.
- Coagulopathy.
- Hepatopulmonary syndrome.
- Portal hypertension and variceal bleeding.
- Ascites.
- Spontaneous bacterial peritonitis.
- Hepatorenal syndrome.
- Pruritus.
- Hepatic osteodystrophy.
- Cirrhotic cardiomyopathy.
- Endocrine dysfunction.
- Hepatocellular carcinoma.

Growth failure and malnutrition

Epidemiology

- Can occur in 50–80% of children with chronic liver disease.

Pathophysiology

There are combined disturbances of intake (anorexia), absorption, metabolism of nutrients, and increased energy expenditure.

- *Fat malabsorption* particularly of the long-chain triglycerides and polyunsaturated fatty acids may also impair absorption of fat-soluble vitamins by up to 50%, although 95% of water-soluble lipids (medium-chain triglycerides) are absorbed. In cholestatic liver disease it is due to reduced delivery of bile salts to the small bowel. Pancreatic exocrine function may also be affected. Hypercholesterolaemia and hypertriglyceridaemia are common as a result of altered lipoprotein synthesis and cholesterol excretion.
- *Carbohydrate metabolism* is abnormal due to peripheral insulin resistance, hyperinsulinaemia, and reduced hepatic glycogen stores.
- *Protein synthesis* is impaired as liver plays a key role in the synthesis of albumin, transferrin, and clotting factors. The metabolism of aromatic amino acids is affected, leading to imbalance of branched-chain amino acids and aromatic amino acids. Inadequate detoxification of nitrogenous waste via urea cycle leads to rise in blood ammonia levels. There is also a resultant increase in muscle protein degradation causing a relatively reduced muscle mass despite nutritional support.
- *Impaired growth hormone (GH)–insulin-like growth factor (IGF)-1 axis* occurs as significant proportion of IGF-1 and insulin-like growth factor binding protein (IGFBP) are synthesized in the liver.
- Increased nutritional requirement up to 140% of normal due to increased resting energy expenditure (REE) and total energy expenditure (TEE).
- *Trace elements* may also be deficient as a result of reduced intake and increased losses.

Clinical features

- Severe deficiency of fat-soluble vitamins may produce clinical signs and symptoms. Increased bruising, epistaxis, coagulopathy due to vitamin K deficiency; osteopenia, rickets and fractures due to vitamin D deficiency; less commonly xerophthalmia and night blindness due to vitamin A deficiency; and peripheral neuropathy, ophthalmoplegia, and haemolysis due to vitamin E deficiency.
- Essential fatty acid deficiency may manifest as desquamation, thrombocytopenia, and poor wound healing.
- Mineral deficiencies may occur (in particular anaemia due to iron deficiency and acrodermatitis due to zinc deficiency).
- In later stages of the disease, protein–energy malnutrition manifests with muscle wasting, stunting, peripheral oedema, and motor developmental delay.

Nutritional assessment and management

See Chapter 68.

Hepatic encephalopathy

Definition
This is defined as a metabolically induced, potentially reversible, functional disturbance of the brain that may occur in acute or chronic liver disease. It is difficult to recognize in children.

Pathophysiology
Precise mechanisms are still not defined.
- Porto-systemic shunting leads to increased blood concentrations of nitrogenous by-products, which are implicated in the alteration of CNS function.
- Hepatocellular dysfunction with poor clearance of nitrogenous metabolites from the intestine.
- Nitrogen metabolites and short-chain fatty acids absorbed from the intestine have been implicated in directly altering CNS function.
- Altered neurotransmitter function leading to imbalance of excitatory and inhibitory functions in particular of the glutamine–nitric oxide system.
- Other proposed mechanisms are increase in false neurotransmitters (octopamine, phenyl methionine), altered ratios of branched chain amino acids and aromatic amino acids, changes in postsynaptic receptor activity, increased permeability of blood brain barrier etc.

Diagnosis
- Requires high index of suspicion and appropriate clinical assessment.
- Hepatic encephalopathy can be clinically graded using the West Haven criteria (see Table 67.1) and conscious level is graded using the Glasgow coma scale.
- Commonest symptoms are irritability and lethargy; subtle presentation may be with neurodevelopmental delay, school problems, sleep pattern reversal, personality changes, delayed reaction times, impaired computation and concentration. Late signs are clouding of consciousness leading to stupor and coma.
- Signs that may be elicited particularly in older children are tremors, incoordination, and asterixis.
- Neuroimaging and electrophysiological studies of brain would give supportive evidence rather than to confirm the diagnosis of hepatic encephalopathy.
- Arterial ammonia concentrations are difficult to interpret in isolation especially in children; serial monitoring may, however, be used as guide to the effectiveness of treatment.
- It is very important to rule out other causes such as infection (encephalitis), hypoglycaemia, acidosis, drug toxicity, and metabolic insults.

Table 67.1 West Haven criteria for grading of mental state

Grade 0	Normal
Grade 1	Euphoria or anxiety
	Impaired performance of addition
	Trivial lack of awareness
	Inverted sleep pattern
Grade 2	Subtle personality change
	Minimal disorientation for time or place
	Impaired performance of subtraction
	Lethargy or slow response
	Tremor and hypoactive reflexes.
Grade 3	Somnolence to semi stupor, but responds to verbal stimuli
	Confusion, gross disorientation
	Inappropriate behaviour
	Brisk reflexes and Babinski's sign
	Muscle rigidity
Grade 4	Deep coma (unresponsive to verbal or noxious stimuli)

Reprinted from Ferenci P. et al. (2002) Hepatic encephalopathy--definition, nomenclature, diagnosis, and quantification: final report of the working party at the 11th World Congresses of Gastroenterology, Vienna, 1998 Hepatology 35(3):716–21 with permission from Wiley.

Treatment
- Identify and treat precipitating factors.
- Lactulose only to achieve 2–3 semi-formed stools per day.
- Rifaximin (gut decontamination) and lactulose given together was found to be more beneficial.
- Branched-chain amino acid enriched nutritional supplements (L-ornithine L-aspartate) have been used but without proven benefit.
- Infants have to be supplemented with 3–4g/kg/day and children with 2g/kg/day of proteins. Protein restriction to 1g/kg/day only in case of encephalopathy.
- Liver transplantation.

Coagulopathy

Definition
Increased risk of bleeding in chronic liver disease due to development of specific disorders of coagulation characterized by prolonged PT, INR, and reduced platelets.

Pathophysiology
- Vitamin K malabsorption leading to deficiency.
- Reduced synthesis of coagulation factors particularly II, VII, IX, X, proteins C and S, and inhibitors of coagulation.
- Thrombocytopenia may occur secondary to portal hypertension, hypersplenism, and immunological destruction; platelet aggregation is also defective.
- Dysfibrinogenemia due to increase in levels of D-dimers and fibrin degradation products.

Diagnosis
- May present as epistaxis, GI bleeding, or bruising.
- Check platelet count, coagulation screen including INR, fibrin degradation products, and D-dimers. NB Fibrinogen concentrations may be normal.
- Therapeutic administration of vitamin K distinguishes vitamin K deficiency from synthetic failure of the liver.

Management
- Vitamin K supplement oral or IV given as 1mg/year of age or maximum of 5mg/day.
- In general, a dose of 10mL/kg of FFP and cryoprecipitate at a dose of 5mL/kg if fibrinogen <100mg/dL is given in case of bleeding episodes or invasive.
- Platelet transfusion if platelet count is 10,000–20,000/mm³ is reached or there is bleeding with platelet count <50,000/mm³. A platelet count of 50,000–70,000/mm³ is usually considered adequate when an invasive procedure is to be performed.
- Persistent severe coagulation disturbances may require factor VII concentrate infusions (40mcg/kg) and desmopressin.
- Evaluate for associated sepsis as it can case thrombocytopenia and worsening of coagulopathy.
- Evaluate for associated sepsis as it can case thrombocytopenia and worsening of coagulopathy.

Portal hypertension and variceal bleeding

See Chapter 70.

Ascites

Definition

Accumulation of fluid in the abdominal cavity in a child with liver disease usually indicates worsening portal hypertension and hepatic insufficiency.

It is a common major complication of decompensated cirrhosis. Onset may be insidious or precipitated by events such as GI bleeding, and infections. Ascites increases the risk of bacterial peritonitis and hepatorenal syndrome, which potentially adds on to the already increased mortality associated with liver decompensation.

Pathophysiology

The factors involved are increased portal venous pressure and decreased plasma oncotic pressure secondary to hypoalbuminemia.

Diagnosis

- Clinical features include distended abdomen, bulging flanks, protrusion of umbilicus, and development of inguinal hernias and hydrocele; percussion of fluid level and shifting dullness may be elicited.
- USS is more sensitive and can detect small volumes of ascites or be employed when clinical examination is difficult.
- Abdominal paracentesis is a rapid and relatively safe procedure with added advantage of ruling out spontaneous bacterial peritonitis.

Management

- Nutritional support.
- Dietary restriction of sodium should be considered.
- Spironolactone at 2–3mg/kg per day to 7mg/kg per day.
- If there is inadequate response, furosemide can be added; chorothiazide is a preferred agent for long-term use.
- Dual therapy at drug dosage ratio of 2(furosemide): 5(spironolactone) has optimal synergistic effect.
- If the ascites is still resistant consider 20% human albumin infusion over 3–4 hours with furosemide cover.
- Monitor weight, serum electrolytes, urea, and creatinine closely. If significant hyponatraemia occurs, consider stopping diuretics and fluid restrict cautiously (50–75% of requirement).
- Therapeutic paracentesis should be considered in resistant ascites especially if compromising respiratory function. Concurrent infusion of albumin is recommended; replace 10% of the removed ascitic fluid volume with 20% albumin IV.
- Surgical intervention apart from liver transplantation is rarely necessary but may include LeVeen shunt (peritoneal to jugular) and transjugular intrahepatic portosystemic shunt (TIPS).

Spontaneous bacterial peritonitis

Definition

Bacterial infection of ascitic fluid in the absence of secondary causes such as bowel perforation or intra-abdominal abscess.

Clinical features

These may be subtle, with fever and irritability.

Diagnosis

- High index of suspicion in a child with ascites and non-specific deterioration is required.
- Abdominal paracentesis and ascitic fluid microscopy and culture is essential. Presence of polymorphonuclear cells >250/mm^3 is diagnostic and usually the infection is mono-microbial.

Treatment

- IV antibiotics, usually third-generation cephalosporins, are the first choice but should be guided by the microbiologist and the culture yield. The duration of treatment is 5–7 days.
- Prophylaxis could be given in the form of cyclical antibiotics
- Recurrent episodes of spontaneous bacterial peritonitis should lead to consideration for liver transplantation.

Hepatorenal syndrome

Definition
Hepatorenal syndrome is a progressive, reversible, functional renal impairment that occurs in patients with advanced liver cirrhosis.

Epidemiology
It occurs in up to 10% of adults with chronic liver disease; mortality rate is 70% without liver transplantation. It is much less common in children and usually associated with refractory ascites.

Pathophysiology
Characterized by intense renal vasoconstriction with coexistent systemic vasodilatation, thereby reducing the renal blood flow despite increased cardiac output and fall in blood pressure.

Diagnosis
- Exclusion of all other potential causes of renal impairment especially hypovolaemia, shock, nephrotoxic drugs, and kidney disease.
- Hereditary tyrosinaemia, Alagille syndrome, and polycystic liver kidney disease are conditions where chronic liver disease and kidney disease occur concomitantly.
- Urine sodium <10 and urine:plasma creatinine ratio <10 help rule out acute tubular necrosis or glomerular disease.
- Glomerular filtration rate is markedly reduced.

Treatment
- Systemic vasoconstrictors including vasopressin analogues (terlipressin and ornipressin), somatostatin analogue (octreotide), and alpha-adrenergic agonists (midodrine and norepinephrine) are helpful in managing hepatorenal syndrome.
- Terlipressin when used alone or with albumin has higher efficacy in reversing the renal function.
- Renal replacement therapy is indicated in failed medical management.
- Liver transplantation usually reverses the condition.

Pulmonary complications

Hepatopulmonary syndrome (HPS)

Definition
The diagnostic criteria for HPS is presence of chronic liver disease along with PaO_2 <70mmHg or alveolar-arterial oxygen gradient >15mmHg and intrapulmonary vascular dilatation.

Epidemiology
The prevalence varies from 0.5% to 20% in adults; a similar prevalence may be expected in children.

Pathophysiology
- Multifactorial with development of intrapulmonary shunts, arteriovenous shunts, V/Q mismatch, and portopulmonary venous anastomosis.
- Extensive dilatation of pre-capillary circulation resulting in V/Q mismatch may be responsible for the milder disease where PaO_2 can be increased with administration of 100% oxygen.
- CT pulmonary angiography could reveal two types of vascular pattern, diffuse (type 1) and focal (type 2). Type 2 has poor reversibility after liver transplantation.

Diagnosis
- Requires high index of suspicion.
- Cyanosis, digital clubbing with or without spider naevi is suggestive. Typically, there may be dyspnoea on standing, improving on lying down (platypnoea) with associated change in PaO_2 (orthodeoxia).
- Suggested diagnostic criteria are (1) presence of chronic liver disease; (2) absence of intrinsic cardiopulmonary disease; (3) pulmonary gas exchange abnormalities; (4) evidence of intrapulmonary vascular shunting.
- Contrast-enhanced echocardiography is the preferred screening test for HPS; technetium-99m macroaggregated albumin (Tc-99m MAA) lung perfusion scan is used to confirm the shunt.

Management
Definitive treatment is by timely liver transplantation. Brain uptake of >5% tracer on Tc-99m MAA is considered to be positive and early liver transplantation should be considered.

Portopulmonary hypertension (PoPH)

Definition
PoPH is defined as presence of mean pulmonary artery pressure (MPAP) >25mmHg along with pulmonary vascular resistance (PVR) >240 dynes.s.cm^{-5} with normal capillary wedge pressure (PCWP) <15mmHg, in the presence of portal hypertension.

Prevalence in children is unknown.

Pathophysiology
Concentric medial hypertrophy with intimal fibrosis in the pulmonary arteries is the hallmark.

Diagnosis
- ECG may show right ventricular hypertrophy, right axis deviation, and right bundle branch block.
- Cardiac catheterization of right heart is essential for diagnosis.

Treatment
- No treatment guideline is available for children.
- Vasodilators such as nitric oxide and calcium channel blockers have been tried in adults.
- Mild to moderate PoPH frequently resolves after liver transplantation while severe uncontrolled PoPH is a contraindication for liver transplantation

Cirrhotic cardiomyopathy

Cardiac dysfunction in chronic liver disease as a discrete phenomenon is called cirrhotic cardiomyopathy:

- All or some these changes can be present:
  - Systolic and/or diastolic dysfunction.
  - Baseline increased cardiac output but blunted response to stimuli.
  - Absence of overt left ventricular failure at rest.
  - Electrophysiological abnormalities including prolonged QT interval on ECG and chronotropic incompetence.
- Liver transplantation remains the only curative therapy in most of the patients.

Pruritus

Definition

A complication of cholestatic liver disease (in particular PFIC); when intense, may affect sleep, feeding, and behaviour.

Management

(See also Chapter 57.)

- Antihistamines are used as first line but are usually ineffective.
- Ursodeoxycholic acid (10mg/kg twice daily) may help by improving bile flow.
- Phenobarbital (15–45mg/day) and colestyramine (one-third to one sachet three times daily) are helpful.
- Rifampicin (4–10mg/kg/day) may improve bile flow.
- Naltrexone (0.1–0.5mg/kg).
- Ondansetron (0.1mg/kg/three times daily—max. 4mg/dose), plasmapheresis, may be used if itching is very intense.
- Partial biliary diversion has been found to be helpful in some children.
- Uncontrollable pruritus with poor quality of life is an indication for liver transplantation.

Hepatic osteodystrophy

Definition
Bone disease with both the components of osteoporosis and osteomalacia in chronic liver disease is termed hepatic osteodystrophy (HO).

Epidemiology
The reported prevalence of fractures due to HO in children is ~10–13%.

Pathophysiology
- Aetiology is still unclear.
- Trabecular bone loss occurs to a much greater degree than cortical bone loss.
- Potential factors directly or indirectly associated are IGF-1 deficiency, hyperbilirubinaemia, hypogonadism (especially adults and adolescents), subnormal levels of vitamin D, and immunosuppressive and corticosteroid therapy.
- In general, the degree of osteopenia correlates with severity of liver disease.

Diagnosis
- Often diagnosed when present with atraumatic fractures and on screening.
- DXA scan to measure bone mass.
- Plain radiographs if there is a suspicion of fracture.

Management
- General measures: avoid long-term use of corticosteroids and loop diuretics; encourage regular weight-bearing exercises.
- Nutritional therapy: early calcium supplementation in particular, together with vitamin D (at a dose of three to ten times the recommended daily allowance), may be useful.
- Hormone replacement therapy may be tried in adolescents especially with delayed puberty under guidance of a paediatric endocrinologist.
- Bisphosphonate therapy is indicated only in the presence of low-impact fractures (≥1 vertebral, or ≥1 lower limb, or ≥2 upper limb) along with low bone mineral density.
- Calcitonin and sodium fluoride have been tried in adults with some benefit.

Endocrine dysfunction

Definition

The regulation and function of multiple endocrine systems is affected in chronic liver disease. These are more frequent and more severe with progression of liver disease and development of portal hypertension.

Pathophysiology

- Although there is an increased secretion of GH, there is reduced synthesis of IGF-1 and IGFBP-3 in the liver. There may therefore be increased GH resistance leading to poor growth and wasting.
- *Feminization and hypogonadism* in males has been studied in adults. There is impairment of hypothalamic–pituitary regulation of testicular function with decrease in serum testosterone and relative increase in oestrone and oestradiol.
- *Hypothyroidism* occurs with increase in thyroxine-binding globulin(TBG) and total T_4 but reduced free T_3 and T_4.
- *Renin–angiotensin–aldosterone* activation occurs due to activation of the hepatorenal reflex contributing to the hepatorenal syndrome.
- Increased *peripheral insulin resistance* has been described leading to glucose intolerance.

Diagnosis

- In adolescent boys, the clinical features may include loss of muscle mass, testicular atrophy, palmar erythema, and spider naevi. Adolescent girls may have amenorrhoea or menstrual irregularities. The features of hypothyroidism may be non-specific.
- Total testosterone and free testosterone and oestrogen levels along with LH and FSH levels may be helpful in older adolescents but are difficult to interpret in early puberty.
- Low free T_3 and high TSH suggest hypothyroidism; when there is uncertainty in diagnosis a thyroid-releasing hormone stimulation test may be required.

Management

- Hypothyroidism is treated with levothyroxine; monitoring of treatment should be based on clinical response and free T_4 and TSH levels.
- There is minimal data on treatment of feminization and hypogonadism in children and adolescents.
- The long-term effects of liver transplant on recovery of endocrine dysfunction are not fully defined.

Hepatocellular carcinoma

See Chapter 66.

Nutritional management of liver disease

Chronic liver disease 584
Causes of malnutrition 585
Nutritional management of chronic liver disease 586
Nutritional assessment and monitoring 590
Methods of feeding 591
Acute liver failure 592
Liver transplantation 596
Nutritional management of common liver conditions 598

Chronic liver disease

- Malnutrition is common and is associated with increased morbidity and mortality.
- Strategies centred on managing symptoms such as malabsorption and reversing malnutrition.
- Optimizing nutrition may prevent further damage to the liver and improve outcomes.

Causes of malnutrition

Malabsorption
- Absent or reduced bile flow causing malabsorption of long-chain fat.
- Bile salt deficiency.
- Pancreatic insufficiency.
- Inflammation and small bowel mucosal oedema due to portal hypertension causing protein malabsorption.

Altered metabolism
- Inefficient use of available substrates.
- Reduced glycogen storage.
- Impaired gluconeogenesis.
- Increased fat and protein oxidation to meet energy requirements.

Decreased nutritional intake
- Pruritus.
- Taste changes due to medications.
- Nausea and vomiting.
- Unpalatable diet.
- Early satiety and discomfort due to ascites or organomegaly.
- Fluid restriction due to ascites.

Increased energy expenditure
- Catabolic stresses such as infection.
- Increased respiratory effort due to organomegaly or ascites.
- Reduced body fat and increased proportion of cells which are metabolically active.

Nutritional management of chronic liver disease

Managing malabsorption

- Energy-dense diet with medium-chain triglycerides (MCTs).
- Give feed with 50% of the fat as MCTs (Table 68.1).
- Hydrolysed protein if inflammation and mucosal oedema in small bowel.
- Pancreatic enzymes if low stool elastase indicates pancreatic insufficiency.
- Supplement fat-soluble vitamins (Table 68.2):
  - Supplementation required by all infants and children with cholestatic liver disease.
  - These are starting doses and should be adjusted according to serum levels.
  - Intramuscular injections may be required.

Table 68.1 MCT formulas and feeds

Feed per 100mL	Age (years)	Standard dilution (%)	Energy (kcal)	Protein (g)	Na (mmol)	MCT (%)	Supplemented with BCAA
Pepti Junior®	0–1	12.8	67	1.8	0.9	50	No
Pregestimil®	0–1	13.5	68	1.9	1.26	54	No
Monogen®	0–1	17.5	74	2	1.5	80	No
Lipistart®	0–1	15%	69	2.1	1.7	80	No
Infatrini Peptisorb®	0–1.5	n/a	100	2.6	1.4	50	No
Heparon Junior®	0–3	18	86.4	2	0.56	49	Yes
Peptamen Junior®	1–6	22	100	3	2.9	60	No
Paediasure Peptide®	1–6	n/a	100	3	3.04	50	No
Nutrini Peptisorb®	1–6	n/a	100	2.8	2.6	46	No
Peptamen AF®	>3	n/a	152	9.4	4.35	50	No
Peptamen HN®	>5	n/a	133	6.6	3.91	70	No
Nutrison MCT®	>6	n/a	100	5	4.3	60	No
Vital 1.5®	> 6	n/a	150	6.75	7.35	64	No

BCAA, branched-chain amino acids.

Table 68.2 Fat-soluble vitamin supplementation

Vitamins	Infants	Children > year
A and D	Abidec® or Dalivit® 0.6mL per day May have additional oral or intra-muscular vitamin D	Abidec® or Dalivit® 1.2mL per day Forceval® 1 capsule per day (if >12 years of age) May have additional oral or intra-muscular vitamin D
E	10mg/kg (up to maximum starting dose of 100mg per day)	100mg/day
K	1mg/day	2mg up to 10mg/day

Managing changes in metabolism

- Avoid periods of fasting.
- IV glucose during periods of fasting or illness.
- Frequent meals or feeds or continuous feeding via pump.
- Supplement with branched-chain amino acids (valine, leucine and isoleucine).
- Starchy carbohydrates and bed time snacks in older children.

Increasing nutrient intake

- Increase concentration of powdered feeds, usually in 2% increments:
  - Adjust concentration cautiously with dietetic guidance to avoid overnutrition, excessive renal solute load, osmolality and error when making up feeds.
- Tube feeding:
  - Bolus feeds.
  - Continuous feeds may be preferable if there is organomegaly, ascites, or hypoglycaemia.
- High-energy, low-volume feeds:
  - Orally or via feeding tube.
  - Not all feeds provide complete nutrition e.g. fat, micronutrients.
  - High-energy sip and tube feeds (Table 68.3).
- Nutrient-dense meals and snacks:
  - Include high-protein and high-energy foods.
  - Fat should not be restricted unless there is evidence of steatorrhoea.
  - Add high-energy products such as cheese, butter, oil, and cream.
  - Energy modules added to foods and drinks.
  - Glucose polymers, fats or a combination of both (Table 68.4).
  - Add in 1% increments and increase daily with tolerance.
  - Adding non-protein energy can affect overall balance of diet.
  - Maintain protein:energy ratio of 7.5–12% for infants and 5–15% for older children.

Managing increase in energy expenditure
- Infants:
  - 120–150kcal/kg.
  - 3–4g/kg protein.
- Older children:
  - 120–160% of the estimated average requirement for age.
  - 3–4g/kg protein.

Table 68.3 High-energy sip and tube feeds

Feed per 100mL	Age (years)	Weight (kg)	Complete nutrition?	Energy (kcal)	Protein (g)	Fat (g)
Infatrini®	0–1.5	<9	Yes	100	2.6	5.4
Paediasure Plus®	1–6	8–30	Yes	150	4.2	7.47
Paediasure Plus Juce®	1–6	8–30	No	150	4.2	0
Scandishake®	>6	n/a	No	200	4	10.1
Fortijuce®	>3	n/a	No	150	4	0
Fortini®	1–6	8–20	Yes	150	3.4	6.8
Frebini Energy®	1–10	8–30	Yes	150	3.75	6.67
Resource Junior®	1–10	>8	Yes	150	3	6.2
Nutrini Energy®	1–6	8–20	Yes	150	4	6.7
Nutrison Energy®	>6	n/a	Yes	150	6	5.8

Nutritional assessment and monitoring

The nutritional assessment and monitoring of patients with liver disease is vital, in order to calculate requirements as well as to see how the patient is progressing. This should be done at regular intervals.

Nutritional assessment

- Feeding history, nutritional intake, estimated requirements, clinical condition.

Biochemistry

- Plasma concentrations of vitamins A, D, and E.
- Levels of, e.g. albumin, reflect the synthesis within the liver and thus liver function rather than nutritional status.

Anthropometry/growth

Weights, lengths, heights, and head circumference should all be plotted on age- and gender-appropriate growth charts up to the age of 18 years:
- Height/length:
  - Marker of long-term nutritional status.
- Weight:
  - Short-term marker of nutritional status.
  - Affected by organomegaly, oedema, and ascites.
- Head circumference:
  - Marker of long-term nutritional status for <2 years.
- Abdominal girth:
  - Useful where there are fluctuating weights due to organomegaly, oedema, or ascites.
- Mid upper arm circumference:
  - Indicator of fat and muscle stores.
  - Sensitive short-term marker of nutritional status.
  - WHO growth charts from 3 months to 5 years and serial measurements if >5 years.
- Triceps skinfold thickness:
  - Distinguishes fat from muscle stores.
  - Marker of medium- to long-term nutritional status.
  - Challenging to measure unless child is cooperative.

Methods of feeding

Oral feeding

- Encourage oral feeding, particularly in infancy when essential skills such as sucking, swallowing, and chewing should be learned.
- Risk of behavioural feeding problems due to tube feeding, vomiting, ascites, organomegaly, or prolonged periods of nil by mouth.
- Weaning should follow standard guidelines, introducing tastes and textures at appropriate times.
- Emotional and social rewards of eating and drinking for the child and family.

Tube feeding

- Nasogastric feeding associated with improvement in body composition.
- May remove pressure on the child and family.
- Useful for administering unpalatable medicines and feeds.
- Can minimize fasting to preserve body stores and promote normoglycaemia.
- Ensure some oral feeding is maintained.
- Gastrostomy (PEG) feeding rarely possible in liver disease:
  - Risk of bleeding during placement due to portal hypertension and varices.
  - Inadequate tract formation due to ascites.
  - PEG feeding may be possible in absence of portal hypertension, varices, and ascites.

Parenteral nutrition

- When it is not possible to feed enterally or where there is severe persistent malabsorption affecting growth.
- May worsen liver function so only used when absolutely necessary.

Acute liver failure

- Often well-nourished initially.
- Aim is to preserve nutritional status and manage complications such as hypoglycaemia and hyperammonaemia.

Management
- Maintain nutritional status:
  - Provide up to 120% of the EAR for energy requirements and at least minimum protein requirements (Table 68.4).
- If inborn error of metabolism suspected e.g. urea cycle disorder, fatty acid oxidation defect:
  - Give emergency regimen (Table 68.5) to meet glucose production rates (Table 68.6) to prevent catabolism.
  - Once diagnosis determined, give specific diet therapy to prevent accumulation of toxic by-products.
  - Protein-free formula (e.g. Energivit®) useful if inborn error of metabolism involving protein metabolism is suspected.
- Prevent hypoglycaemia.
- Manage hyperammonaemia:
  - Provide minimum protein requirements initially to reduce ammonia production in the gut.
  - Avoid prolonged protein restriction as this leads to increased muscle breakdown, which may increase ammonia and worsen malnutrition.
  - No evidence that protein restriction or branched-chain amino acids reduce encephalopathy.

Table 68.4 Minimum safe levels of protein intake

Age		Protein (g/kg)	
Months	1	1.77	
	2	1.5	
	3	1.36	
	4	1.24	
	6	1.14	
Years	1	1.14	
	1.5	1.03	
	2	0.97	
	3	0.90	
	4	0.86	
	5	0.85	
	6	0.89	
	7	0.91	
	8	0.92	
	9	0.92	
	10	0.91	
		Males	Females
	11	0.91	0.9
	12	0.90	0.89
	13	0.90	0.88
	14	0.89	0.87
	15	0.88	0.85
	16	0.87	0.84
	17	0.86	0.83
	18	0.85	0.82

Table 68.5 Emergency regimen

Age	Weight (kg)	Carbohydrate concentration (%)	Volume (mL) 2-hourly	Super Soluble Maxijul® recipes	SOS®-10,15,20,25 recipes
Newborn	3–5	10	40–65	3 yellow scoops* made up with 120mL water	1 sachet SOS-10 made up with 200mL water
3 months	5.5–7	10	70–90		
6 months	7.5–8	10	95–100		
9–12 months	9 – 10	10	100		
1–2 years	11	15	95	2 yellow scoops* made up with 55mL water or 200mL juice	1 sachet SOS-15 made up with 200mL water or 500mL juice
2–3 years	13–15	20	100–110	4 yellow scoops* made up with 85mL water or 200mL juice	1 sachet SOS-20 made up with 200mL water or 400mL juice
4–6 years	17–22	20	115–130		
7–10 years	24–33	20	135–155		
11–14 years	35–54	25	175–200	2 large blue scoops* made up with 190mL water or 7 yellow scoops* made up with 200mL juice	1 sachet SOS-25 made up with 200mL water or 350mL juice
15–18 years	>55	25	220		

*SHS scoops available in the UK.

Table 68.6 Glucose production rates

Age	Glucose mg/kg/min	Glucose g/kg/hour
Infants	8–9	0.5
Children	5–7	0.3–0.4
Adolescents	2–4	0.2–0.25

Liver transplantation

- Feeding within 3–5 days.
- Tube feeding may be used until oral feeds can be established.
- A normal diet for age is often achieved relatively quickly.
- High-energy feeds used if catch-up growth required.
- There is generally catch-up growth in the 2 years after transplant but final height may be below genetic potential.
- PN used if there is severe under-nutrition pre transplant or where there are complications such as bowel perforation post transplant.
- Tube feeding may continue where there are pre-existing behavioural feeding difficulties.
- Avoid Seville oranges and grapefruit due to interference with immunosuppressants.
- Strict food hygiene as increased vulnerability to food poisoning when on high-dose immunosuppressant medication. Avoid:
  - Unpasteurized milk and cheese, live yoghurt, soft cheeses, pâté, deli meats, unwashed salad, shellfish, raw fish, raw egg.

Nutritional management of common liver conditions

Conjugated hyperbilirubinaemia in infancy
- MCT formula or fat emulsion alongside breastfeeding.
- Two-thirds MCT formula to one-third breast milk.
- Increase proportion of MCT formula if growth poor.
- If galactosaemia not excluded, temporarily stop breastfeeding and use MCT feed containing only trace amounts of galactose (e.g. Pregestimil®).
- Encourage expressing of breast milk so that breastfeeding can be resumed once galactosaemia excluded.

Extrahepatic biliary atresia
- Presentation with excessive feeding due to malabsorption.
- Initial treatment as described previously for conjugated jaundice.
- Following Kasai, build up MCT feeds from day 3 to day 5 and then reintroduce one-third breast milk.
- Careful monitoring of growth and feeding following discharge.
- Standard weaning.
- MCT formula until jaundice clears and then replace with standard or high energy formula.

Non-alcoholic fatty liver disease
- Disease severity ranges from benign hepatic steatosis to forms that may progress to cirrhosis in childhood.
- Most common cause of paediatric liver disease.
- Treatment:
  - Address associated metabolic abnormalities: treating insulin resistance, reducing central obesity, and treating oxidative stress.
  - Lifestyle measures in the form of dietary modifications and physical activity.
  - Vitamin E to reduce oxidative stress.

Wilson disease
- Treatment involves chelating agents that bind dietary copper for excretion, as well as a low-copper diet.
- Avoid excessive amounts of the following foods which have a high concentration of copper: shellfish, offal, nuts, dried fruit, dried beans, dried peas and lentils, some grains such as whole wheat, barley and millet, soya products, chocolate, and mushrooms.

Progressive familial intrahepatic cholestasis
- MCT feeds or supplements due to fat malabsorption.
- Poor intake and appetite due to pruritus.
- Short stature is common but may improve after liver transplantation.
- Consider tube feeding.

Alagille syndrome

- Malabsorption, poor growth, fussy eating, renal acidosis, and itching.
- Pancreatic insufficiency may occur.
- MCT feeds or supplements.
- Maximize energy density of diet.
- Fussy eating may be treated through specialist feeding clinics.
- Consider tube feeding.

Intestinal failure-associated liver disease

- Can progress from cholestasis to fibrosis and cirrhosis.
- Risk factors include prematurity, short bowel syndrome, sepsis, intestinal bacterial overgrowth, and a lack of enteral nutrition.
- Maximize enteral nutrition.
- Specialist multidisciplinary management and avoidance of sepsis.
- SMOF (soybean oil, MCT, olive oil, fish oil) may reduce PN-related cholestasis.

Chylous ascites

- Complication of transplant.
- Restrict long-chain triglycerides (LCTs) for up to 3 weeks to reduce flow of lymph.
- Infants:
  - Give feed containing >75% of fat as MCT.
- Older children:
  - Low LCT diet.
  - Fat-free supplement drinks (Table 68.3, p. 588).
  - MCT emulsions or oils (Table 68.7).
- Essential fatty acid deficiency risk if using feed with >75% of the fat as MCT. Supplement with walnut oil at 1mL/100kcal if using for prolonged time

Table 68.7 Energy supplementation

Per 100g/mL	Kcal	Glucose (g)	Fat (g)	Protein (g)	Comments
Carbohydrates					
Super Soluble Maxijul®	380	100	0	0	
Polycal®	380	100	0	0	
Fat					
Calogen®	450	0	50	0	100% LCT
Liquigen®	450	0	50	0	100% MCT
MCT Oil®	855	0	95	0	99% MCT
Carbohydrate and fat combined					
Super Soluble Duocal®	492	72.7	22.3	0	100% LCT
MCT Duocal®	497	72	23.2	0	75% MCT

Acute liver failure

Definition *602*
Aetiology *604*
Therapy *610*
Complications *612*
Transplantation *616*
Liver support system *616*
Prognosis *617*
References and resources *617*

Definition

Acute liver failure (ALF) in children is defined as 'a rare multisystem disorder in which severe impairment of liver function, with or without encephalopathy, occurs in association with hepatocellular necrosis in a patient with no recognized underlying chronic liver disease'. Hepatic-based coagulopathy not correctable by vitamin K is used as surrogate marker of severe impairment of liver function. PT >15 seconds or INR >1.5 in the presence of hepatic encephalopathy or a PT >20 seconds or INR >2.0 in the absence of hepatic encephalopathy, is being used as a cut off.

Aetiology

The aetiology of ALF varies depending on the age of the child, with metabolic liver disease and infections being most common in those <1 year of age. The aetiology largely remains indeterminate in older children; however, of the known aetiologies viral infections, drug-induced hepatitis, autoimmune hepatitis, and Wilson disease (WD) are the commonest causes (Table 69.1). The aetiology of ALF not only provides indication of prognosis but also dictates specific management options.

Viral hepatitis

- Hepatotropic viruses are probably the most identifiable cause of ALF worldwide.
- Hepatitis A (HAV) and hepatitis E (HEV) are amongst the most common causes in Asia and Africa.
- Risk of developing ALF with HAV infection is 0.1–0.4% and HEV is 0.6–2.8%
- Hepatitis B infection can lead to ALF during acute infection or reactivation of chronic HBV infection in immunocompromised patients, co-infection or superinfection with hepatitis D virus, or during the seroconversion from hepatitis e antigen positive state to hepatitis B e antibody positive state. Rarely infants born to HbeAb positive mothers can develop ALF around 6 weeks to 6 months of age.
- Heterotropic viruses such as HSV, CMV, EBV, and varicella zoster virus can cause severe hepatitis especially in immunocompromised state leading to ALF.

Table 69.1 Aetiologies of ALF in children in a tertiary referral unit (King's College Hospital, London)

Aetiology	
Indeterminate cause (non-A–E hepatitis)	68 (31%)
Drug/toxins	51 (23%)
Viral	23(11%)
NH	17(8%)
Metabolic	15 (7%)
Autoimmune	13 (6%)
Wilson disease	10(5%)
Haem Malig	8(4%)
Miscellaneous	10 (5%)
Total	215 (100%)

Haem Malig, haematological malignancy; NH, neonatal haemochromatosis.

Data sourced from Dhawan A. Etiology and prognosis of acute liver failure in children. Liver Transpl 2008;14(Suppl 2):S80–4.

- HSV-induced ALF in the newborn carries a high mortality; it should be considered in every sick neonate with coagulopathy and raised transaminases even if there are no vesicular lesions on the skin. Treatment with IV aciclovir should begin immediately.
- Parvovirus B19 infection also causes severe hepatitis or ALF and bone marrow failure in children.
- Viruses such as echovirus, coxsackievirus, and other enteroviruses can cause ALF.
- ALF of indeterminate aetiology encompasses viruses and metabolic disorders yet to be identified as there is associated bone marrow failure in a proportion of children.

Metabolic diseases

- Inherited disorders of metabolism are an important cause of ALF in the paediatric population, especially in the neonatal period; diagnosis requires a high degree of suspicion because overt signs and symptoms of liver disease are usually absent.
- Galactosaemia, which usually presents with conjugated hyperbilirubinaemia, hypoglycaemia, and Gram-negative septicaemia, can progress to liver failure; immediate exclusion of lactose from the diet and medications usually lead to recovery except in severe cases.
- Tyrosinaemia can present with severe coagulopathy, jaundice, and sometimes rickets; dietary management and the use of nitisinone (NTBC) have improved the survival of these children.
- A history of administration of fructose as in fruit juice, honey, or sugar coinciding with the onset of symptoms suggests the diagnosis of hereditary fructose intolerance.
- Recently, mitochondrial respiratory chain disorders such as Pearson syndrome, mitochondrial DNA depletion syndrome, nuclear DNA defect, and mitochondrial enzyme complex deficiency, have been implicated as aetiological factors for ALF in children. They usually present with hypoglycaemia, vomiting, coagulopathy, acidosis, and raised lactate with or without neurological symptoms. However, usually not all the features are present; hence diagnosis should be considered in every child with ALF. Diagnosis is based on quantitative assessment of the respiratory chain enzyme complexes in muscle, liver, or skin fibroblasts.
- Rarely, fatty acid oxidation defects and inborn errors of bile acid synthesis can present as ALF.

Neonatal haemochromatosis

- Neonatal haemochromatosis (NH) is a disease of intrauterine onset associated with hepatic and extrahepatic siderosis that spares reticuloendothelial system.
- Current hypothesis suggest NH to be an alloimmune process where maternal antibody is directed towards fetal liver cells resulting in hepatocyte loss. High ferritin is non-specific and seen in other cause of ALF.
- The diagnosis could be safely confirmed by labial salivary gland biopsy, showing extra hepatic iron deposits with reticuloendothelial system sparing.

- Exchange transfusion and IV immunoglobulin has become the first line of treatment and transplantation is only in cases which do not respond.
- Antenatal weekly IV immunoglobulin as prophylaxis (1g/kg) from the 18th week of gestation until term in high-risk mothers (who had babies with NH) has been shown to prevent or reduce the severity of disease.

Wilson disease (WD)

(See Chapter 62.)

- WD, an autosomal recessive disorder, is an uncommon cause of ALF in older children.
- It can present acutely with Coombs-negative haemolytic anaemia, mixed hyperbilirubinaemia (both conjugated and unconjugated), and liver failure.
- Kayser–Fleischer rings, present in about 50% of cases of WD, are diagnostic in a patient presenting with ALF.
- Serum caeruloplasmin is typically low but may be normal in about 15% of cases, and serum free copper concentration may be normal or raised.
- Very low serum alkaline phosphatase or uric acid levels or a high bilirubin (μmol/dL) to alkaline phosphatase (IU/L) ratio of >2 are indirect indicators of WD as a cause of ALF.
- Treatment depends on the severity of illness. ALF in WD with encephalopathy is an indication for emergency liver transplantation. Children with ALF due to WD but without encephalopathy may respond to chelation treatment. Liver assist devices such as MARS® can act as a bridge, while the patient awaits transplant.

Drugs and toxins

- Drug-induced hepatotoxicity can be a dose-dependent response, an idiosyncratic, or a synergistic reaction
- Detailed history should be taken with name of all medications used, the time period of their use, and the quantities ingested as sometimes it is a diagnosis of exclusion.
- The Councils for International Organizations of Medical Sciences/ Roussel Uclaf Causality Assessment Method (CIOMS/RUCAM) scale is helpful in establishing a causal relationship between an offending drug and liver damage. Using the scoring system, a suspected drug could be categorized into 'definite or highly probable' (score >8), 'probable' (score 6–8), 'possible' (score 3–5), 'unlikely' (score 1–2), and 'excluded' (score ≤0).
- Paracetamol, the most common over-the-counter medicine, is a dose-dependent hepatotoxic agent causing ALF. Commonly, paracetamol hepatotoxicity is either due to intended suicidal overdose or the inadvertent use of a supratherapeutic dose. Serum paracetamol levels 4 hours after ingestion are useful to identify high-risk patients but these levels may not be informative if toxicity is due to chronic administration. Activated charcoal may be useful for GI decontamination in suspected or known paracetamol overdose, especially if administered within 4–6 hours of ingestion. Acetylcysteine has been shown to be quite an

effective antidote even if patients have presented quite late after the overdose. In acute paracetamol overdose the dose of acertylcysteine is 150mg/kg in 5% glucose over 15 minutes followed by 50mg/kg given over 4 hours followed by 100mg/kg over 16 hours. If the patient has any evidence of coagulopathy then NAC should be continued at a dose of 100mg/kg per day till the INR is <1.5.

- 'Mushroom' (*Amanita phalloides*) poisoning as a cause of ALF has been reported from Europe, the US, and South Africa. It usually presents with severe diarrhoea with or without vomiting a few hours after ingestion and progresses to overt liver failure in 3–4 days. Benzylpenicillin (300,000–1 million units/kg per day) and silibinin (30–40mg/kg per day I/V or orally) have been used as an antidote.
- Sodium valproate can lead to ALF by unmasking an underlying mitochondrial cytopathy, hence detailed investigations should be carried out for the same.
- Other common hepatotoxic agents are antituberculous drugs, antiepileptics, or antibiotics (sulfonamides, erythromycin, co-amoxiclav etc.).
- There are no specific antidotes for idiosyncratic drug reactions but corticosteroids have been used in suspected drug hypersensitivity reaction.

Autoimmune hepatitis

- Autoimmune hepatitis can rarely present with ALF; the diagnosis may be difficult since autoantibodies may be negative.
- Patients with fulminant hepatic failure due to autoimmune hepatitis need emergency liver transplantation.

Ischaemic injury

- Ischaemic injury due to aetiologies such as heart failure, hypotensive/ hypovolaemic/septic shock can lead to ALF.
- Usually the typical features of ischaemia are over by the time the patient presents with ALF; hence a careful history is important.

Vascular causes

- Any conditions causing obstruction of hepatic venous outflow (Budd–Chiari syndrome, veno-occlusive disease, cardiomyopathies) can also present as ALF.
- Abdominal pain, ascites, and significant hepatomegaly are useful clinical clues.
- Doppler USS, CT, or MR venography is usually diagnostic.

Malignancies

- Haemophagocytic lymphohistiocytosis (HLH) could be primary (familial) or secondary to infection, and can present with fever, cutaneous rash, hepatosplenomegaly, pancytopenia, and, in severe cases, with ALF. HLH is due to paradoxical inefficient overactivation of natural killer cells and of CD8+ T-cell lymphocytes, invariably leading to clinical and haematological alterations. Either molecular diagnosis or fulfilment of five out of eight diagnostic criteria is essential for making the diagnosis.

- Leukaemia or lymphoma can rarely present with ALF due to massive infiltration of the liver. Presence of high fever with hepatosplenomegaly, high alkaline phosphatase, high lactate dehydrogenase, and abnormalities on peripheral blood film are the diagnostic clues and bone marrow examination is confirmatory.
- It is essential to rule out haematological malignancy in ALF as it is a contraindication for liver failure.
- Table 69.2 lists disease-specific tests.

Table 69.2 Diagnostic tests

Cause	Test
Infections	Hepatitis A: anti-HAV IgM antibody
	Hepatitis B: HBsAg, HBcAb(IgM), HBcA
	Hepatitis C: anti-hep C antibody, hep C PCR
	Hepatitis E: anti-HEV IgM antibody
	Cytomegalovirus PCR
	Epstein–Barr virus PCR
	Human immunodeficiency virus (HIV) PCR
ALF of indeterminate cause	
Metabolic disorders	Galactosaemia; galactose-1-phosphate uridyl transferase level in blood
	Tyrosinaemia; urinary succinylacetone
	Fatty acid oxidation defect: serum fatty acid profile
	Urea cycle defects/defect in amino acid metabolism: serum amino acid profile, ammonia
Neonatal haemochromatosis	Buccal mucosal biopsy, high ferritin, high transferrin saturation
Mitochondrial hepatopathies	Muscle and liver biopsies for quantitative assay of respiratory chain enzyme
Wilson disease	Urinary copper, Kayser–Fleischer rings, Coombs-negative haemolytic anaemia
Drugs and toxins	History, urine toxicology
Autoimmune hepatitis	Immunoglobulins (IgG, IgA, and IgM)
	Tissue antibodies (anti-SMA, GPC, mitochondrial, liver-kidney microsomal and antinuclear antibodies)
Vascular causes	Doppler USS/CT scan/MR venography
Malignancies	Haemophagocytic lymphohistiocytosis, leukaemia/lymphoma : bone marrow aspiration, perforin expression, genetics
Non A to E	Diagnosis by exclusion (all tests)

Therapy

General measures

- All children with ALF should be nursed in a quiet environment with as little stimulation as possible to minimize acute increase in the intracranial pressure (ICP).
- Children with encephalopathy or an INR >4 (without encephalopathy) should be admitted to an intensive care unit for continuous monitoring.
- Sedation is contraindicated unless the patient is to be mechanically ventilated because of the possibility of aggravating the encephalopathy or precipitating respiratory failure.
- Vital parameters (heart rate, blood pressure, respiratory rate, oxygen saturation, neurological observations), urine output should be monitored each 4–6 hours, while metabolic parameters (electrolytes, blood sugar) and coagulation studies (INR), should be monitored twice daily.
- Controlled trials in adults have failed to substantiate any beneficial effect of corticosteroids, interferon, insulin and glucose, prostaglandin E1, bowel decontamination, and charcoal haemoperfusion in patients with ALF.
- Maintenance of nutrition is crucial and hypoglycaemia should be avoided; a protein intake of 1g/kg is well tolerated and should be provided.
- Total fluid intake is usually restricted to two-thirds of the maintenance.
- Maintaining serum sodium concentrations of 145–155mmol/L has a cerbroprotective effect
- Routine surveillance and treatment of infection is essential. Use of prophylactic broad-spectrum antibiotics and antifungal have decreased the incidence of infection significantly and improved survival.

Complications

Neurological

- The most serious complications of ALF are cerebral oedema with resultant intracranial hypertension and hepatic encephalopathy. It is rarely present in grade I–II encephalopathy but the risk increases to 25–35% in grade III and 65–75% or more in grade IV encephalopathy. Arterial ammonia of >150mmol increases the risk of cerebral oedema.
  - Clinical features of raised ICP include systemic hypertension, brady-cardia, hypertonia, hyperreflexia, and in extreme cases decerebrate or decorticate posturing.
  - Mannitol is an osmotic diuretic commonly used to treat intracranial hypertension. A rapid bolus of 0.5g/kg as a 20% solution over a 15-minute period is recommended, and the dose can be repeated if the serum osmolarity is <320mOsm/L. Similarly, 3% saline could be given as bolus (3mL/kg) during raised intracranial hypertension.
  - In ventilated patients, hyperventilation provides no role and $PaCO_2$ should be kept between 4 and 4.5kPa. Studies have shown sodium thiopental, mild cerebral hypothermia (32–35◦C) and hypernatrae-mia (serum sodium >145 mmol/L) improves cerebral perfusion.
- Grade II encephalopathic but agitated patients and grade III–IV encephalopathic patients should be electively intubated and transferred to a liver transplantation centre.
- Normocapnia should be maintained and excessive hyperventilation should be avoided as it can cause cerebral vasoconstriction and paradoxically decrease the cerebral perfusion pressure
- ICP monitoring with intracranial bolts:
  - There are no clear-cut guidelines on candidate selection for intra-cranial bolts in ALF, but in general those patients who are ventilated with grade III or IV encephalopathy who are at high risk of coning would benefit from intracranial bolts.
  - Aim of ICP monitoring is to maintain ICP <20–25mmHg and cere-bral perfusion pressure (mean arterial blood pressure – ICP) should be maintained at >50mmHg and might require use of ionotropic agents to increase mean arterial blood pressure.
  - Helps in accurate monitoring of ICP but overall survival is not affected; there is a 10% risk of intracranial bleeding.
  - Other measures include sodium thiopental infusion, phenytoin infu-sion for subclinical seizure activity.
- Ammonia-lowering measures such as dietary protein restriction, bowel decontamination, or lactulose are of limited or no value in rapidly advancing encephalopathy.

Infection

- Infection can lead to development and progression of multiorgan failure; about 60% of deaths in ALF have been attributed to sepsis.
- Active uncontrolled infection is a relative contraindication for liver transplantation.
- Most common bacterial infections are due to *Staphylococcus aureus*, but streptococci or Gram-negative organisms such as coliforms are also isolated.
- Prophylactic IV antibiotics have been shown to reduce the incidence of culture-positive bacterial infection from 61.3% to 32.1%.
- *Candida* spp. are the most common fungal infections and often unrecognized; fluconazole is the preferred prophylactic agent.
- Deterioration of hepatic encephalopathy after initial improvement, a markedly raised leucocyte count, pyrexia unresponsive to antibiotics, and established renal failure are strong indicators of fungal infection.

Coagulopathy

- ALF is characterized by decreased synthesis of clotting factors (factors II, V, VII, IX, X), accelerated fibrinolysis, and impaired hepatic clearance of activated clotting factors and fibrin degradation products.
- The PT expressed as an INR is markedly elevated and is used as an indicator of the severity of the liver damage.
- Significant disseminated intravascular coagulation is unusual in ALF.
- Clinically, bleeding tends to be less severe than might be expected from the degree of INR prolongation, although the risk of haemorrhage correlates with thrombocytopenia (platelet count $<450 \times 10^9$/L).
- Common sites of haemorrhage include the GI tract, nasopharynx, lungs, and retroperitoneum; intracranial haemorrhage is uncommon.
- The presence of significant disseminated intravascular coagulation usually indicates sepsis or secondary haemophagocytic lymphohistiocytosis.
- Since coagulopathy is a very good tool for assessment of prognosis and monitoring of disease progression, correction of coagulopathy is indicated only if the patient is already listed for transplant, in premature babies, or before an invasive procedure such as insertion of a central venous catheter or ICP monitor (please discuss with the tertiary referral centre before correcting coagulopathy).
- Prophylactic ranitidine (H_2 blocker) or PPIs have been shown to decrease the incidence of gastric bleeding.

Haemodynamic changes

- In ALF, there is a state of hyperdynamic circulation with decreased systemic peripheral vascular resistance and increased cardiac output (similar to systemic inflammatory response syndrome).
- Circulatory failure is a common mode of death in patients with ALF, often complicating sepsis or multiorgan failure.
- Invasive devices such as pulse contour cardiac output (PiCCO) and lithium dilutional cardiac output (LiDCO) monitoring, which can measure various body water compartments, are good devices to rationalize fluid management and the choice of vasopressors.
- Newer non-invasive cardiac output monitoring devise such as USCOM (ultrasonic cardiac output monitor) could help with decision-making in rationalizing fluid management.
- In the presence of persistent hypotension despite normal filling pressure, vasopressors such as adrenaline are the inotropic agents of choice.
- Cardiac arrhythmias of most types may occur in the later stages and are usually caused by electrolyte disturbances (e.g. hypo- or hyperkalaemia, acidosis, hypoxia, or cardiac irritation by a central venous catheter).

Renal failure

- In the paediatric population, the incidence of renal failure is lower (10–15%) than in the adult population.
- Renal failure could be due either to the direct toxic effect on kidneys, as in paracetamol overdose, or to a complex mechanism such as hepatorenal syndrome or acute tubular necrosis secondary to complications of ALF (sepsis, bleeding, and/or hypotension).
- Blood urea estimation is unreliable as a marker of renal dysfunction because GI haemorrhage may increase urea disproportionately.
- Serum creatinine is a better indicator of kidney function.
- Intravascular hypovolaemia, if present, needs correction.
- Low-dose dopamine is not only ineffective but can have deleterious effects especially in the setting of profound vasodilatation, which is seen typically in ALF.
- Renal replacement therapy:
  - Haemodiafiltration and haemodialysis should be instituted when the urine output is <1mL/kg/hour.
  - Continuous filtration or dialysis systems are associated with less haemodynamic instability and consequently less risk of aggravating latent or established encephalopathy than intermittent haemodialysis.
  - Epoprostenol infusion at a rate of 5ng/kg per minute has been found to be superior to heparin anticoagulation with respect to functional duration of the filters and the haemorrhagic complications.

Metabolic derangements

- Hypoglycaemia in ALF can be present in 40% of patients.
- Classic signs and symptoms of hypoglycaemia are often masked specially in the presence of encephalopathy, hence regular blood glucose monitoring is important.
- Metabolic acidosis is associated with poor outcome; 50% of patients with grade III or IV encephalopathy can have lactic acidosis due to inadequate tissue perfusion.
- Other metabolic disturbances include respiratory alkalosis, hypokalaemia, hyponatraemia, hypophosphataemia, hypocalcaemia, and hypomagnesaemia.

Others

- Acute pancreatitis:
  - Rare in ALF but mild elevation of serum amylase may be present.
  - Should be suspected if patient has abdominal pain and hypocalcaemia.
  - Precipitating factors are sodium valproate, shock, causative virus, etc.
  - Treatment is supportive.
- Adrenal suppression:
  - Seen in about 60% of adults with ALF.
  - Should be investigated with short tetracosactide test.
  - Corticosteroid replacement should be considered in patients with poor tetracosactide response or intractable hypotension.

Transplantation

- Liver transplantation is the only definitive treatment available.
- Contraindications are permanently fixed and dilated pupils, uncontrolled active sepsis, and severe respiratory failure (acute respiratory distress syndrome). Relative contraindications are accelerating inotropic requirements, infection under treatment, cerebral perfusion pressure of <40mmHg for >2 hours, and a history of progressive or severe neurological problems in which the ultimate neurological outcome may not be acceptable.
- In very unstable patients, a two-stage procedure with hepatectomy, while waiting for donor liver followed by liver transplant has been tried with some success.
- Auxiliary liver transplantation:
  - Due to the potential of regeneration of native liver if given sufficient time to recover, auxiliary liver transplantation has been used to provide liver function while the native liver regenerates.
  - The advantage of this procedure is that once the native liver shows signs of recovery, immunosuppression can be weaned and eventually stopped.
  - 60% of children who had auxiliary liver transplantation in our institution (King's College Hospital, London, UK) have shown regeneration of their own liver and have stopped immunosuppression.
- Hepatocyte transplantation:
  - To provide a functioning hepatic mass while the native liver regenerates; has shown some encouraging results as a bridge to transplantation and in one child, liver transplant was avoided; however, the technique remains experimental.

Liver support system

- Liver support devices are either cleansing devices or a bioartificial liver support system.
- Cleansing devices perform only the detoxifying function of the liver, whereas bioartificial liver support systems have a theoretical advantage of providing the synthetic and detoxifying properties.
- A recent meta-analysis, considering all forms of devices together, demonstrated no efficacy for bioartificial liver devices for the treatment of ALF.

Prognosis

- The prognosis of ALF varies greatly with the underlying aetiology.
- PT is the best predictor of survival.
- Factor V concentration has been used as a prognostic marker, especially in association with encephalopathy (Clichy criteria). In children, a factor V concentration of <25% of normal suggests a poor outcome.
- Liver biopsy is rarely helpful in ALF and is usually contraindicated because of the presence of coagulopathy. Hepatic parenchymal necrosis of >50% is associated with a reduced survival but the potential for sampling error is considerable.
- A small liver, or more particularly a rapidly shrinking liver, is an indicator of a poor prognosis. CT volumetry of the liver has been used to assess both the size of the liver and its functional reserve.
- Fulminant WD is invariably fatal, and emergency liver transplantation is the only effective treatment.
- There is no single criterion that can predict the outcome with absolute certainty and be universally applicable for all patients with ALF with different aetiologies. However, prediction of a low chance of survival (<20%) is clinically useful in deciding whether to list the patient for orthotopic liver transplant, which has a 1-year survival rate of 75%.

References and resources

Dhawan A. Etiology and prognosis of acute liver failure in children. Liver Transpl 2008;14 (Suppl 2):S80–4.

Portal hypertension

Definition 620
Pathophysiology 620
Clinical features 621
Management 622
Management of acute variceal bleeding 626
Conclusion 628
References and resources 628

Definition

Portal hypertension (PHT) is the term used for increased pressure of >10mmHg within the portal venous system. Normal pressure within the portal system ranges normally between 5 and 10mmHg.

The increase in portal pressure results from altered blood flow at (i) pre-hepatic level (e.g. portal vein or superior mesenteric vein thrombosis); (ii) intrahepatic subdivided into presinusoidal (e.g. congenital hepatic fibrosis, schistosomiasis) sinusoidal (cirrhosis), post sinusoidal; and at (iii) post hepatic (e.g. Budd–Chiari Syndrome, hepatic vein occlusion, right heart failure).

Pathophysiology

Varices are abnormal venous communications between portal and systemic circulations that develop to decompress the portal venous system once PHT is established. The varices commonly develop in the lower oesophagus, stomach, and rectum. Gastro-oesophageal varices are more prone to bleeding due to their position and exposure to food and acid, while varices in other sites such as splenorenal or retroperitoneal are less likely to bleed but can present rarely with compression symptoms of adjacent organs. The hepatic venous pressure gradient (HVPG) (normally 1–4mmHg), measured via interventional venography, is the current widely acceptable surrogate marker of PHT in adults. HVPG can also differentiate the origin of PHT as it is normal in presinusoidal PHT and raised >5mm of Hg in sinusoidal and post sinusoidal PHT. A pressure gradient >10mmHg is associated with development of varices and >12mmHg predicts the risk of variceal bleeding. The invasive nature of the procedure is a major limitation in its application in children.

Variceal classification

The accepted current classification of varices is:
- Grade 0: no oesophageal varices.
- Grade 1: small and non-tortuous oesophageal varices.
- Grade 2: tortuous oesophageal varices but occupying less than one-third of the distal oesophageal radius.
- Grade 3: large and tortuous oesophageal varices covering more than one-third of the distal oesophageal radius.
  - The presence of red spots and wheals markings along with gastric varices either at the fundal or the lesser/great curve of the stomach is considered to be associated with higher risk of GI bleeding.
  - Other endoscopic signs of PHT include presence of gastropathy manifesting with vascular congestion, oedema and gastric antral vascular ectasia (GAVE).

Clinical features

GI bleeding from ruptured varices is the most common and severe complication of PHT. GI bleeding may present as haematemesis or melaena; this is commonly the first symptom of previously undiagnosed PHT. The risk of GI bleeds in children with PHT can be as high as 75% over a period of a decade without treatment. In children with biliary atresia (BA) oesophageal varices are found in 30–50% by 10 years of age with their native liver. The mortality associated with first variceal bleed has recently been reported as 1–3% increasing to 20% in cirrhotic patients. The overall mortality of children following a GI bleed with an underlying chronic liver disease (CLD), such as BA, is higher due to decompensation of their liver disease while children with PVT if adequately managed have a much better outcome. Variceal bleeding in children with CLD usually is an indication for liver transplantation. Other complications include splenomegaly and thrombocytopenia, hepatic encephalopathy, hepatopulmonary syndrome and portopulmonary hypertension, growth failure, ascites, vascular coagulation, biliopathy, and poor quality of life.

Management

PHT therapy is aimed mainly at trying to manage and reduce the likelihood of any GI bleed from ruptured varicose veins. This may be achieved with pharmacological agents (non-selective beta blockers (NSBBs) with evidence of raised hepatic venous pressure gradient, endoscopic variceal band ligation (EVL) and sclerotherapy (EST) or shunt surgery such as creating a bypass to reduce the pressure in the portal system. Both EST and EVL have been shown to eradicate varices with a 90% success rate. Therefore they are currently the gold standard of treatment for active GI bleeding. EVL is the preferable mode of endoscopic treatment, as it is proven to be easier and safer but applicable only to older children due to technical limitations. A randomized trial comparing the two treatment methods showed significantly lower mortality and fewer complications in EVL, while providing similar efficacy for active bleeding and recurrent haemorrhaging.

Prediction tools of PHT

The pathophysiology of PHT involves a complex relationship between the liver, the spleen, and the connecting vascular structures. This means that biochemical changes associated with each aspect of the pathophysiology may provide useful information for the diagnosis and monitoring of PHT. Several potential non-invasive markers have been studied as possible predictors of PHT, including biomarkers and imaging techniques. In order to be clinically useful, the ideal marker would be one that could not only predict the presence of PHT but could also differentiate between severities.

The process of liver cirrhosis results from chronic tissue damage and subsequent inflammation, which leads to fibrosis and impaired architecture of the liver. In liver cirrhosis, PHT is the result of impaired blood flow through a cirrhotic liver. Therefore, various markers of inflammation (interleukins, TNF-β, CD163, hemeoxygenase-1), endothelial dysfunction (circulating endothelial cells), fibrosis (hyaluronic acid, laminin, collagen), haemostasis (platelet count, von Willebrand factor antigen), King's Variceal Prediction Score (KVaPS), Variceal Prediction Rule (VPR), clinical prediction rule, and aspartate aminotransferase-to-platelet ratio (APRI), are some of the parameters which have been investigated as potential markers for the development of PHT secondary to CLD. In addition to laboratory biomarkers a number of imaging techniques have been used including USS to measure spleen size, portal vein dilatation, and vascular resistance with Doppler; FibroScan® measuring liver and spleen stiffness and MRI.

Endoscopic therapy

According to recent recommendations, children with PHT should be considered for surveillance OGD on the basis of splenomegaly and thrombocytopenia with intention to treat if oesophageal varices grade ≥2 with mucosal stigmata are identified. 70% of children undergoing primary prophylaxis with varices grade ≥2 with mucosal stigmata of PHT can achieve eradication of varices with >84% probability of 10-year survival without liver transplantation. There is a 28% relapse rate of varices after eradication suggesting that a long-term surveillance OGD programme with aggressive treatment of recurrent varices may be beneficial.

There are two options for treatment including EST or EVL. EST involves intravariceal or perivariceal injection with a sclerosing agent causing it to stop haemorrhaging and thrombose. Sclerosing agents such as ethanolamine and tissue adhesive (cyanoacrylate) or thrombin can be used. EVL involves cutting off the blood supply to the varix by applying a rubber band tightly around it with subsequent thrombosis of the varix but it may be only applicable to children >10kg in weight. Both EST and EVL have been shown to eradicate varices with a 90% success rate. EVL is more commonly used, as it an easier and safer modality. Both procedures are associated with some risk and a small procedural mortality. EVL appears to have higher risk in young children because of the risk of entrapping the full oesophageal wall thickness in the band causing ischaemia. EST has been reported to potentially cause major complications such as ulceration and stricture formation also with a risk of bacteraemia. Following endoscopic therapy, patients should fast for at least 4 hours and solid feeding withheld until liquids are tolerated. Sucralfate or antacid medication should be given for 5–7 days. It is recommended to carry out EVL or EST every 2–4 weeks following the first variceal bleed to ablate gastro-oesophageal varices. Subsequent follow-up endoscopies are recommended at 6–12-monthly intervals with recurrent varices being ablated where indicated.

Pharmacological therapy

Pharmacological treatment involves NSBBs (often propranolol or more recently carvedilol), in order to decrease the pressure within the portal system. NSBBs work by reducing cardiac output through β_1 receptor blockage and increasing splanchnic vasoconstriction via β_2 blockage. The use of NSBBs is well established in adults with confirmation of potential therapeutic effect following HVPG measurements aiming to reduce HVPG below 12mmHg or by 20% from initial pre-treatment measurement. In children, the combination of NSBB and secondary endoscopic prophylaxis has not shown any significant benefit when studied in a small number of children.

Shunt surgery

The management of PHT via surgical procedures has not been well standardized and fully adopted by paediatric liver centres worldwide. Children with extrahepatic PVT may be considered for meso-Rex bypass procedure involving the surgical connection via intrapositional autologous vascular graft (usually internal jugular vein) between the superior mesenteric vein and the Rex recessus, a remnant of the ductus venosus. Meso-Rex bypass can be considered once these children achieve a body weight >8kg depending always on local surgical expertise. The patients have to fulfil specific criteria including absence of an underlying liver disease, patency of the intrahepatic portovenous system demonstrated on axial imaging and/or portal venography, and absence of prothrombotic tendencies. The procedure can be considered as part of treatment or prophylactic management.

In children with refractory PHT due to CLD, rarely a transjugular portosystemic shunt (TIPSS) may be considered with direct transhepatic portal vein puncture via the transjugular route and insertion of a shunt to establish portosystemic communication with reduction in portal vein pressure. There is a risk of shunt thrombosis and development of hyperammonaemia and hepatic encephalopathy. There are limited studies in children and only short-term follow-up where TIPSS is utilized as a bridge to liver transplantation.

Other treatment options

Balloon tamponade via Sengstaken–Blakemore tube is highly effective and has been shown to control bleeding in up to 90% of patients but the risk of recurrence is extremely high once the balloon is deflated. Sengstaken–Blakemore tamponade should only be used in an intubated and sedated child where there is failure to control active bleeding, as a bridge to definitive treatment or to facilitate transfer to a specialist liver centre. Haemostatic spray is a simple technique where powder is sprayed under direct vision through the endoscope onto actively bleeding lesions and subsequently forms a mechanical haemostatic barrier. Haemostatic spray is not an alternative to EVL or EST but can be useful in gastric erosions or oozing portal gastropathy particularly if experienced interventional endoscopists are not immediately available. Recombinant factor VIIa may also be considered in intractable cases resistant to conventional treatment.

Management of acute variceal bleeding

Airway, breathing, and circulation (ABC)

- ABC patient assessment:
  - *Airway*: ensure airway is patent.
  - *Breathing*: visually assess patient for breathing efficacy and effort. Obtain respiratory rate and oxygen saturation. Administer oxygen via a face mask if required.
  - *Circulation*: obtain heart rate, manual pulse, capillary refill, and blood pressure.
- Obtain initial observations. Continue with regular observations. Consider referral to a more acute setting.
- Patient must remain on monitoring to assess heart rate and oxygen saturations (consider cardiac monitoring), in anticipation of acute deterioration/shock.
- Assess Glasgow coma scale level ± neuro-observations.
- Grade encephalopathy if patient is considered to be encephalopathic.

Bloods and IV access

- Minimum of two wide-bore peripheral IV cannulas.
- Cross-match 2 units of packed red cells (×1 unit if patient <1 year).
- Obtain blood gas (processed urgently) and blood sugar.
- Bloods: full blood count, urea and electrolytes, INR, renal, liver, and bone profiles and blood cultures. Consider sending ammonia sample (stored on ice) if patient is encephalopathic.

Fluid resuscitation and fluids

- A blood transfusion must be administered as soon as possible; transfuse up to 90g/L.
- If no blood group-matched blood is available, *O-negative* can be obtained from the emergency blood fridge. A '*code red*' blood should be requested clearly from blood bank.
- Commence blood transfusion slowly; transfusing rapidly will increase portal pressure and risk further bleeding.
- Other blood products can also be considered such as FFP, cryoprecipitate, and platelets where indicated. Administer platelet transfusion if level <100 × 10^9/L. If INR >1.5 and bleeding is not controlled, administer FFP.
- Do not give a fluid bolus unless clinically indicated to maintain haemodynamic stabilities or in the process of obtaining blood products.
- Commence patient on two-thirds maintenance IV fluids (0.45% saline and 5% glucose).
- Monitor blood sugars 2–4-hourly. Aim for a blood sugar of 4–8mmol. Consider changing to 10% glucose IV fluids if patient is hypoglycaemic.
- Keep patient nil by mouth.
- Correct any electrolyte or pH abnormalities.
- Strict fluid balance (monitor input and output).

Pharmacological therapy

- Vasoactive drugs must be used in combination with endoscopic therapy. Patient to commence octreotide—25mcg/hour in 0.9% N/S. Octreotide is prescribed as 500mcg in 40mL N/S to infuse at a rate of 2mL/hour.
- This dose could be increased to 50mcg/hour (4mL/hour) if there is no response.
- Octreotide needs dedicated IV access in order to support a continuous infusion.
- Wean for 12–24 hours post OGD and following discussion with endoscopist.
- Commence the following IV medications:
  - Antibiotics (piptazobactam 90mg/kg three times daily) as per microbiology guidelines.
  - Ranitidine (1mg/kg three times daily) or pantoprazole (child <12 years: 500mcg/kg; max. 20mg once daily. Child >12 years: 40mg once daily)
  - Vitamin K (<1 year: 1mg, 1–4 years: 2mg, 5–12 years: 5mg, >12years: 10mg).

Additional management

- If a NGT is *in situ*, it may be used to aspirate and be put on free drainage. Do not insert a new NGT due to risk of further bleeding.
- If bleeding continues and the patient is not responsive to all of the above management, consider placing a Sengstaken–Blackmore tube. Patient must be intubated and transferred to intensive care setting prior to Sengstaken–Blackmore tube insertion.
- Consider terlipressin acetate if uncontrolled bleeding and patient is not responding to above management as per British National Formulary guidelines. Child 12–18 years, 2mg every 4 hours until bleeding controlled (after initial dose, may reduce to 1mg every 4 hours if not tolerated or bodyweight <50kg). With respect to smaller children, suggested dosing from data on refractory septic shock in paediatric series is 0.02mg/kg.
- Monitor for side effects and discontinue after a maximum of 48 hours
- On-call PHT consultant to be contacted urgently for advice and to schedule an OGD, ideally within 24 hours of bleed as per adjusted international recommendations for adults.
- Ensure patient's care is managed in a suitable environment. Consider high-dependency setting transfer if patient's condition deteriorates, based on observations.
- Consider starting NSBBs such as propranolol or carvedilol as part of second-stage management. No indication as first-line management.
- Consider discussing surgical intervention (i.e. bypass) at a next stage depending on severity of bleed and underlying condition.

Conclusion

PHT is a significant complication of chronic liver disease or altered blood flow at a pre- or post-hepatic level. Children with PHT carry a risk of variceal bleeding which can be life-threatening, albeit rare. Recent advances in prediction, surveillance, and treatment options have been helpful in optimizing the PHT care pathway. Management of children with PHT in a specialized paediatric liver centre is highly recommended to achieve optimum outcome.

References and resources

de Franchis R, Baveno VI Faculty. Expanding consensus in portal hypertension: report of the Baveno VI Consensus Workshop: stratifying risk and individualizing care for portal hypertension. J Hepatol 2015;63:743–52.

Duché M, Ducot B, Ackermann O, Guérin F, Jacquemin E, Bernard O. Portal hypertension in children: High-risk varices, primary prophylaxis and consequences of bleeding. J Hepatol 2017;66:320–7.

Paediatric liver transplantation

Indications *630*
Contraindications *630*
Timing *630*
Survival rates *631*
Pre-transplant assessment *632*
Types of liver transplantation *634*
Initial post-transplant management *636*
Post-transplant complications *638*
Quality of life and growth *642*
References and resources *642*

Indications

Liver transplantation is now a standard treatment for:
• Decompensated chronic liver disease.
• Acute liver failure.
• Non-cirrhotic liver-based metabolic disorders.
• Selected liver tumours.

Liver transplant should be considered in these scenarios if:
• The likelihood of death secondary to liver disease is 18 months or less.
• There is unacceptable quality of life secondary to liver disease.
• Growth failure due to liver disease exists, that is not responsive to maximal medical therapy.
• Reversible neurodevelopmental impairment due to liver disease exists.
• There is likelihood of irreversible other end-organ damage that is remediable by liver transplantation.

Contraindications

There are few absolute contraindications to liver transplant. All cases should be discussed in a multidisciplinary setting. The following scenarios would be considered high risk and unsuitable for transplantation:
• Overwhelming bacterial, fungal, or viral infection outside of the liver.
• Severe cardiovascular disease.
• Extrahepatic malignancy.
• Inherited diseases with multisystemic involvement, e.g. mitochondrial.

Timing of transplantation

Timing of liver transplantation is important. The risks of imposing surgical morbidity on an unwell child should be balanced against the risk of death on the waiting list. The following clinical features can inform the decision-making process:
• Synthetic liver dysfunction (prolonged INR, low serum albumin, ascites).
• Disordered metabolism (jaundice, encephalopathy, loss of muscle mass, osteoporosis, intractable pruritus).
• Portal hypertension (variceal bleeding, intractable ascites).
• Profound lethargy.
• Spontaneous bacterial peritonitis, recurrent cholangitis.
• Hepatorenal or hepatopulmonary syndrome.

Survival rates

Both graft and patient survival have improved over the past four decades. Increased mortality is seen in acute liver failure versus chronic liver disease.

Table 71.1 shows survival rates for liver transplantation.

Table 71.1 Liver transplantation: survival*

	1 year	5 years	10 years
Patient survival (%)	85–95	75–85	75–85
Graft survival (%)	85–90	70–80	70–80

* Data sourced from the NHS Blood and Transplant (NHSBT) annual reports 2016/17 © NHS Blood and Transplant 2017.

Pre-transplant assessment

Prior to transplantation, the patient meets with members of the multidisciplinary team to undergo rigorous assessment to help:

- Identify pre-existing co-morbidities that may preclude transplantation or may impact management after transplantation.
- Optimize the health status of the patient pre-transplantation.

Table 71.2 shows a systematic approach to the pre-transplant assessment procedure, which is led by the transplant coordinators.

Table 71.2 Pre-transplant assessment

Cardiac	12-lead ECG
	Echocardiogram
	Selected patients may need further cardiac studies, e.g. pressure studies, exercise tolerance
Pulmonary	Pulse oximetry to detect intrapulmonary shunts. If oxygen saturation in room air <95%, needs macro-aggregated albumin scan or contrast echocardiogram
	Chest radiograph
	Formal pulmonary functional assessment if pre-existing pulmonary disease, e.g. cystic fibrosis
Renal	Urea, creatinine. Cystatin C, a low-molecular-weight protein has been shown to be an accurate marker for glomerular filtration
	If there is evidence of renal dysfunction, glomerular filtration rate is required
	If renal dysfunction, nephrotoxic effects of calcineurin inhibitors post transplant are minimized by addition of renal-sparing immunosuppression (mycophenolate mofetil or sirolimus)
Nutritional	Height, weight, skinfold thickness, mid-arm circumference
	Optimal nutritional support pre transplant is essential to improve post-transplant outcomes
Vascular	Doppler ultrasound to assess vascular anatomy
	Axial imaging in selected patients with anomalous vascular anatomy
Infection immune status	Hepatitis A, B, C, E
	EBV, CMV
	Herpes simplex, varicella zoster, measles
	Human immunodeficiency virus
	Adenovirus, toxoplasmosis
Immunization	All routine vaccinations should be administered prior to transplantation
	In addition, varicella, hepatitis A and B, influenza (inactivated) should be given
	Live vaccines are not given post transplant
Dental	Optimal dental hygiene is recommended for patients going on to long-term immunosuppression
Social	Patient/family meets with the social work team to identify potential social, financial, and medical burdens of a liver transplant and to aim to formulate a plan prior to transplant
Psychology	Patient/family meets with a clinical psychologist to identify any psychosocial stressors which may interact with the transplant process and to enable the appropriate support to be put in place
Pharmacy	Patient/family meets with the pharmacist to discuss optimization of medications prior to transplant and the benefits and side effects of medications post transplant
Education	Education for the patient/family is a key part of pre-transplant assessment, and will be discussed by the members of the multidisciplinary team, led by the transplant coordinators. The importance of medication compliance, recognition of complications, and follow-up post transplant are key issues

Types of liver transplantation

Liver transplantation can either be from a deceased or a living donor. The liver from a deceased donor can be obtained after brainstem death (DBD) or from a donor after cardiac death (DCD). Both donor and recipient should be ABO compatible, but preferably an identical ABO is used. HLA typing is not routinely used in paediatric transplantation.

Whole liver transplantation

The deceased liver is removed and replaced by a donor liver. The hepatic artery, portal vein, and hepatic vein are then anastomosed to their corresponding structure. The bile duct is usually anastomosed to a Roux-en-Y loop created from the small bowel. It is relatively uncommon in children <5 years of age.

Partial liver graft transplantation

The use of partial liver grafts was the solution to both organ shortage and size restriction in transplanting young children. Hence, surgical techniques have been developed to reduce the size of an adult liver to fit within the morphological restrictions of a paediatric recipient.

- Reduced liver transplantation—the donor liver can be cut down to provide smaller grafts, based on the segmental anatomy of the liver. Patients as small as 2.5kg may be transplanted with the use of a monosegmental graft.
- Split graft transplantation—the donor liver is divided and shared between two recipients. The smaller left lateral segment or left lobe usually goes to a paediatric recipient and the larger right lobe to an adult.

Living related transplantation

The mortality of patients on waiting lists for deceased donor transplantation has led to techniques involving living donor transplantation. This involves transplanting the left lateral segment of a family member (usually a parent) into the child. Potential donors are rigorously screened to assess their suitability for donation. Good graft and recipient survival figures are seen with living donation; however, there is a small risk of donor morbidity and mortality.

Auxiliary transplantation

Auxiliary transplantation is the implantation of a donor partial or whole liver graft, while retaining all or part of the native liver. This can be an effective technique for acute liver failure and selected non-cirrhotic liver-based metabolic disorders. The key aim is to provide sufficient functioning liver mass to allow for native liver recovery in acute liver failure and to provide adequate metabolic function in metabolic disorders. Liver regeneration occurs in the majority of acute liver failure patients and immunosuppression may be withdrawn in two-thirds of long-term survivors

Hepatocyte transplantation

Hepatocyte transplantation is an alternative or bridge to transplantation in a select group of children with non-cirrhotic liver-based metabolic disorders and acute liver failure. This technique involves the infusion of isolated hepatocytes, preferably into the portal venous system, but alternative sites are the spleen and the peritoneal cavity. The injected hepatocytes aim to integrate into the liver plates and repopulate the recipient liver. The donated cells are maintained by immunosuppression. There is accumulating promising experience for clinical hepatocyte transplantation and further research to improve this technique continues.

Initial post-transplant management

All liver transplant recipients are admitted to the paediatric intensive care unit and monitored very closely in the immediate post-transplant period (see Table 71.3).

Table 71.3 Initial post-transplant management

Respiratory	Patients return from the operating theatre ventilated. Early extubation is preferred if USS Doppler scan within normal limits and no other contraindications
Cardiovascular	It is essential to maintain good central venous pressure and blood pressure.
	Blood transfusions are avoided post transplant due to the risk of haemoconcentration and thrombosis
Fluids	IV fluids are initially restricted to 2/3 of the daily maintenance fluid allowance. Intravascular sufficiency is measured by central venous pressure (5–6mmHg) and urine output (>1mL/kg/hour)
Infection	All patients receive broad-spectrum antibiotics (piptazobactem and gentamicin). Selected high-risk patients should receive prophylactic antifungals
	Patients who are CMV naive who receive a liver from a CMV-positive donor are treated with a 2-week course of IV ganciclovir
Standard immunosuppression (see Table 71.4)	Methylprednisolone: 10mg/kg in theatre followed by 2mg/kg per day (max. dose 60 mg) the day after transplant for 5 days. Thereafter doses are weaned to a maintenance dose of approx. 0.1mg/kg oral prednisolone (rounded to 1mg, 2.5mg, or 5mg)
	Calcineurin inhibitor: tacrolimus is preferred over ciclosporin due to a lower side effect profile and lower level of steroid resistant rejection and chronic rejection. It is started on the first day of transplant (0.15 mg/kg/day) and the doses are adjusted according to trough monitoring levels.
	Renal sparing: renal-sparing immunosuppressive agent (e.g. mycophenolate mofetil) may be commenced soon after transplant to reduce tacrolimus-induced toxicity in patients with renal dysfunction. Induction therapy with anti-IL2 antibody, basiliximab, can also be considered

Tacrolimus levels are described in Table 71.4.

Table 71.4 Tacrolimus levels

Time post-transplant	Trough level (ng/L)
0–3 months	10–12
3 months–1 year	5–8
1 year on	3–5

Post-transplant complications

Surgical

Primary non-function of the graft (PNF; 2%)

- PNF presents as haemodynamic instability, metabolic acidosis, coagulopathy, and rising liver transaminases.
- Mortality is high. Treatment is emergency re-transplantation.

Postoperative bleeding (5–10%)

- Correction of coagulopathy or thrombocytopenia will often lead to haemostasis or else, exploratory laparotomy may be needed.

Hepatic artery thrombosis (HAT; 5–10%)

- Early HAT may result in ischaemia of the graft. Early recognition and immediate surgical revascularization may salvage the graft.
- If too late for surgical intervention, patient is monitored carefully to ensure sufficient collateral arterial supply.

Portal vein thrombosis (PVT; 5%)

- PVT can present with transaminitis, INR prolongation, gastrointestinal bleeding, and signs of portal hypertension.
- Early surgical intervention to restore portal venous flow will usually rescue the graft.

Risk factors for HAT and PVT include hypercoagulability, elevated haematocrit, severe acute rejection, small vessel size, whole graft transplantation, and surgical technique.

Biliary complications (5–30%)

- Bile leaks may occur from the anastomosis or cut surface of a partial graft and can present insidiously with fever or mild graft dysfunction. Biliary strictures usually occur at the anastomosis and can present with cholestasis, cholangitis, or features of biliary obstruction on liver function tests or histology.
- Endoscopic or percutaneous cholangiography and stenting (for leak) and balloon dilatation ± stenting (for stricture) usually lead to resolution. Surgical reconstruction may be required if these procedures do not succeed.

Caval obstruction

- Caval complications are rare. Percutaneous venous angioplasty and stenting have good results.

Intestinal complications

- Bowel perforation and diaphragmatic herniae are rare complications.

Rejection

Acute cellular rejection (ACR)

- 50–75% of patients have an episode of ACR in the first 3 months after transplant, despite immunosuppression. The rate is lower in infants.
- ACR is detected by a rise in the blood levels of aspartate and alanine transaminases (AST, ALT). Doppler USS is performed and diagnosis is confirmed on liver biopsy.

- Treatment is with 3 days of methylprednisolone (10mg/kg/day) followed by weaning oral prednisolone (initial dose 2mg/kg/day; max. dose 60mg).
- 75% of patients are steroid responsive. If steroid non-responsive, immunosuppressive treatment may be escalated with additional agents:
  - Monoclonal antibodies (e.g. basiliximab).
  - Adjuvant agents (e.g. mycophenolate mofetil, sirolimus).
  - Anti-lymphocyte agents (antithymocyte globulin; ATG).

Chronic rejection
- Chronic rejection presents as cholestatic liver disease. It presents in 5% of patients.
- Histological features include loss of bile ducts and graft arteriopathy.
- Treatment guidelines are not fully defined and re-transplantation rates are high. Some grafts can be rescued with adjuvant immunosuppressive agents (e.g. sirolimus, mycophenolate mofetil).

Immunosuppression

All patients should be monitored for possible complications of immunosuppression (see Table 71.5).

Post-transplant lymphoproliferative disorder

- PTLD is characterized by uncontrolled proliferation of lymphoid lineage cells (typically B cells), usually in association with EBV infection, in the context of post-transplant immunosuppression.
- It affects 5% of children by the first year post transplant.
- PTLD represents a spectrum of disorders ranging from benign hyperplasia to high-grade lymphoma.
- Risk factors include young age (<5 years old), EBV-naive transplant recipients, high-level immunosuppression.
- There is no pathognomonic symptom for PTLD, but a high level of suspicion should be held if there are any of the following; lymphadenopathy, unexplained fever, unexplained anaemia, gastrointestinal symptoms including microscopic or macroscopic blood in stool, high EBV viral load, high lactate dehydrogenase.
- Diagnosis of PTLD is histological. Lymphadenopathy requires radiological assessment (CT chest, abdomen) and subsequent lymph node biopsy. If gastrointestinal symptoms, upper and lower gastrointestinal endoscopies with biopsies should be performed. If bone marrow involvement, biopsy ± trephine should be considered and if neurological involvement, a lumbar puncture may be needed.
- Treatment is dependent on the grade/severity of histological disease:
  - Reduction or cessation of immunosuppression is first-line therapy.
  - Immunotherapy with anti-CD20 monoclonal antibody (rituximab) and chemotherapy are therapeutic modalities.
  - Antiviral agents (e.g. ganciclovir) may be considered.
  - Careful monitoring for graft rejection while on no/reduced immunosuppression.

Table 71.5 Immunosuppressants: mechanisms and possible complications

Drug	Mechanism	Complications
Prednisolone	Multiple	Acute: hypertension Hyperglycaemia Psychosis
Tacrolimus	Calcineurin inhibitor IL2 gene transcription inhibitor	Hypertension Hyerglycaemia Renal impairment Neurotoxicity PTLD
Ciclosporin	Calcineurin inhibitor IL2 gene transcription inhibitor	Hirsutism Gingival hyperplasia PTLD
*Sirolimus	IL2 post receptor signalTransduction inhibition	Hyperlipidaemia Leucopenia Thrombocytopenia Poor wound healing Hepatic artery thrombosis
Basiliximab*/**	Anti-IL-2 antibody	Infections PTLD
Mycophenolate mofetil*	Purine synthesis inhibitor	Bone marrow suppression Gastrointestinal
Azathioprine	Antimetabolite of DNA and RNA synthesis	Bone marrow suppression Hepatotoxic
Anti-thymoglobulin**	Anti-T-cell antibody	Allergic reaction Infections PTLD

* Renal-sparing immunosuppressive agent.

** Rescue therapy

Infection

Patients on immunosuppression are at increased risk of infections, often presenting as fever, and raised transaminases:

- CMV: this is the commonest early transplant viral infection. The highest risk patients are those who are CMV naïve at the time of transplant and receive a CMV-positive graft. These patients are treated with prophylactic ganciclovir for 14 days.
- EBV: see details for PTLD.
- Hepatitis E: there has been a recent emergence of hepatitis E post-transplant; antiviral agents (e.g. ribavirin) should be considered.
- Adenovirus: this can be treated with antivirals if severe, disseminated.

- Varicella: patients who are varicella IgG negative and have a significant contact with primary or secondary varicella infection should receive IV immunoglobulin within 3 days of contact. Oral aciclovir has also been shown to be of prophylactic benefit. If patients develop clinical illness, IV aciclovir or oral valganciclovir should be given until the illness has resolved.
- Herpes simplex: patients in contact with herpes simplex or who develop clinical illness can respond to antiviral treatment.
- Fungal: fungal infections should be considered in all post-transplant patients not responding to antimicrobial treatment.

Renal function

Renal dysfunction is common and multifactorial in liver transplantation. Risk factors include:
- Calcineurin inhibitors.
- Hypertension.
- Suboptimal fluid management.
- Pre-existing renal dysfunction.

Management includes optimizing fluid intake, reduction of calcineurin inhibitor dosing, and/or addition of renal-sparing immunosuppression and treatment of hypertension.

Hypertension

Hypertension occurs in 10–20% of patients post transplantation and is multifactorial. Risk factors include:
- Corticosteroids.
- Calcineurin inhibitors.
- Renal impairment.

First-line management includes calcium channel antagonists (amlodipine, nifedipine).

Haematology

Bone marrow suppression post transplant may represent immunosuppressant side effects, hypersplenism, infection, or immune-mediated effects.

Skin malignancy

The risk of all types of cutaneous malignancy is increased. All post-transplant patients are advised skin protection.

De novo autoimmune liver disease

- Development of autoimmune liver disease occurs in 2–5% of liver transplant recipients, irrespective of initial diagnosis.
- It is characterized by elevated liver transaminases and the presence of autoantibodies (anti-nuclear, smooth muscle, liver kidney microsomal).
- Treatment includes long-term prednisolone.

Quality of life and growth

Although patient and graft survival after liver transplantation has improved, children can continue to exhibit chronic health problems throughout their life. Health-related quality of life (HrQoL) in children has been reported from multicentre studies, using standardized tools. Data demonstrates lower physical and psychosocial functioning compared to matched peers but equivalent functioning to children with other chronic conditions. HrQoL depends on multiple factors, such as graft function and post-transplant complications.

Liver transplant recipients exhibit catch-up growth after transplantation. Most patients achieve normal height after transplant, except patients with syndromes associated with poor growth, e.g. Alagille syndrome and PFIC1 disease. Successful liver transplantation is not associated with pubertal delay.

References and resources

Kohli R, Cerisuelo MC, Heaton N, Dhawan A. Liver transplantation in children: state of the art and future perspectives. Arch Dis Child 2018;103:192–8.
NHS Blood and Transplant: http://www.nhsbt.nhs.uk

Index

A

Aagenaes syndrome 475, 478
abdominal
    migraine 342, 343
abdominal pain
    acute 335
    functional 342, 343
    recurrent 339–54
abdominal tuberculosis 379
abdominal wall defects 3
abetalipoproteinaemia 297
abscess, liver 555–6
achalasia 225–7
acid suppressors 252
acidosis 512
acute cellular
    rejection 138–9, 638–9
acute gastroenteritis, see gastroenteritis
acute liver failure 601–17
    adrenal suppression 615
    aetiology 604–8
    coagulopathy 613
    complications 612–15
    definition 602
    drug-induced 488, 606–7
    haemodynamics 614
    infection 613
    liver support system 616
    liver transplantation 616
    metabolic derangement 615
    metabolic disease 508–10, 605, 608
    neurological complications 612
    nutrition 592–5
    pancreatitis 615
    prognosis 615
    renal function 614
    therapy 610
adalimumab 392–3
adefovir 542
adenomas 292, 294
adolescent rumination syndrome 242
adrenal suppression 615
adrenaline injection 162
adrenoleucodystrophy, neonatal 510
Alagille
    syndrome 467–72, 599
alanine aminotransferase (ALT) 438
albumin 438

alkaline phosphatase (ALP) 438
allergen 158
allergy, definition 158
    See also food allergy
alpha-1 antitrypsin deficiency 463–6
aluminium hydroxide 253
Amanita phalloides 607
5-aminosalicylic acid derivatives 389–90
aminotransferases 438
ammonia 438
amoebiasis 560
co-amoxiclav 492
amylopectin 166
amylose 166
anaemia
    iron deficiency 72
    pernicious 79
anal fissure 289, 372
ankyloglossia 45
anorectal malformations 10
anorectal manometry 360
anorexia nervosa 146–7
anthropometry 12, 36–7, 590
antibody-mediated rejection 139
anti-HBc IgG 538, 539
anti-HBc IgM 538, 539
anti-HBe 538, 539
anti-HBs 538, 539
anti-HCV 547
antineoplastic drugs 492
antioxidants 527
anti-thymoglobulin 640
anti-tumour necrosis factor therapy
    Crohn's diseases 392–3
    ulcerative colitis 412
antivirals 542–3, 548–9
antral gastritis 260–1, 262
anus, imperforate 10
appendicitis 337
appetite 153
ascariasis 561
ascites
    chronic liver disease 575
    chylous 599
    liver biopsy 441
    neonatal 511
aspartate aminotransferase (AST) 438

aspiration, enteral feeding 102
aspirin 492
atopy 158
autoimmune enteropathy 127, 299
autoimmune hepatitis 503, 607, 608
autoimmune hepatitis/sclerosing cholangitis overlap syndrome 504
autoimmune liver disease 499–504, 641
autoimmune pancreatitis 435
avoidant-restrictive food intake disorder 149
azathioprine
    Crohn's disease 390
    drug-induced liver injury 492
    mechanisms and complications 640
    ulcerative colitis 411–12

B

bacterial gastroenteritis 237, 238
bacterial overgrowth 129, 332–3
bacterial peritonitis 576
bacterial sepsis 554–7
Bannayan–Riley–Ruvalcaba syndrome 293
bariatric surgery 197
barium radiology 246
Barrett's oesophagus 254
basal metabolic rate 22
basiliximab 640
battery ingestion 273
Behçet syndrome 379
beriberi 78
bile acid synthesis defect 510
bile salt export pump deficiency 475, 477, 478–9, 484
biliary atresia 459–62, 598
biliary diversion 482–3
bilirubin 448
binge eating disorder 148
biopsychosocial model of pain 344
biotin
    deficiency 79
    recommended intake 87

bisacodyl 365
blenderized feeds 177
blind loop
    syndrome 332–3
body composition 37
body mass index (BMI) 12,
    37, 192
Boix-Ochoa score 246
borreliosis 558
bottle-feeding 48–50
bowel obstruction, distal 7
bowel transit studies 360
breast engorgement 41
breast milk jaundice 450
breastfeeding 39–45
    benefits 40
    common problems 41
    contraindications 43
    poor weight gain 41
    positions 42
    promotion 44
    successful 42
    tongue tie 45
    WHO
        recommendations 40
BRIC1/BRIC2 477
brucellosis 557
buffering agents 253
bulimia nervosa 148
bulking agents 363
butterfly vertebrae 468
button
    gastrostomy 96, 187

C
C-13 breath test 260–1
calciferol 79–80
calcium
    deficiency 82
    neonates 58
    recommended intake 24
calories 22
capillary refill time 234
carbamazepine 492
carbohydrate
    intolerance 165–71
    diagnosis 170
    fructose intolerance/mal-
        absorption 169, 605
    glucose–galactose malab-
        sorption 169, 297
    hypolactasia/lactose
        intolerance 168,
        320
    post-gastroenteritis
        101, 239
    sucrase–isomaltase
        deficiency 168,
        170, 308
carbohydrates
    dietary 166

digestion 167
metabolism in chronic
    liver disease 571
ceftriaxone 492
cerebral oedema 612
cerebral palsy 257
cholangitis
    bacterial 556
    neonatal sclerosing 477
    neonatal sclerosing with
        ichthyosis 477
cholecalciferol 79–80
cholestasis
    benign recurrent 477,
        480, 484
    drug-associated 481
    infantile 477, 509–10
    pathophysiology 478–9
    pregnancy 477, 480
    progressive familial
        intrahepatic 475, 477,
        478, 598
    progressive
        intrahepatic 480
    pruritus 483
    sepsis-induced 554
chromium deficiency 84
chronic constipation, see
    constipation
chronic granulomatous
    disease 379
chronic idiopathic intestinal
    pseudo-obstruction 126
chronic liver disease
    570–72, 574, 577–78,
    580–82
    ascites 575
    cirrhosis 570
    cirrhotic
        cardiomyopathy 580
    coagulopathy 574
    endocrine
        dysfunction 582
    growth failure 571
    hepatic
        encephalopathy 572–3
    hepatic
        osteodystrophy 581
    hepatopulmonary
        syndrome 578
    hepatorenal
        syndrome 577
    malnutrition 571, 585
    nutritional manage-
        ment 584, 586–8
    portopulmonary
        hypertension 578–9
    pruritus 580
    pulmonary
        complications 578–9
    spontaneous bacterial
        peritonitis 576

chronic rejection 139, 639
chylous ascites 599
ciclosporin 492, 640
ciliopathies 477
cirrhosis 570
cirrhotic
    cardiomyopathy 580
CLO test 261
cloacal anomaly 10
Clonorchis sinensis 562
Clostridium difficile
    232
coagulopathy
    acute liver failure 613
    chronic liver disease 574
    conjugated hyperbilirubin-
        aemia 456
cobalt deficiency 84
coeliac disease 312
    coeliac crisis 314
    compliance to diet 329
    diagnosis 318, 319
    follow-up 322
    gluten challenge
        321, 325
    gluten-free diet 320,
        324, 326–7
    gluten-free products 327
    growth faltering 69
    high-risk screening 314
    HLA testing 316
    investigations 316
    monitoring 328
    non-GI
        manifestations 315
    nutritional
        management 323–9
    oat consumption 326–7
    predisposing
        conditions 315
    prescribable foods 327
    presentation 314
    serology 316
    small bowel biopsy 316
    support group (Coeliac
        UK) 322, 327
    treatment 320
colitis 376
    acute toxic 408–10
    distal 411
    eosinophilic 421
    indeterminate 376
    infectious 289
    See also ulcerative colitis
complementary
    feeding 51
compound alginates 252
congenital anomalies 1–10
congenital chloride
    diarrhoea 297
congenital disorders of
    glycosylation 509

congenital
  hypopituitarism 509–10
congenital
  hypothyroidism 509–10
congenital microvillus
  atrophy 298
congenital sodium
  diarrhoea 297
congenital syphilis 558
congenital
  toxoplasmosis 562
conjugated hyperbiliru-
  binaemia 452–6, 598
constipation 355–70
  clinical assessment 359
  definition 356
  differential diagnosis 358
  disimpaction 363–4
  enemas 366
  examination 359
  functional 358
  history 359
  investigation 360
  laxatives 363,
    364, 365
  management 362
  outcome 368
  PACCT group
    terminology 356, 357
  pathogenesis 358
  pharmacotherapy 196,
    363, 364
  red flags 369
copper deficiency 84
corticosteroids 389
cow milk challenge 162
cow milk protein
  allergy 160–1
Cowden syndrome 293
Coxiella burnetii 559
Creon® 212
Crigler–Najjar (type I/II)
  451
Crohn's disease 376, 382
  5-aminosalicylic acid
    derivatives 389–90
  anti-TNF therapy 392–3
  azathioprine 390
  clinical course 386
  clinical features 382
  complications 385
  corticosteroids 389
  exclusive enteral
    nutrition 388–9,
    398, 400–1
  extraintestinal
    manifestations 385
  food reintroduction
    403
  growth failure
    69, 385
  investigation 384

management 388–91
  methotrexate 390–1
  monitoring 402
  nutritional
    requirements 399
  nutritional status 398
  nutritional support 404
  oesophagitis 393
  oral disease 393
  perianal 393
  presenting symptoms 382
  refeeding 402
  remission 389–91
  surgery 393
cyclical vomiting
  syndrome 263–6
cyclical vomiting syndrome
  plus 264
cystic fibrosis 202
  distal intestinal obstruc-
    tion syndrome
    204–5
  enteral feeding 210
  growth assessment 208
  intestinal disease
    204–5
  liver disease 215–19
  management of
    gastrointestinal
    symptoms 206
  meconium ileus 7,
    204–5
  nutrition 208–11
  nutritional
    supplements 210
  pancreatic disease 204
  pancreatic enzyme
    replacement
    therapy 212
  sodium deficiency 211
  vitamins 210–11

D

D-lactic acidosis 332–3
DCDC2
  defects 477, 478
dehydration 234, 235
DeMeester score 246
diarrhoea
  chronic 239, 301–6
  chronic non-specific
    306
  congenital chloride 297
  congenital sodium 297
  enteral feeding 102
  factitious 306
  intractable 295–9
  osmotic 296
  phenotypic 298
  secretory 296
  toddler's 306

dietary protein-induced
  enterocolitis of
  infancy 420
dietary protein-induced
  proctocolitis of
  infancy 418–19
dietary reference
  value 22–3, 34
dietary supplements 490
distal bowel obstruction 7
distal colitis 411
distal intestinal obstruction
  syndrome 204–5
domperidone 253
drug-induced
  cholestasis 481
drug-induced liver
  injury 487–98
  acute liver
    failure 488, 606–7
  cholestatic 491
  clinical features 490–1
  cytotoxic 489
  epidemiology 488
  hepatocellular 491
  herbal and dietary
    supplements 490
  immune-mediated 489
  investigation 494
  management 496
  mixed hepatocellular-
    cholestatic 491
  pathophysiology 489
  prevention 498
  prognosis 498
drug-induced
  pancreatitis 428–9
dumping syndrome 103
duodenal atresia 6
duodenal haematoma 275
duodenal juice
  culture 332–3
duodenal
  ulcer 260–1, 262
dyspepsia,
  functional 342, 343

E

eating disorders 143–50
  anorexia nervosa 146–7
  avoidant-restrictive food
    intake disorder 149
  binge eating disorder 148
  bulimia nervosa 148
echinococcosis 561
elemental iron 73
embryology 2
Emerade® 162
encopresis 356
endocrine
  dysfunction 582

endoscopy 269–76
  bowel preparation 274
  chronic diarrhoea 305
  complications 275
  contraindications 274
  diagnostic 272
  duodenal
    haematoma 275
  environment 271
  equipment 271
  food bolus
    impaction 273
  foreign bodies 273
  gastrointestinal
    bleeding 284–5
  Helicobacter pylori
    261
  indications 272–3
  infection risk 275
  perforation risk 275
  safety 275
  surveillance 272
  therapeutic
    272, 623
energy
  balance 22
  estimated average
    requirement 24
  increasing intake 155
  metabolism 22
  neonatal intake 58
Entamoeba histolytica 560
entecavir 543
enteral nutrition 93–104
  access routes 96–8
  aspiration 102
  bolus feeding 101
  complications 102
  continuous feeding 101
  Crohn's disease 388–9,
    398, 400–1
  cystic fibrosis 210
  diarrhoea 102
  gastrostomies 96, 178
  hygiene 101
  jejunal feeding 101
  jejunostomies 96
  liquid feed composition
    and choice 100–1
  medicine
    administration 98
  nasogastric
    tubes 96, 97, 98
  premature
    newborn 56–7
  regurgitation 102
  See also tube feeding
enterocolitis
  eosinophilic 420
  Hirschsprung-associated 9
eosinophilic disorders 416
  colitis 421

enterocolitis of
  infancy 420
  gastritis 421
  gastroenterocolitis 421
  gastroenteropathies 421
  oesophagitis 256,
    421, 422
  proctitis 289
  proctocolitis of
    infancy 418–19
EPHX1 deficiency 477
EpiPen® 162
ergocalciferol 79–80
erythrocyte
  protoporphyrin 72
erythromycin 492
Escherichia coli O157
  infection 239
estimated average requirement 22–3, 24, 34
exomphalos 3

F

faddy eating 153
faecal A1-antitrypsin 304
faecal calprotectin
  304, 384
faecal elastase 304
faecal incontinence 357
failure to thrive 67–70
familial adenomatous
  polyposis coli 294
familial intrahepatic
  cholestatic
  syndromes 473–84
  biliary diversion 482–3
  definition 474
  epidemiology 476
  liver transplantation 483
  management 482–4
  natural history 481
  nomenclature 475
  pathophysiology 478–9
  presentation 480
Fasciola hepatica 561
fat
  malabsorption 571
  neonatal intake 58
fatty acid oxidation
  disorders 508–9
feeding history 35
feeding problems
  breastfeeding 41
  young children 154
FibroScan® 217
fluconazole 492
fluids, normal
  requirements 24
fluoride deficiency 84
focal nodular
  hyperplasia 567

folic acid
  deficiency 81
  recommended intake 87
follow-on milks 50
food allergy 157–64, 423
  adrenaline injection 162
  cow milk protein 160–1
  definitions 158
  diagnosis 160–2
  food challenge 161
  IgE-mediated
    reactions 158, 159
  management 160–2
  non-IgE
    reactions 158, 159
  oral allergy
    syndrome 159
  prevention 161
  pseudo-intolerance/
    allergy 161
food bolus
  impaction 273
food challenge 161
food refusal 152, 154
foreign bodies 273
formula feed 48
  number and volume of
    feeds 49
  types of 50
  WHO International Code
    of Marketing Breast
    milk Substitutes 44
Francisella tularensis 557
frenotomy 45
fructosaemia 509–10
fructose 166
  intolerance/malabsorp-
    tion 169, 605
functional abdominal
  pain 342, 343
functional constipation 358
functional
  dyspepsia 342, 343
functional faecal
  incontinence 357
fungal liver infections 559

G

galactosaemia 508–9,
  605, 608
gallstones 130
gamma-glutamyl transferase
  (GGT) 438
Gardener syndrome 294
gastric ulcer 260–1, 262
gastritis
  antral 260–1, 262
  eosinophilic 421
gastroenteritis 229–40
  aetiology 230
  antibiotics 237

assessment 234, 235
bacterial 230, 231
carbohydrate intolerance after 239, 308
clinical features 231
complications 239
dehydration 234, 235
differential diagnosis 232
feeding 237
hospital admission 236
investigations 236
management 236, 237
oral rehydration solutions 236–7
parasitic 230
pathogenesis 230
post-enteritis syndrome 239, 305, 308, 317, 318
prevention 238
probiotics 237
rehydration 236–7
starvation 237
stool samples 236
viral 230, 231
gastroenterocolitis, eosinophilic 421
gastrointestinal bleeding 277–90
assessment 280–1
differential diagnosis 288–9
endoscopy 284–5
examination 282
history 280–1
imaging 284
investigation 284–5
lower 286, 289
obscure 279
portal hypertension 619
rectal 278, 279, 294
resuscitation 280
upper 279, 285, 288
gastrointestinal endoscopy, see endoscopy
gastrointestinal polyposis 289, 291
gastro-oesophageal reflux 244
assessment 244
Barrett's oesophagus 254
cerebral palsy 257
differential diagnosis 244
investigation 246–8
management 244, 250
milk exclusion 250
obstructive apnoea 244
pharmacotherapy 252–3

physiological reflux 244
respiratory disease 244
sleeping position 250
surgical treatment 253–4
symptoms and signs 243
gastro-oesophageal reflux disease 242
neurodisability 177
gastro-oesophageal scintigraphy 247
gastroschisis 3, 126
gastrostomies 96, 178–88
Gaucher type II 511
Gaviscon® Infant 252
Giardia lamblia 232
Gilbert syndrome 450
glucose 166
malabsorption 239
glucose–galactose malabsorption 169, 297
gluten challenge 321, 325
gluten-free diet 320, 324, 326–7
glycogen storage disease type IV/VI 510
glycosylation disorders 509
GM1 gangliosidosis 511
granulomatous hepatitis 564
growth
charts 12–13, 14–19
factors influencing 69
faltering 67–70
normal 13
potential 12
rate 12–13
velocity 12
growth hormone–insulin-like growth factor-1 axis 571

H

haemangiomata, infantile 566
haematemesis 279
haematochezia 279
haematoma, duodenal 275
haemochromatosis, neonatal 508–9, 605–6, 608
haemolysis 450
haemolytic uraemic syndrome 239
haemophagocytic lympho-histiocytosis 508–9, 607–8
haemoptysis 279
haemostatic spray 624
hamartomas 292, 293, 567

Harvoni® 548
HBeAg 538, 539
HBsAG 538, 539
HBV DNA 538, 539
HCV RNA 547
head circumference measurement 36, 590
normal growth 13
height
estimation 12, 175
measurement 36, 590
Helicobacter pylori 260–1
Henoch–Schönlein purpura 338
hepatic amoebiasis 560
hepatic artery thrombosis 638
hepatic encephalop-athy 572–3, 612
hepatic osteodystrophy 581
hepatic venous pressure gradient 620
hepatitis
autoimmune 502–3, 607, 608
autoimmune/sclerosing cholangitis overlap syndrome 504
granulomatous 564
hypoxic 554–7
idiopathic neonatal 458
hepatitis A 604–5
hepatitis B 535–44
acute 537, 539
acute liver failure 604–5
antivirals 542–3
chronic 537, 539, 542–3
clinical features 537
complications 540
epidemiology 536
immunoprophylaxis 541
postexposure prophylaxis 541
prevention 541
serology 538, 539
transmission 537
hepatitis C 545–50
antivirals 548–9
chronic 547
clinical features 547
diagnosis in infants born to infected mothers 547
epidemiology 546
management 548–9
subtypes 546
transfusion-acquired 547
transmission risk 546
viral tests 547
hepatitis E 604–5
hepatoblastoma 568

hepatocellular
   carcinoma 484, 568
hepatocyte
   transplantation 616, 635
hepatopulmonary
   syndrome 578
hepatorenal syndrome 577
heterotaxy 4–5
Hirschsprung
   disease 8–9, 289
histamine H₂ receptor
   blockers 252
HLA testing 316
hydatid disease 561
hydrogen breath
   test 305, 332–3
hyperammo-
   naemia 511, 517
hyperbilirubinaemia
   conjugated 452–6, 598
   unconjugated 448, 450–1
hypernatraemic
   dehydration 234
hyperplastic
   polyps 292, 294
hypersensitivity 158
hypogonadism 582
hypolactasia 168
hypopituitarism 509–10
hypothyroidism 509–10, 582

idiopathic neonatal
   hepatitis 458
IgA deficiency 317
IgG antibody test 260–1
immunodeficiency,
   diarrhoea 309
immunosuppression
   intestinal
      transplantation 137
   liver transplantation 640
imperforate anus 10
incontinence, faecal 357
indeterminate colitis 376
infantile
   cholestasis 477, 509–10
infantile
   haemangiomata 566
infantile hypertrophic pyloric stenosis 268
infantile Refsum disease 510
infection
   catheter-related 114–15, 129
   colitis 289
   complication of acute
      liver failure 613
   endoscopy 275
   inflammatory bowel
      disease 378
   intestinal transplant 139

liver transplant 640–1
   See also liver infections
inflammatory bowel disease
   diagnostic work-up 385
   differential diagnosis
      378
   infective 378
   non-infective 378
   perianal involvement
      374
   unclassified 376
   very early onset 299
   See also Crohn's disease;
      ulcerative colitis
inflammatory
   polyps 284–5, 292
infliximab 412, 492
insulin resistance 523, 521
interferon 542, 549
intestinal epithelial
   dysplasia 127
intestinal failure 121–32
   -associated liver dis-
      ease 115–16,
      129, 599
   complications 129–30
   management 128
   mucosal
      disorders 122, 127
   neurodisability 190
   neuromuscular motility
      disorders 122, 126
   short bowel
      syndrome 122, 124–5
   surgery 128
intestinal lymphangiectasia
   309
intestinal transplantation
   133–42
   acute cellular
      rejection 138–9
   antibody-mediated
      rejection 139
   chronic rejection 139
   combined liver
      intestine 136
   complications 138–40
   contraindi-
      cations 132, 135
   immunosuppression 137
   indications 132, 135
   infection 139
   isolated intestinal 136
   malignancy 140
   modified
      multivisceral 136
   multivisceral 136
   nomenclature 135
   nutrition 137
   outcomes 142
   postoperative
      management 137

quality of life 140
intolerance 158
intracranial
   hypertension 612
intrauterine growth
   retardation 20
intussusception 289, 338
iodine deficiency 84
IPEX syndrome 299
iron
   deficiency 71–4, 84
   medication
      (elemental) 73
   neonates 58
   recommended intake 24
irritable bowel syn-
   drome 306, 342, 343
ischaemic injury 607
isomaltose 166
isoniazid 492
isovaleric acidaemia 512

J

jaundice 445–58
   bacterial sepsis 554–7
   breast milk 450
   breastfeeding 41
   conjugated
      hyperbilirubina-
         emia 452–6, 598
   epidemiology 446
   haemolysis 450
   physiological 450
   unconjugated
      hyperbiliru-
         binaemia 448,
         450–1
jejunal feeding 101
jejuno-ileal atresia 6
jejunostomies 96
juice drinking,
   excessive 154
juvenile polyposis 293
juvenile polyps 293

K

keratomalacia 78
ketosis 512
kwashiorkor 27

L

lactose-free
   diet 320, 326–7
lactose intolerance
   168, 308
lactulose 365
Ladd's procedure 4–5
lamivudine 542
lansoprazole 252

laxatives 363, 364, 365
length
  measurement 36, 590
  normal growth 13
leptospirosis 558
leukaemia 608
liquid paraffin 365
listeriosis 557
liver abscess 555–6
liver biopsy 439–44
  ascites 441
  clotting abnormalities 441
  complications 443
  contraindications 441
  indications 440
  laparoscopy/
    laparotomy 443
  metabolic liver
    disease 514–15
  monitoring 443
  non-alcoholic fatty liver
    disease 522
  percutaneous 443
  post-biopsy care 444
  preparation 442
  transjugular 443
liver disease
  alpha-1 antitrypsin
    deficiency 464, 466
  autoimmune 499–504,
    641
  chronic (see chronic liver
    disease)
  cystic fibrosis 215–19
  intestinal failure-
    associated 115–16,
    129, 599
  malnutrition 571, 585
  metabolic (see metabolic
    liver disease)
  non-alcoholic fatty liver
    (see non-alcoholic
    fatty liver disease)
  nutritional assessment
    and monitoring 590
  nutritional
    management 583–99
  Wilson disease 530
liver failure (see acute liver
  failure)
liver function tests 437–8
liver infections 552
  bacterial 554–7
  fungal 559
  granuloma 564
  parasitic 560–2
  rickettsial 559
  spirochaetal 558
liver
  transplantation 629–42
  acute cellular
    rejection 638–9

acute liver failure 616
  auxiliary 616, 634
  biliary
    complications 638
  bone marrow
    suppression 641
  chronic rejection 639
  combined liver
    intestine 136
  complications 638–41
  contraindications 630
  cystic fibrosis 218
  de novo autoimmune liver
    disease 641
  donor ABO
    compatibility 634–5
  familial intrahepatic
    cholestatic
    syndromes 483
  growth 642
  hepatic artery
    thrombosis 638
  hepatocyte transplant-
    ation 616, 635
  hypertension 641
  immunosuppressants
    640
  indications 630
  infection risk 640–1
  intestinal
    complications 638
  living related 634
  nutrition 596
  partial 634
  portal vein
    thrombosis 638
  postoperative
    bleeding 638
  post-transplant
    lymphoproliferative
    disorder 639
  post-transplant
    management 636
  pre-transplant
    assessment 632, 633
  primary non-function of
    graft 638
  quality of life 642
  renal dysfunction 641
  skin malignancy 641
  split graft 634
  survival rates 631
  timing 630
  whole liver 634
  Wilson disease 534
liver tumours 565–8
Looser's zones 80
lower gastrointestinal
  bleeding 286, 289
lubricants 363
Lyme disease 558
lymphoma 608

M

McBurney's point 337
magnesium
  deficiency 82
  neonates 58
magnesium hydroxide 253
magnet ingestion 273
malabsorption 585, 586
malaena 279
malignancy
  acute liver failure 607–8
  bile salt export pump
    deficiency 484
  chronic diarrhoea 304
  liver tumours 565–8
  post-intestinal
    transplant 140
  skin, post-liver
    transplant 641
  ulcerative colitis 413
Mallory–Weiss
  syndrome 289
malnutrition 106,
  26–9, 90
  chronic liver
    disease 571, 585
  classification 26, 27
  risk factors for
    undernutrition 33
  tube feeding 27
  WHO definition 26
  WHO
    recommendations
    for treatment 26–9
malrotation 4–5
maltose 166
manganese deficiency 84
mannitol 612
marasmic kwashiorkor 27
marasmus 27
mastitis 41
MDR3
  deficiency 477, 478–9
Meckel's diverticulum 289
Meckel's scan 284
meconium ileus 7,
  204–5
medium-chain triglyceride
  (MCT) feeds 586,
  599
6-mercaptopurine 412
mesenchymal
  hamartoma 567
meso-Rex bypass
  623
metabolic liver
  disease 505–18
  acidosis 512
  acute hypoglycaemic
    event 517
  acute illness 516

metabolic liver disease
(*Contd.*)
acute liver failure 508–10,
605, 608
catabolic states 516
clinical features 507
clinical
presentations 508–12
emergency regimen 516
hyperammo-
naemia 511, 517
infantile
cholestasis 509–10
investigation 514–15
ketosis 512
liver enzymes 511
management 516–17
neonatal ascites 511
metabolic syndrome 198
methotrexate 390–1, 492
methylmalonic
acidaemia 512
micronutrients 76
microvillus inclusion
disease 127, 298
midparental height 12
mid-upper arm circumfer-
ence 12, 36, 590
milk
excessive drinking 154
refusal 154
mineral oil 365
minerals
deficiency 76, 82
supplements 86
mitochondrial
hepatopathies 508–9,
605, 608
molybdenum deficiency 85
monosaccharide
intolerance 239
motility disorders,
neuromuscular 122, 126
mucosal
disorders 122, 127
multiple intraluminal
impedance/pH
monitoring 246–7
mushroom poisoning 607
mycophenolate
mofetil 640

N

nasogastric tubes 96, 97, 98
nausea and vomiting,
enteral feeding 102
necrotizing
enterocolitis 61–6, 289
neonatal adrenoleucodystrophy 510
neonatal ascites 511

neonatal haemochro-
matosis 508–9,
605–6, 608
neonatal jaundice 445–58
breast milk 450
conjugated hyperbilirubinaemia 452–6, 598
epidemiology 446
haemolysis 450
physiological 450
unconjugated hyperbiliru-
binaemia 448, 450–1
neonatal nutrition 58
neonatal sclerosing
cholangitis 477
Neuhauser's sign 7
neurodisability 173–90
assessment 175
feeding 177
gastro-oesophageal reflux
disease 177
intestinal failure 190
tube feeding 176
neuromuscular motility
disorders 122, 126
nicotinic acid (niacin)
deficiency 78
recommended intake 87
Niemann–Pick type C 511
NISCH syndrome 477
nodular regenerative
hyperplasia 567
non-alcoholic fatty liver
disease 519–28
antioxidants 527
biomarkers 523
clinical
presentation 522–4
definition 520
diagnosis 522–4
dietary intervention 527
epidemiology 520
insulin
resistance 523, 521
lifestyle interventions 527
liver biopsy 523
management 527
monitoring 527
natural history 526
nutritional
management 598
obesity 198
pathophysiology 521
pharmacotherapy 527
probiotics 527
PUFAs 527
risk factors 520
two-hit hypothesis 521
non-alcoholic
steatohepatitis 520
non-allergic
hypersensitivity 158

non-selective beta
blockers 622, 623
non-steroidal anti-
inflammatory drugs 492
North American Indian
cholestasis 475, 478
nutrient requirements
healthy children 22–3, 24
neonates 58
nutritional
assessment 31–8
feeding history 35
liver disease 590
neurodisability 175
nutritional intake 34
premature newborn 57
nutritional screening 38
nutritional support
teams 90, 91

O

obesity 191–200
aetiology 192
complications 198
definitions 27, 192
epidemiology 193
evaluation 194
metabolic
syndrome 198
non-alcoholic fatty liver
disease 198
orlistat therapy 197
prevention 193
surgery 197
treatment 196–7
unusual causes 194
obstructive apnoea
244
oesophageal biopsy 248
oesophageal
manometry 247
oesophageal pH
monitoring 246, 247
oesophagitis
Crohn's disease 393
eosinophilic 256,
421, 422
reflux 243
oesophagoscopy 248
omeprazole 252
oral allergy syndrome 159
oral contraceptive pill
492
oral rehydration
solutions 236–7
orlistat 197
osmotic agents 363
osteodystrophy,
hepatic 581
osteomalacia 79–80
overweight 27

P

paediatric NAFLD fibrosis index 523
Paediatric Ulcerative Colitis Activity Index (PUCAI) 410
pain
  biopsychosocial model 344
  pancreatitis 432
pancolitis 406
pancreas, anatomy and physiology 426
pancreatic enzyme replacement therapy 212, 432–3
pancreatic enzymes 426
pancreatic exocrine insufficiency 204, 304
pancreatitis 428–9
  acute 428–9, 615
  acute recurrent 429
  autoimmune 435
  chronic 429
  drug-induced 428–9
  hereditary 434
  investigation 430
  management 432–3
  nutrition 432–3
  pain control 432
  pancreatic enzyme replacement therapy 432–3
  pancreatic rest 432–3
pantothenate, recommended intake 87
paracetamol overdose 492, 496, 497, 606–7
parasitic infections
  gastroenteritis 230
  liver 560–2
parenteral
  nutrition 109–19
  catheter-related complications 114–15, 129
  estimating calorie requirement 110
  home-based 118
  indications 111
  infections 114–15, 129
  intestinal failure-associated liver disease 115–16
  liver disease 591
  metabolic complications 116, 129
  monitoring 112
  occlusion of CVC 114–15
  premature newborn 55

renal complications 116, 129
  social implications 116, 130
  urokinase infusion 115
  urokinase lock 115
  vascular access 110
partial villous atrophy 315
pegylated interferon 542, 549
pellagra 78
penicillamine 532
  challenge 531
peptic ulcer 260–1, 262
percutaneous endoscopic gastrostomy (PEG) 96
  with jejunal insert (PEGJ) 96
perianal disorders
  anal fissure 289, 372
  Crohn's disease 393
  examination 372
  inflammatory bowel disease 374
  rectal prolapse 373
  solitary rectal ulcer syndrome 374
  streptococcal infection 373
  threadworm 373
peritonitis, spontaneous bacterial 576
pernicious anaemia 79
peroxisomal disorders 510
personality type 344–5
Peutz–Jeghers syndrome 293
PFIC1 disease 475, 477, 478, 483
phenobarbital 492
phenotypic diarrhoea 298
phenytoin 492
phosphate, neonates 58
phosphorus deficiency 82
physiological jaundice 450
physiological reflux 244
picky eating 153
polyethylene glycol 363, 365
polyposis 289, 291
polyunsaturated fatty acids 527
porphyria 338
portal hypertension 619
  balloon (Sengstaken–Blakemore) tamponade 624
  clinical features 621
  definition 620
  endoscopic therapy 622

haemostatic spray 624
  management 622
  meso-Rex bypass 623
  pathophysiology 620
  pharmacotherapy 623
  prediction tools 622
  shunt surgery 623
  transjugular portosystemic shunt 623
portal vein thrombosis 638
portopulmonary hypertension 578–9
post-enteritis syndrome 239, 305
post-transplant lymphoproliferative disorder 639
potassium
  neonates 58
  recommended intake 24
prednisolone 640
pregnancy-associated cholestasis 477, 480
premature newborn 53–60
  enteral feeding 56–7
  necrotizing enterocolitis 61–6
  nutritional assessment 57
  nutritional requirements 58
  parenteral nutrition 55
primary hyperoxaluria type I 510
probiotics
  gastroenteritis 237
  non-alcoholic fatty liver disease 527
proctitis, eosinophilic 289
proctocolitis, eosinophilic 418–19
progressive familial intrahepatic cholestasis 475, 477, 478, 598
progressive intrahepatic cholestasis 480
prokinetics 253
propionic acidaemia 512
protein
  minimum safe intake levels 593
  neonates 58
  recommended intake 24
  synthesis in chronic liver disease 571
prothrombin time 438
proton pump inhibitors 252
pruritus 470, 471, 483, 580

pseudo-intolerance/
   allergy 161
psychological therapy 346
psychologically based
   food reaction
   (aversion) 158
puberty 20, 21
pyloric stenosis 268
pyogenic liver
   abscess 555–6
pyridoxine
   deficiency 78
   recommended intake 87

Q

Q fever 559

R

rachitic rosary 80
ranitidine 252
rapid urease test 261
recommended daily
   amount 22–3
recommended nutrient
   intake 22–3, 24
recto-perineal fistula 10
recto-urethral fistula 10
recto-vestibular fistula 10
rectum
   bleeding
      278, 279, 294
   prolapse 373
   ulcer 374
refeeding syndrome 106–7
reference nutrient
   intake 34
reflux oesophagitis 243
Refsum disease 510
regurgitation 222, 242
   enteral feeding 102
renal dysfunction
   acute liver failure 614
   parenteral
      nutrition 116, 129
   post-liver transplant 641
renal replacement 614
renal tubular acidosis 69
renin–angiotensin–
   aldosterone
   system 582
retinoids 492
ribavirin 549
riboflavin
   deficiency 78
   recommended intake 87
rickets 79–80, 80
rickettsial liver
   infections 559
rotavirus 230
rumination 222, 242

S

schistosomiasis 561
Schwalbe's ring 468
screening
   coeliac disease
      314, 315
   nutritional risk 38
Screening Tool for Risk of
   Impaired Nutritional
   Status and Growth
   (STRONG_kids) 38
Screening Tool for
   the Assessment
   of Malnutrition in
   Paediatrics (STAMP)
   38
scurvy 79
selenium deficiency 85
Sengstaken–Blakemore
   tamponade 624
senna 364, 365
sensory homunculus 351
sepsis 554–7
serology
   coeliac disease 316
   Helicobacter
      pylori 260–1
   hepatitis B 538, 539
serum iron 72
short bowel
   syndrome 122, 124–5
Shwachman–Diamond
   syndrome 308
sirolimus 640
skin malignancy, post-liver
   transplant 641
skinfold thickness 12,
   37, 590
small bowel
   atresia 6
   bacterial
      overgrowth 129, 332–3
   biopsy 316
sodium
   cystic fibrosis 211
   neonates 58
   recommended intake 24
sodium docusate 365
sodium picosulfate 364,
   365
sodium valproate 607,
   492
soiling 356, 359
solitary rectal ulcer
   syndrome 374
Sovaldi® 548
soy formula 50
spirochaetal liver
   infections 558
spontaneous bacterial
   peritonitis 576

stagnant loop
   syndrome 332–3
STAMP 38
steatosis, differential
   diagnosis 522
stimulant laxatives
   363, 365
stool antigen test 260–1
stool osmotic gap 296,
   304
stool softeners 363
streptococcal perianal
   infection 373
stress 342, 344–5
STRONG_kids 38
sub-scapular skinfold
   thickness 37
sucralfate 253
sucrase–isomaltase
   deficiency 168, 170
sucrose 166
sulfasalazine 492
syphilis 558

T

tacrolimus 637, 640
tenofovir 543
thiamine
   deficiency 78
   recommended intake 87
thiopurine
   derivatives 390, 411–12
threadworm 373
TJP2 defects 477, 478
toddler's diarrhoea 306
tongue tie 45
total energy
   expenditure 22
total iron binding
   capacity 72
toxic megacolon 408
toxocariasis 561
toxoplasmosis 562
trace element
   deficiency 76, 84–5
transferrin receptor 72
transferrin saturation 72
transgastric double lumen
   jejunostomy (GJ
   button) 96
transient elastography
   217
transjugular portosystemic
   shunt 623
transplantation, see intestinal transplantation;
   liver transplantation
triceps skinfold
   thickness 37, 590
tricho-hepato-enteric
   syndrome 298